Breast Cancer in Young Women

Oreste Gentilini • Ann H. Partridge
Olivia Pagani

Editors

Breast Cancer in Young Women

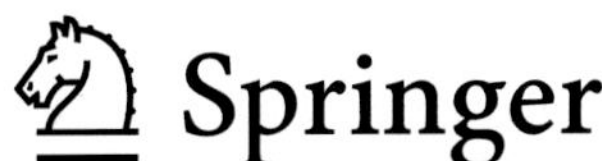
Springer

Editors
Oreste Gentilini
Breast Unit, San Raffaele University and
Research Hospital
Milan
Italy

Olivia Pagani
Geneva University Hospitals
Swiss Group for Clinical
Cancer Research (SAKK)
Institute of Oncology
of Southern Switzerland
Bellinzona
Switzerland

Ann H. Partridge
Dana–Farber Cancer Institute
Department of Medical Oncology
Harvard Medical School
Boston, MA
USA

ISBN 978-3-030-24764-5   ISBN 978-3-030-24762-1   (eBook)
https://doi.org/10.1007/978-3-030-24762-1

This Springer imprint is published by the registered company Springer Nature Switzerland AG
The registered company address is: Gewerbestrasse 11, 6330 Cham, Switzerland

Contents

Contributors

Banu Arun Department of Breast Medical Oncology and Clinical Cancer Genetics Program, The University of Texas MD Anderson Cancer Center, Houston, TX, USA

Hamdy A. Azim Department of Clinical Oncology, Cairo University Hospital, Cairo, Egypt

Hatem A. Azim Jr Division of Hematology/Oncology, Department of Internal Medicine, American University of Beirut (AUB), Beirut, Lebanon

Soley Bayraktar Biruni Univeristy School of Medicine, Protokol Yolu, Istanbul, Turkey

Sharon Bober Dana–Farber Cancer Institute, Boston, MA, USA

Fatima Cardoso Breast Unit, Champalimaud Clinical Center/Champalimaud Foundation, Lisbon, Portugal

Maria João Cardoso Breast Unit, Champalimaud Clinical Center/ Champalimaud Foundation, Lisbon, Portugal

Giuseppe Curigliano IEO, European Institute of Oncology IRCCS, Milano, Italy

Department of Oncology and Hemato-Oncology, University of Milano, Milan, Italy

Ella Evron Sackler School of Medicine, Tel Aviv University, Tel Aviv, Israel

Tanja Gagliardi University of Aberdeen, Aberdeen, UK

Karen A. Gelmon BC Cancer Agency, Vancouver Cancer Centre, Vancouver, BC, Canada

Oreste Gentilini Breast Unit, San Raffaele University and Research Hospital, Milan, Italy

Clara Hungr Cambridge Health Alliance, Cambridge, MA, USA

Bella Kaufman Breast Oncology Institute, Sheba Medical Centre, Ramat Gan, Israel

Assia Konsoulova Medical Oncology Clinic, University Hospital Sveta Marina, Varna, Bulgaria

Matteo Lambertini Department of Medical Oncology, Clinica di Oncologia Medica, Policlinico San Martino-IST, University of Genova, Genoa, Italy

Nathalie Levasseur BC Cancer Agency, Vancouver Cancer Centre, Vancouver, BC, Canada

Sibylle Loibl German Breast Group, Neu-Isenburg, Germany

Centrum für Hämatologie und Onkologie Bethanien, Frankfurt am Main, Germany

Rosa Di Micco Breast Unit, San Raffaele University and Research Hospital, Milan, Italy

Department of Clinical Medicine and Surgery, University of Naples Federico II, Naples, Italy

Bastien Nguyen Breast Cancer Translational Research Laboratory (BCTL), Institut Jules Bordet, UniversitéLibre de Bruxelles (ULB), Brussels, Belgium

Olivia Pagani Institute of Oncology of Southern Switzerland, Geneva University Hospitals, Swiss Group for Clinical Cancer Research (SAKK), and International Breast Cancer Study Group (IBCSG), Lugano, Viganello, Switzerland

Shani Paluch-Shimon Breast Oncology Unit, Shaare Zedek Medical Centre, Jerusalem, Israel

Ann H. Partridge Dana–Farber Cancer Institute and Harvard Medical School, Boston, MA, USA

Fedro A. Peccatori Fertility and Procreation Unit, Division of Gynecologic Oncology, European Institute of Oncology, Milan, Italy

Philip D. Poorvu Dana–Farber Cancer Institute and Harvard Medical School, Boston, MA, USA

Joana Mourato Ribeiro Breast Unit, Champalimaud Clinical Center/ Champalimaud Foundation, Lisbon, Portugal

Julia H. Rowland Smith Center for Healing and the Arts, Washington, DC, USA

Department of Psychiatry, Georgetown University School of Medicine, Washington, DC, USA

Sabine Seiler German Breast Group, Neu-Isenburg, Germany

Elżbieta Senkus Department of Oncology & Radiotherapy, Medical University of Gdańsk, Gdańsk, Poland

Dario Trapani IEO, European Institute of Oncology IRCCS, Milano, Italy

Department of Oncology and Hemato-Oncology, University of Milano, Milan, Italy

Luzia Travado Psycho-Oncology, Neuropsychiatry Unit, Champalimaud Clinical Center, Champalimaud Foundation, Lisbon, Portugal

Simona Volovat Breast Unit, Champalimaud Clinical Center/Champalimaud Foundation, Lisbon, Portugal

Rinat Yerushalmi Davidoff Cancer Center, Rabin Medical Center, Petah Tikva, Israel

Epidemiology

Philip D. Poorvu and Ann H. Partridge

1.1 Incidence and Time Trends

Breast cancer is the most common malignancy among women, with more than 1.3 million new breast cancers diagnosed annually worldwide, and the second leading cause of cancer death among women [1]. The disease is largely diagnosed in older women, with a median age at diagnosis of 61 [2], and less than 7% of cases are diagnosed among young women, including about 1% prior to age 30 and 2.5% prior to age 35 [3]. The risk to an individual woman is about 1 in 1500 by age 30 and 1 in 200 by age 40 [3]. Although there is a higher incidence among young women in developed countries, there is fairly limited variation across the world, particularly as compared with older women among whom the incidence varies more widely (Fig. 1.1) [1, 2, 4, 5]. Yet, there are 10,500 young women diagnosed annually in the USA, greater than the incidence of both Hodgkin lymphoma and testis cancer [2, 6].

Due to changing reproductive patterns, implementation of breast cancer screening, and the use of peri- and postmenopausal hormone replacement therapy (HRT), the overall incidence of breast cancer rose in the second half of the twentieth century. As HRT use diminished abruptly in the early 2000s, rates of breast cancer subsequently declined [7]. While some figures have suggested a slight increase of 0.6% per year from 1994 to 2012 [2], the incidence of breast cancer among young women has remained mostly stable over the past several decades, presumably because young women were not subject to the factors that drove changes in incidence among older women [3, 4]. While one SEER analysis found a small increase in the incidence of de novo metastatic breast cancer (1.5–2.9 cases/100,000 women from 1976 to 2009), this may be explained by improvements in the ability to detect distant disease using cross-sectional imaging and differential use of such imaging in young women in particular over time [8].

1.2 Risk Factors

1.2.1 Reproductive and Hormonal Factors

Several large cohort studies have identified risk factors for the development of breast cancer, many specifically for premenopausal breast cancer and fewer for breast cancer among young women. Younger age at menarche and older age at first-term pregnancy are more strongly associated with premenopausal than postmenopausal

P. D. Poorvu · A. H. Partridge (✉)
Dana–Farber Cancer Institute and Harvard Medical School, Boston, MA, USA
e-mail: ann_partridge@dfci.harvard.edu

© Springer Nature Switzerland AG 2020
O. Gentilini et al. (eds.), *Breast Cancer in Young Women*,
https://doi.org/10.1007/978-3-030-24762-1_1

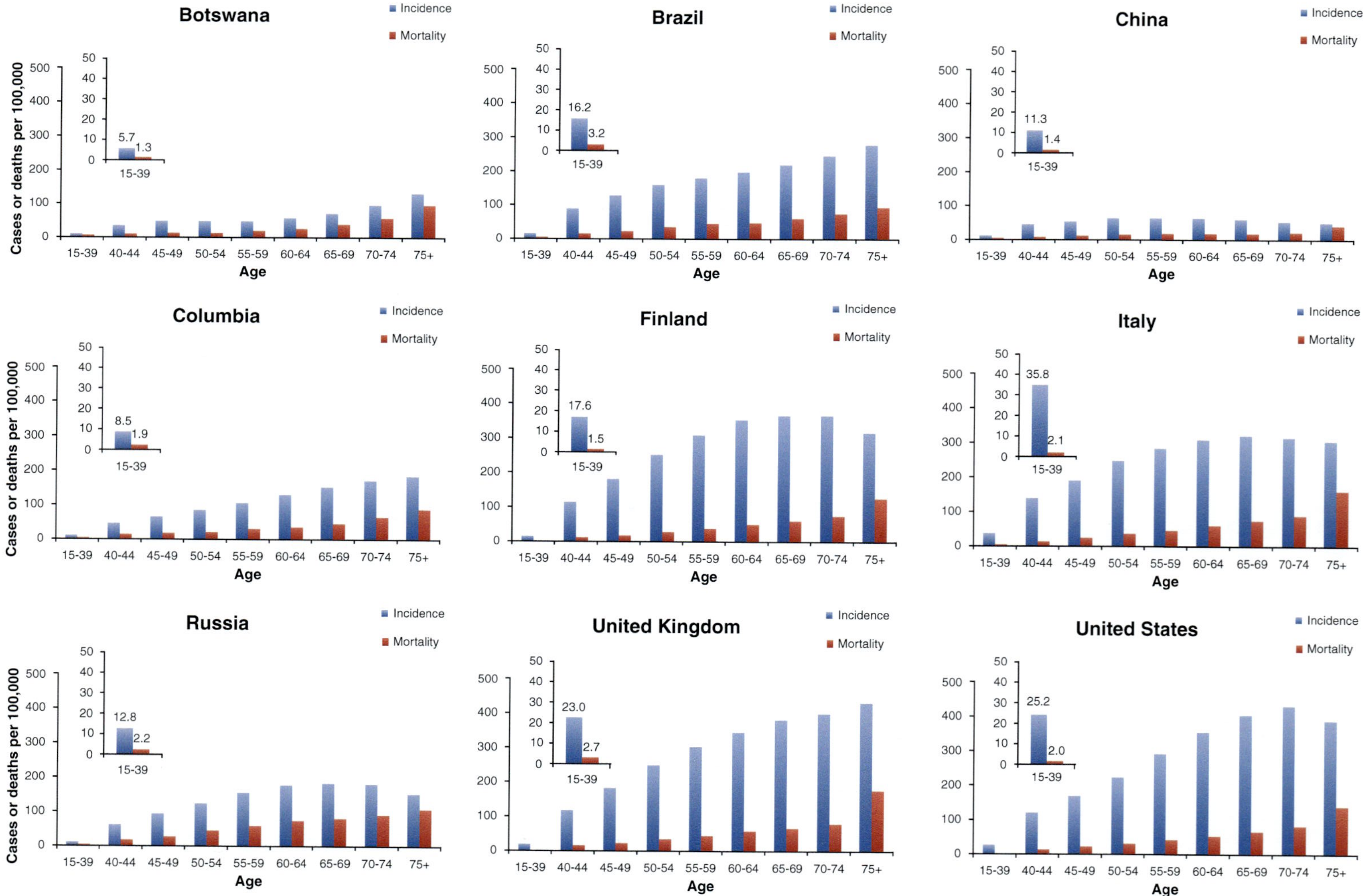

Fig. 1.1 Breast cancer incidence and mortality by age across nine countries. Source: GLOBOCAN 2012: Estimated Cancer Incidence, Mortality and Prevalence Worldwide in 2012, International Agency for Research on Cancer, World Health Organization

breast cancer, though the incremental risks of each are low regardless of menopausal status [9], and data from the Nurses' Health Study further showed that the impact is similar among premenopausal women diagnosed at age<40 or ≥40 [9, 10]. However, the protective effect of parity appeared stronger in one study for postmenopausal breast cancer (~12% overall reduction for each full-term pregnancy) than premenopausal breast cancer (~3% overall reduction for each full-term pregnancy) [9], potentially because of the small increase in risk of breast cancer in the period immediately following pregnancy, and pregnancy-associated breast cancer largely occurs among women age<40 [4, 9, 11, 12]. Interestingly, the risk attributable to pregnancy appears slightly greater with later age at first pregnancy and is also greater and peaks later for uniparous women than biparous women [13]. The mechanisms by which pregnancy exerts this "dual effect" of risk followed by protection are not well-defined [14]. Breastfeeding is well-known to reduce the risk of breast cancer and has been found specifically among young women to be protective, with an RR of 0.85 compared to women who did not breastfeed in a Nurses' Health Study analysis [10].

While pregnancy may represent a short-term risk, oral contraceptives (OCs) have also been associated with a very modest increase in risk of breast cancer. One analysis of data aggregated from 54 studies found that risk is elevated among current OC users (RR 1.24), but returns to baseline 10 years after discontinuing OCs [15]. A subsequent systematic review and meta-analysis also confirmed a small increase in risk among current OC users that progressively decreases after discontinuing [16]. Importantly, multiple large prospective studies have failed to demonstrate an increase in risk of breast cancer following in vitro fertilization and non-IVF fertility medication use [17–20]. Several physiologic parameters, including higher endogenous estradiol and testosterone levels, birth weight, growth rate, and peak height, have been associated with premenopausal breast cancer, but not specifically among young women [21–26].

1.2.2 Health Behaviors and Environmental Factors

Interestingly, weight and BMI are inversely associated with premenopausal breast cancer but positively associated with postmenopausal breast cancer, suggesting that the effect of obesity is not mediated only through an increase in circulating endogenous estrogen [24, 26, 27]. Exercise has been associated with a dose-dependent protective effect on the risk of premenopausal breast cancer, with inconsistent findings regarding differential impact for the breast cancer subtypes [28–31].

There is great interest in identifying dietary patterns or specific foods that could be associated with either a protective or harmful effect on breast cancer risk in young women. Prior studies have established what appears to be a dose-dependent association between alcohol intake and breast cancer risk, with no apparent difference in risk among pre- and postmenopausal women [32–35]. Work on adolescent dietary patterns has identified an inflammatory dietary pattern, described as high in soft drinks, refined grains, and red meat and low in vegetable and coffee intake [36] and butter consumption (RR 1.06) as small risk factors for premenopausal breast cancer, while high dietary fiber (RR 0.78) and vegetable fat intake (0.85) were associated with a modest protective effect [37]. Additional data demonstrated that high intake of low-fat dairy products is associated with a lower risk of premenopausal breast cancer (RR 0.68), as was dairy calcium intake (RR 0.69) and total vitamin D (0.72), whereas there was no association with postmenopausal breast cancer [38]. The Mediterranean-style diet has been associated with a lower risk of premenopausal breast cancer than a Western diet and is often recommended, particularly since it may be more conducive to weight loss [39–41].

Mantle radiation, once used frequently in the treatment of Hodgkin lymphoma but now administered rarely, is a strong risk factor for breast cancer among young women and, in one study, was associated with an estimated cumulative risk of 15% by age 40, which is on par with the risk in BRCA1 mutation carriers [42]. Therefore, HL survivors previously treated with mantle radiation may warrant more intensive screening and risk reduction strategies.

1.2.3 Race

In the USA, the burden of breast cancer among young women is not distributed proportionally across demographic subgroups. African-American women account for 14% of cases among women age≤40 and 8% >40, whereas Caucasian women account for 76% of cases among women ≤40 and 85% among women >40 [43]. Across age groups, including young women, African-American women are diagnosed with a higher rate of triple-negative and later-stage breast cancers than other racial groups [44–47].

1.2.4 Genetic Risk Factors

Breast cancer patients are enriched for deleterious germline mutations, with a prevalence of 10% among unselected patients, 60% of which occur in the BRCA1 or BRCA2 genes and 40% in lower-penetrance genes, including ATM, BRIP1, CHEK2, and PALB2 [48, 49]. The cumulative incidence of developing breast cancer is greater for BRCA1 than BRCA2 mutations: 0.02 vs.0 by age 30, 0.17 vs.0.04 by age 40, 0.35 vs.0.09 by age 50, 0.41 vs.0.26 by age 60, and 0.52 vs.0.32 by age 70 for BRCA1 and BRCA2 mutation carriers, respectively [50]. Because these germline mutations predispose to early-onset cancers, young women have an even greater prevalence of about 16%, ¾ of which are mutations in BRCA1 or BRCA2 and the remaining ¼ in other lower-penetrance genes [49]. BRCA1 and BRCA2 mutations are more common among Ashkenazi Jewish women with a prevalence of 1 in 40 unaffected women [51, 52]. However, BRCA mutations are not limited to higher-risk populations as evidenced by data from the Florida Cancer Registry, which demonstrated that 13% of black women diagnosed at age<50 have a BRCA1 or BRCA2 mutation[53], and another series that found BRCA mutations in 24% of young Mexican women with triple-negative breast cancer[54].

1.3 Features of Breast Cancer in Young Women

1.3.1 Stage, Grade, and Tumor Subtypes

Young women have more extensive disease involvement at diagnosis relative to their older counterparts, with a greater proportion presenting with larger tumors (50% vs. 36% T2–T4), lymph node involvement (39% vs. 25% node positive and 29% vs. 18% with >3 nodes involved), and higher stage (56% vs. 40% stage II or higher), in one study[43]. Although many patients and clinicians may assume that a breast abnormality in a young woman is more likely to represent a benign entity, diagnostic delays are uncommon and do not appear to be the primary driver of the greater disease burden at presentation for most patients[55]. The differences in extent of disease are due in part to the lack of breast cancer screening for young women but also due at least in part to known differences in the frequency of the various breast cancer subtypes between age groups. Relative to older women, young women more frequently have high-grade tumors (43% vs. 26%, in one study), which are associated with a worse prognosis and often require more intensive systemic therapy [43]. Young women are also more likely to have triple-negative and HER2+ disease [56, 57]. Of cancers diagnosed among young women, about 60–66% are ER-positive and 25–33% HER2+ [43, 57–59]. One study found that 49% were HR+/HER2−, 23% HR−/HER2−, 18% HR+/HER+, and 10% HR−/HER2+ [57]. A large prospective cohort study also found that young women appear to have a greater incidence of luminal B subtype cancers (35%) and lower incidence of luminal A subtype cancers (33%), relative to published data for older women [58]. In one very large dataset, among women with ER-positive disease for whom genomic testing was sent presumably for clinical testing, young women appeared to have a right-shifted distribution of Oncotype Dx Recurrence Scores, with 48%, 38%, and 14% having low, intermediate, and high risk scores, respectively, vs. 60%, 33%, and 7% among women age 40–49 [60]. Molecular analysis of breast cancers from The Cancer Genome Atlas (TCGA) has found that GATA3 mutations are more common among young women, though the significance of this finding in breast cancer development is not yet clear [61].

1.3.2 Independent Risk of Young Age

Even accounting for the greater incidence of poor prognostic features, several studies have confirmed that young age is an independent risk factor for disease recurrence and death [43, 56, 62]. Interestingly, this increase in risk appears to be subtype-dependent, with young age particularly prognostic for women with luminal A (HR 2.1) and luminal B (1.4) tumors and less so for triple-negative and HER2-positive tumors [63], perhaps due to less effective endocrine therapies for young premenopausal women and a less robust chemohormonal effect from adjuvant chemotherapy [64]. Similarly, the independent risk of young age on breast cancer-specific mortality appears limited to women with stage I (HR 1.4) and II (HR 1.1) disease, but not stage III (HR 1.0) disease [43]. Inadequate approaches to endocrine therapy along with poor adherence (see endocrine therapy and adherence section later in chapter) have been issues for young women [65]. Given recent data supporting the use of ovarian function suppression for young patients, it will be important to assess patterns of care for young women to ensure optimization of their endocrine therapy and hopefully address excess risk in young women with luminal subtype cancers [66, 67]. While young age is predictive of greater chemotherapy benefit in terms of breast cancer-specific and overall mortality, breast cancer is still a very heterogeneous disease among young women, and therapies must be tailored to the individual's disease features [68]. Young women are at particular risk for over-treatment and stand to suffer the greatest burden of toxicities from chemotherapy. Hopefully, the effect of age will fade with improved tumor subtyping and more effective targeted approaches.

Disparities exist in outcomes as well, as demonstrated by relatively poor 5-year disease-specific survival rates of 79% for black women vs. 90% for white women [69]. Furthermore, the rate of improvement in survival outcomes has been slower for young black women with a hazard of death in 2005 relative to 1990 of 0.68 for young black women and 0.55 for young white women [69]. Decreased rates of adherence to endocrine therapy contribute to these disparities, and additional research efforts are needed to identify and address other drivers [70, 71].

1.3.3 Unique Treatment

The general approach to treatment of young women with breast cancer, outside of endocrine therapy, is similar to that of middle-aged women. However, differences in local and systemic therapy may be driven not only by concerns about higher risk in young patients but also by the unique psychosocial and reproductive issues, as well as the more common genetic predisposition that young women face, which is discussed in greater detail in subsequent chapters [72]. It is important to note that young women generally do participate in clinical trials as much if not more than older women. However, unless a study is focused on young women, they usually only represent a small minority of participants. Thus, clinicians may not feel comfortable adopting newer treatment paradigms for young patients, particularly those that aim to de-escalate treatment, given the natural inclination to treat young, otherwise healthy individuals more aggressively.

Young women have historically faced a higher risk of locoregional recurrence (LRR) with breast-conserving surgery (BCS) relative to older women, with studies demonstrating up to a fivefold higher risk; however, BCS is not associated with worse overall survival relative to mastectomy in women of all ages [72–77]. The risk of locoregional recurrence is felt to be acceptably low, and BCS has therefore remained the standard approach for appropriate candidates [72]. LRR rates have declined substantially over the past decades likely due to improvements in diagnostic and surgical techniques and the development of effective targeted therapies (i.e., anti-HER2 antibodies) [78–80]. The higher incidence of lymph node involvement and resultant need for post-mastectomy radiation among young women makes BCS even more desirable for suitable candidates, given the effects of radiation on the reconstructed breast. However, BCS rates fell by more than 15% and the rate of bilateral mastectomy rose from 3.6% to 33% between 1998 and 2011 [74]. This phenomenon is complex and driven by multiple factors, including the uptake of preoperative MRI and misperceptions about risk reduction from contralateral prophylactic mastectomy [75, 81–83].

Young women also receive more adjuvant chemotherapy than older women, both within and outside the USA. In a Swedish registry, chemotherapy usage was 65%, 61%, 46%, and 27% among women age 20–34, 35–39, 40–49, and 50–69, with only a small proportion of the variability due to differences in disease characteristics and suitability for treatment [56]. Within large prospective cohorts in the UK, South Korea, and Saudi Arabia, the rate of chemotherapy usage has exceeded 85% [59, 84, 85].

Over the past decade, multiple genomic assays have been implemented that are both prognostic and predictive of disease recurrence and better inform selection for adjuvant chemotherapy in HR+/HER2− breast cancer [86–88]. A retrospective, population-based study found that chemotherapy usage was more frequent for young women with intermediate risk scores (age<40, 55%; age 40–49, 46%; age 50–59, 37%) and low risk scores (node negative, age<40, 18%; age 40–49, 12%; age 50–59, 7%; node positive, age<40, 55%; age 40–49, 37%; age 50–59, 27%) [89].

1.3.4 Adherence

Endocrine therapy (ET) improves disease-free and overall survival in women of all ages, therefore ensuring optimal access, and adherence to

ET is an important aspect of breast cancer care [68]. The converse is also true—poor adherence has been associated with increased rates of breast cancer recurrence and poorer survival (HR 1.2) [90]. Young women are more likely than older women to be non-adherent to endocrine therapy, with about a third discontinuing ET early and another quarter using ET inconsistently, yielding only about half of women who are fully adherent through the 5 years of treatment [91, 92]. A large prospective study found that of 515 premenopausal women, including some age 41–45, 13% did not initiate tamoxifen, 16% discontinued tamoxifen prior to 5 years, and 71% persisted with tamoxifen through 5 years [93]. Women concerned about future fertility were significantly more likely not to initiate ET (OR 5.0) or discontinue early (OR 1.8) [93]. Therefore, attention to fertility, including counseling on risks of treatment and age-related decline in ovarian reserve as well as fertility preservation options, may be an important strategy for improving adherence among young women [94]. Vasomotor, gynecologic, and sexual side effects and the fear of developing side effects, particularly in young women, are important drivers of nonadherence, including both non-initiation and non-persistence, and proactive counseling and early management of ET side effects with behavioral and pharmacologic approaches are critical and may address this source of nonadherence [93, 95, 96].

1.4 Special Considerations for Young Women

Breast cancer not only threatens a patient's physical well-being, but for a young woman it also threatens several aspects of life that are integral to role functioning. The diagnosis comes at a time when many are interested in building a family, and the recommended treatment may impair future fertility. Most young women are treated with gonadotoxic chemotherapy and the risk of amenorrhea, a frequently used surrogate for fertility, is heavily dependent upon age and treatment regimen [97]. Prospective studies have found that the risk of chemotherapy-related amenorrhea (CRA) is low for women under age 35 (15%) and even lower for women age<30 [98, 99]. Ovarian reserve naturally starts to decline more rapidly around age 35 and the risk of CRA thereafter increases to about 30% for women age 35–40 and>50% for women age>40 [98, 99]. Fertility is a primary issue for young women and, at the time of diagnosis, the majority report being concerned about the risk of becoming infertile with treatment, particularly those who are nulliparous, very young, and receiving chemotherapy [100]. Pregnancy after breast cancer, including the impact on breast cancer outcomes and fertility preservation techniques, is discussed in greater detail in Chap. 17.

Gonadotoxic chemotherapy and endocrine therapy also place young women at risk for premature menopause and associated short-term side effects, such as vasomotor symptoms and sexual dysfunction, as well as long-term side effects, such as osteoporosis, heart disease, and cognitive side effects [101–104]. Menopausal symptoms are prevalent among young women, including hot flashes (40%), dyspareunia (40%), vaginal dryness (50%), and breast sensitivity (50%) [105]. About 60% of women also report cognitive side effects, including difficulty concentrating and forgetfulness, and the performance on neurocognitive testing of survivors is worsened by chemotherapy and further by the addition of endocrine therapy to chemotherapy, though reported symptoms do not necessarily correlate to performance [104, 105]. While menopausal symptoms are more prevalent among postmenopausal and perimenopausal patients, women who are premenopausal at diagnosis and subsequently undergo a menopausal transition as a result of adjuvant therapy experience an even greater burden of vasomotor symptoms [106]. Sexual health is frequently a concern for young women, with up to 40% of women reporting issues with sexual interest and 60% with physical sexual function (see Chap. 16) [107].

Young women with breast cancer are also at greater risk of gaining weight than other age-matched women and older patients, with up to 50% of women reporting weight gain during treatment [108–110]. A very high proportion of young survivors (~70%) also report dissatisfaction with their physical appearance [111]. Obesity has been associated with worse survival outcomes, particularly among premenopausal women [108, 112]. Young women may become less physically active early in treatment, likely contributing to the increase in weight gain experienced by those undergoing chemotherapy, but activity levels subsequently increase over the following year [113]. Exercise is associated with a dose-dependent reduction in risk of breast cancer death among survivors and is discussed in greater detail in Chap. 16 [114].

Due at least in part to these unique issues, young women experience a greater detriment to their psychosocial functioning and quality of life, both physical and mental [115, 116]. Given their developmental stage, young women also often need to try to balance their education or early career goals and also manage parenting issues for young children at a time of significant stress. Young women are more likely to report depressive symptoms and for their symptoms to reach the threshold of clinical depression [116, 117]. Factors associated with worse quality of life include a greater burden of symptoms (i.e., pain, menopausal symptoms) as well as relationship and body image issues, whereas improved social support and functioning (i.e., employment) are associated with improved quality of life and exercise with improved health-related quality of life [104, 109, 116, 118, 119]. These issues along with approaches to psychosocial support are discussed in Chap. 17.

1.5 Summary

Young women are a minority population of women diagnosed with breast cancer. However, their unique concerns and disparate outcomes warrant focused attention. Dedicated psychosocial and clinical programming as well as research designed to address questions important to this population should help to provide additional support and information to improve care and outcomes for young women with breast cancer.

References

1. Ferlay J, Shin H-R, Bray F, Forman D, Mathers C, Parkin DM. Estimates of worldwide burden of cancer in 2008: GLOBOCAN 2008. Int J Cancer. 2010;127(12):2893–917.

2. DeSantis CE, Fedewa SA, Goding Sauer A, Kramer JL, Smith RA, Jemal A. Breast cancer statistics, 2015: convergence of incidence rates between black and white women. CA Cancer J Clin. 2016;66(1):31–42.

3. Anders CK, Johnson R, Litton J, Phillips M, Bleyer A. Breast cancer before age 40 years. Semin Oncol. 2009;36(3):237–49.

4. Narod SA. Breast cancer in young women. Nat Rev Clin Oncol. 2012;9(8):460–70.

5. GLOBOCAN. Estimated cancer incidence, mortality and prevalence worldwide in 2012. International Agency for Research on Cancer. [cited August 10, 2017]. 2012. http://globocan.iarc.fr/Pages/age-specific_table_sel.aspx.

6. Siegel RL, Miller KD, Jemal A. Cancer statistics, 2016. CA Cancer J Clin. 2016;66(1):7–30.

7. Toriola AT, Colditz GA. Trends in breast cancer incidence and mortality in the United States: implications for prevention. Breast Cancer Res Treat. 2013;138(3):665–73.

8. Johnson RH, Chien FL, Bleyer A. Incidence of breast cancer with distant involvement among women in the United States, 1976–2009. JAMA. 2013;309(8):800–5.

9. Clavel-Chapelon F, Gerber M. Reproductive factors and breast cancer risk. Do they differ according to age at diagnosis? Breast Cancer Res Treat. 2002;72(2):107–15.

10. Warner ET, Colditz GA, Palmer JR, Partridge AH, Rosner BA, Tamimi RM. Reproductive factors and risk of premenopausal breast cancer by age at diagnosis: are there differences before and after age 40? Breast Cancer Res Treat. 2013;142(1):165–75.

11. Talamini R, Franceschi S, La Vecchia C, Negri E, Borsa L, Montella M, et al. The role of reproductive and menstrual factors in cancer of the breast before and after menopause. Eur J Cancer. 1996;32(2):303–10.

12. Lambe M, Hsieh C-c, Trichopoulos D, Ekbom A, Pavia M, Adami H-O. Transient increase in the risk of breast cancer after giving birth. N Engl J Med. 1994;331(1):5–9.

13. Liu Q, Wuu J, Lambe M, Hsieh S-F, Ekbom A, Hsieh C-C. Transient increase in breast cancer risk after giving birth: postpartum period with the highest risk (Sweden). Cancer Causes Control. 2002;13(4):299–305.

14. Shakhar K, Valdimarsdottir HB, Bovbjerg DH. Heightened risk of breast cancer following pregnancy: could lasting systemic immune alterations contribute? Cancer Epidemiol Biomark Prev. 2007;16(6):1082–6.

15. Collaborative Group on Hormonal Factors in Breast Cancer. Breast cancer and hormonal contraceptives: collaborative reanalysis of individual data on 53 297 women with breast cancer and 100 239 women without breast cancer from 54 epidemiologic studies. Lancet. 1999;347(9017):1713–27.

16. Gierisch JM, Coeytaux RR, Urrutia RP, Havrilesky LJ, Moorman PG, Lowery WJ, et al. Oral contraceptive use and risk of breast, cervical, colorectal, and endometrial cancers: a systematic review. Cancer Epidemiol Biomark Prev. 2013;22(11):1931–43.

17. van den Belt-Dusebout AW, Spaan M, Lambalk CB, Kortman M, Laven JS, van Santbrink EJ, et al. Ovarian stimulation for in vitro fertilization and long-term risk of breast cancer. JAMA. 2016;316(3):300–12.

18. Venn A, Watson L, Lumley J, Giles G, King C, Healy D. Breast and ovarian cancer incidence after infertility and in vitro fertilization. Lancet. 1995;346(8981):995–1000.

19. Brinton LA, Trabert B, Shalev V, Lunenfeld E, Sella T, Chodick G. In vitro fertilization and risk of breast and gynecologic cancers: a retrospective cohort study within the Israeli Maccabi Healthcare Services. Fertil Steril. 2013;99(5):1189–96.

20. Sergentanis TN, Diamantaras A, Perlepe C, Kanavidis P, Skalkidou A, Petridou ET. IVF and breast cancer: a systematic review and meta-analysis. Hum Reprod Update. 2014;20(1):106–23.

21. Eliassen AH, Missmer SA, Tworoger SS, Spiegelman D, Barbieri RL, Dowsett M, et al. Endogenous steroid hormone concentrations and risk of breast cancer among premenopausal women. J Natl Cancer Inst. 2006;98(19):1406–15.

22. Kaaks R, Berrino F, Key T, Rinaldi S, Dossus L, Biessy C, et al. Serum sex steroids in premenopausal women and breast cancer risk within the European Prospective Investigation into Cancer and Nutrition (EPIC). J Natl Cancer Inst. 2005;97(10):755–65.

23. Hankinson SE, Willett WC, Manson JE, Colditz GA, Hunter DJ, Spiegelman D, et al. Plasma sex steroid hormone levels and risk of breast cancer in postmenopausal women. J Natl Cancer Inst. 1998;90(17):1292–9.

24. Ahlgren M, Melbye M, Wohlfahrt J, Sørensen TIA. Growth patterns and the risk of breast cancer in women. N Engl J Med. 2004;351(16):1619–26.

25. Gunnell D, Okasha M, Davey Smith G, Oliver SE, Sandhu J, Jolly JMP. Height, leg length, and cancer risk: a systematic review. Epidemiol Rev. 2001;23(2):313–42.

26. Friedenreich CM. Review of anthropometric factors and breast cancer risk. Eur J Cancer Prev. 2001;10(1):15–32.

27. Carmichael AR, Bates T. Obesity and breast cancer: a review of the literature. Breast. 2004;13(2):85–92.

28. Steindorf K, Ritte R, Eomois P-P, Lukanova A, Tjonneland A, Johnsen NF, et al. Physical activity and risk of breast cancer overall and by hormone receptor status: the European prospective

investigation into cancer and nutrition. Int J Cancer. 2013;132(7):1667–78.

29. Maruti SS, Willett WC, Feskanich D, Rosner B, Colditz GA. A prospective study of age-specific physical activity and premenopausal breast cancer. J Natl Cancer Inst. 2008;100(10):728–37.

30. Rockhill B, Willett WC, Hunter DJ, Manson JE, Hankinson SE, Coldtiz GA. A prospective study of recreational physical activity and breast cancer risk. Arch Intern Med. 1999;159(19):2290–6.

31. Baer HJ, Tworoger SS, Hankinson SE, Willett WC. Body fatness at young ages and risk of breast cancer throughout life. Am J Epidemiol. 2010;171(11):1183–94.

32. Liu Y, Colditz GA, Rosner B, Berkey CS, Collins LC, Schnitt SJ, et al. Alcohol intake between menarche and first pregnancy: a prospective study of breast cancer risk. J Natl Cancer Inst. 2013;105(20):1571–8.

33. Willett WC, Stampfer MJ, Colditz GA, Rosner BA, Hennekens CH, Speizer FE. Moderate alcohol consumption and the risk of breast cancer. N Engl J Med. 1987;316(19):1174–80.

34. Chen WY, Rosner B, Hankinson SE, Colditz GA, Willett WC. Moderate alcohol consumption during adult life, drinking patterns, and breast cancer risk. JAMA. 2011;206(17):1884–90.

35. Bowlin SJ, Leske MC, Varma A, Nasca P, Weinstein A, Caplan L. Breast cancer risk and alcohol consumption: results from a large case-control study. Int J Epidemiol. 1997;26(5):915–23.

36. Harris HR, Willett WC, Vaidya RL, Michels KB. An adolescent and early adulthood dietary pattern with inflammation and the incidence of breast cancer. Cancer Res. 2017;77(5):1179–87.

37. Frazier AL, Ryan CT, Rockett H, Willett WC, Colditz GA. Adolescent diet and risk of breast cancer. Breast Cancer Res. 2003;5(3):R59–64.

38. Shin M, Holmes MD, Hankinson SE, Wu K, Colditz GA, Willett WC. Intake of dietary products, calcium, and vitamin D and risk of breast cancer. J Natl Cancer Inst. 2002;94(17):1301–11.

39. Castello A, Pollan M, Buijsse B, Ruiz A, Casas AM, Baena-Canada JM, et al. Spanish Mediterranean diet and other dietary patterns and breast cancer risk: case-control EpiGEICAM study. Br J Cancer. 2014;111(7):1454–62.

40. Hirko KA, Willett WC, Hankinson SE, Rosner BA, Beck AH, Tamimi RM, et al. Healthy dietary patterns and risk of breast cancer by molecular subtype. Breast Cancer Res Treat. 2016;155(3):579–88.

41. Schwingshackl L, Hoffmann G. Adherence to Mediterranean diet and risk of cancer: an updated systematic review and meta-analysis of observational studies. Cancer Med. 2015;4(12):1933–47.

42. Moskowitz CS, Chou JF, Wolden SL, Bernstein JL, Malhotra J, Novetsky Friedman D, et al. Breast cancer after chest radiation therapy for childhood cancer. J Clin Oncol. 2014;32(21):2217–23.

43. Gnerlich JL, Deshpande AD, Jeffe DB, Sweet A, White N, Margenthaler JA. Elevated breast cancer mortality in women younger than age 40 years compared with older women is attributed to poorer survival in early-stage disease. J Am Coll Surg. 2009;208(3):341–7.

44. Morris GJ, Naidu S, Topham AK, Guiles F, Xu Y, McCue P, et al. Differences in breast carcinoma characteristics in newly diagnosed African-American and Caucasian patients: a single-institution compilation compared with the National Cancer Institute's Surveillance, Epidemiology, and End Results database. Cancer. 2007;110(4):876–84.

45. Amirikia KC, Mills P, Bush J, Newman LA. Higher population-based incidence rates of triple-negative breast cancer among young African-American women: implications for breast cancer screening recommendations. Cancer. 2011;117(12):2747–53.

46. Carey LA, Perou CM, Livasy CA, Dressler LG, Cowan D, Conway K, et al. Race, breast cancer subtypes, and survival in the Carolina Breast Cancer Study. JAMA. 2006;295(21):2492–502.

47. Copson E, Maishman T, Gerty S, Eccles B, Stanton L, Cutress RI, et al. Ethnicity and outcome of young breast cancer patients in the United Kingdom: the POSH study. Br J Cancer. 2014;110(1):230–41.

48. Cancer Genome Atlas N. Comprehensive molecular portraits of human breast tumours. Nature. 2012;490(7418):61–70.

49. Tung N, Lin NU, Kidd J, Allen BA, Singh N, Wenstrup RJ, et al. Frequency of germline mutations in 25 cancer susceptibility genes in a sequential series of patients with breast cancer. J Clin Oncol. 2016;34(13):1460–8.

50. Gabai-Kapara E, Lahad A, Kaufman B, Friedman E, Segev S, Renbaum P, et al. Population-based screening for breast and ovarian cancer risk due to BRCA1 and BRCA2. Proc Natl Acad Sci U S A. 2014;111(39):14205–10.

51. Roa BB, Boyd AA, Volcik K, Richards CS. Ashkenazi Jewish population frequencies for common mutations in BRCA1 and BRCA2. Nat Genet. 1996;14(2):185–7.

52. Warner E, Foulkes W, Goodwin P, Meschino W, Blondal J, Paterson C, et al. Prevalence and penetrance of BRCA1 and BRCA2 gene mutations in unselected Ashkenazi Jewish women with breast cancer. J Natl Cancer Inst. 1999;91(14):1241–7.

53. Pal T, Bonner D, Cragun D, Monteiro ANA, Phelan C, Servais L, et al. A high frequency of BRCA mutations in young black women with breast cancer from Florida. Cancer. 2015;121(23):4173–80.

54. Villarreal-Garza C, Weitzel JN, Llacuachaqui M, Sifuentes E, Magallanes-Hoyos MC, Gallardo L, et al. The prevalence of BRCA1 and BRCA2 mutations among young Mexican women with triple-negative breast cancer. Breast Cancer Res Treat. 2015;150(2):389–94.

55. Ruddy KJ, Gelber S, Tamimi RM, Schapira L, Come SE, Meyer ME, et al. Breast cancer presentation

and diagnostic delays in young women. Cancer. 2014;120(1):20–5.

56. Fredholm H, Eaker S, Frisell J, Holmberg L, Fredriksson I, Lindman H. Breast cancer in young women: poor survival despite intensive treatment. PLoS One. 2009;4(11):e7695.

57. Keegan TH, DeRouen MC, Press DJ, Kurian AW, Clarke CA. Occurrence of breast cancer subtypes in adolescent and young women. Breast Cancer Res. 2012;14:R55.

58. Collins LC, Marotti JD, Gelber S, Cole K, Ruddy K, Kereakoglow S, et al. Pathologic features and molecular phenotype by patient age in a large cohort of young women with breast cancer. Breast Cancer Res Treat. 2012;131(3):1061–6.

59. Copson E, Eccles B, Maishman T, Gerty S, Stanton L, Cutress RI, et al. Prospective observational study of breast cancer treatment outcomes for UK women aged 18–40 years at diagnosis: the POSH study. J Natl Cancer Inst. 2013;105(13):978–88.

60. Swain SM, Nunes R, Yoshizawa C, Rothney M, Sing AP. Quantitative gene expression by recurrence score in ER-positive breast cancer, by age. Adv Ther. 2015;32(12):1222–36.

61. Azim HA Jr, Nguyen B, Brohee S, Zoppoli G, Sotiriou C. Genomic aberrations in young and elderly breast cancer patients. BMC Med. 2015;13:266.

62. Han W, Kim SW, Park IA, Kang D, Kim SW, Youn YK, et al. Young age: an independent risk factor for disease-free survival in women with operable breast cancer. BMC Cancer. 2004;4:82.

63. Partridge AH, Hughes ME, Warner ET, Ottesen RA, Wong YN, Edge SB, et al. Subtype-dependent relationship between young age at diagnosis and breast cancer survival. J Clin Oncol. 2016;34(27):3308–14.

64. Swain SM, Jeong J, Geyer CE Jr, Costantino JP, Pajon ER, Fehrenbacher L, et al. Longer therapy, iatrogenic amenorrhea, and survival in early breast cancer. N Engl J Med. 2010;362(22):2053–65.

65. Bellet M, Gray KP, Francis PA, Lang I, Ciruelos E, Lluch A, et al. Twelve-month estrogen levels in premenopausal women with hormone receptor-positive breast cancer receiving adjuvant triptorelin plus exemestane or tamoxifen in the Suppression of Ovarian Function Trial (SOFT): the SOFT-EST substudy. J Clin Oncol. 2016;34(14):1584–93.

66. Francis PA, Regan MM, Fleming GF, Lang I, Ciruelos E, Bellet M, et al. Adjuvant ovarian suppression in premenopausal breast cancer. N Engl J Med. 2015;372(5):436–46.

67. Saha P, Regan MM, Pagani O, Francis PA, Walley BA, Ribi K, et al. Treatment efficacy, adherence and quality-of life among very young women (age <35 years) in the IBCSG TEXT and SOFT Adjuvant Endocrine Therapy Trials. J Clin Oncol. 2017;35:3113–22.

68. Early Breast Cancer Trialists' Collaborative Group. Effects of chemotherapy and hormonal therapy for early breast cancer on recurrence and 15-year sur-

vival: an overview of the randomised trials. Lancet. 2005;365(9472):1687–717.

69. Ademuyiwa FO, Gao F, Hao L, Morgensztern D, Aft RL, Ma CX, et al. US breast cancer mortality trends in young women according to race. Cancer. 2015;121(9):1469–76.

70. Wheeler SB, Reeder-Hayes KE, Carey LA. Disparities in breast cancer treatment and outcomes: biological, social, and health system determinants and opportunities for research. Oncologist. 2013;18(9):986–93.

71. Roberts MC, Wheeler SB, Reeder-Hayes K. Racial/ethnic and socioeconomic disparities in endocrine therapy adherence in breast cancer: a systematic review. Am J Public Health. 2015;105(S3):e4–e15.

72. Paluch-Shimon S, Pagani O, Partridge AH, Bar-Meir E, Fallowfield L, Fenlon D, et al. Second international consensus guidelines for breast cancer in young women (BCY2). Breast. 2016;26:87–99.

73. Kroman N, Holtveg H, Wohlfahrt J, Jensen MB, Mouridsen HT, Blichert-Toft M, et al. Effect of breast-conserving therapy versus radical mastectomy on prognosis for young women with breast carcinoma. Cancer. 2004;100(4):688–93.

74. Mahmood U, Morris C, Neuner G, Koshy M, Kesmodel S, Buras R, et al. Similar survival with breast conservation therapy or mastectomy in the management of young women with early-stage breast cancer. Int J Radiat Oncol Biol Phys. 2012;83(5):1387–93.

75. Kurian AW, Lichtensztajn DY, Keegan TH, Nelson DO, Clarke CA, Gomez SL. Use of and mortality after bilateral mastectomy compared with other surgical treatments for breast cancer in California, 1998–2011. JAMA. 2014;312(9):902–14.

76. Braunstein LZ, Taghian AG, Niemierko A, Salama L, Capuco A, Bellon JR, et al. Breast-cancer subtype, age, and lymph node status as predictors of local recurrence following breast-conserving therapy. Breast Cancer Res Treat. 2017;161(1):173–9.

77. Arvold ND, Taghian AG, Niemierko A, Abi Raad RF, Sreedhara M, Nguyen PL, et al. Age, breast cancer subtype approximation, and local recurrence after breast-conserving therapy. J Clin Oncol. 2011;29(29):3885–91.

78. Aalders KC, Postma EL, Strobbe LJ, van der Heiden-van der Loo M, Sonke GS, Boersma LJ, et al. Contemporary locoregional recurrence rates in young patients with early-stage breast cancer. J Clin Oncol. 2016;34(18):2107–14.

79. Radosa JC, Eaton A, Stempel M, Khander A, Liedtke C, Solomayer EF, et al. Evaluation of local and distant recurrence patterns in patients with triple-negative breast cancer according to age. Ann Surg Oncol. 2017;24(3):698–704.

80. Kuijer A, King TA. Age, molecular subtypes and local therapy decision-making. Breast. 2017;34:S70–7.

81. King TA, Sakr R, Patil S, Gurevich I, Stempel M, Sampson M, et al. Clinical management factors contribute to the decision for contralateral prophylactic mastectomy. J Clin Oncol. 2011;29(16):2158–64.

82. Rosenberg SM, Sepucha K, Ruddy KJ, Tamimi RM, Gelber S, Meyer ME, et al. Local therapy decision-making and contralateral prophylactic mastectomy in young women with early-stage breast cancer. Ann Surg Oncol. 2015;22(12):3809–15.

83. Rosenberg SM, Partridge AH. Management of breast cancer in very young women. Breast. 2015;24(Suppl 2):S154–8.

84. Han W, Kang SY, Korean Breast Cancer Society. Relationship between age at diagnosis and outcome of premenopausal breast cancer: age less than 35 years is a reasonable cut-off for defining young age-onset breast cancer. Breast Cancer Res Treat. 2010;119(1):193–200.

85. Elkum N, Dermime S, Ajarim D, Al-Zahrani A, Alsayed A, Tulbah A, et al. Being 40 or younger is an independent risk factor for relapse in operable breast cancer patients: the Saudi Arabia experience. BMC Cancer. 2007;7(1):222.

86. Paik S, Shak S, Tang G, Kim C, Baker J, Cronin M, et al. A multigene assay to predict recurrence of tamoxifen-treated, node-negative breast cancer. N Engl J Med. 2004;351:2817–26.

87. Paik S, Tang G, Shak S, Kim C, Baker J, Kim W, et al. Gene expression and benefit of chemotherapy in women with node-negative, estrogen receptor-positive breast cancer. J Clin Oncol. 2006;24(23):3726–34.

88. Sparano JA, Gray RJ, Makower DF, Pritchard KI, Albain KS, Hayes DF, et al. Prospective validation of a 21-gene expression assay in breast cancer. N Engl J Med. 2015;373(21):2005–14.

89. Petkov VI, Miller DP, Howlader N, Gliner N, Howe W, Schussler N, et al. Breast-cancer-specific mortality in patients treated based on the 21-gene assay: a SEER population-based study. NPJ Breast Cancer. 2016;2:16017.

90. Makubate B, Donnan PT, Dewar JA, Thompson AM, McCowan C. Cohort study of adherence to adjuvant endocrine therapy, breast cancer recurrence and mortality. Br J Cancer. 2013;108(7):1515–24.

91. Partridge AH, Wang PS, Winer EP, Avorn J. Nonadherence to adjuvant tamoxifen therapy in women with primary breast cancer. J Clin Oncol. 2003;21(4):602–6.

92. Hershman DL, Kushi LH, Shao T, Buono D, Kershenbaum A, Tsai WY, et al. Early discontinuation and nonadherence to adjuvant hormonal therapy in a cohort of 8,769 early-stage breast cancer patients. J Clin Oncol. 2010;28(27):4120–8.

93. Llarena NC, Estevez SL, Tucker SL, Jeruss JS. Impact of fertility concerns on tamoxifen initiation and persistence. J Natl Cancer Inst. 2015;107(10):djv202.

94. Rosenberg SM, Partridge AH. New insights into nonadherence with adjuvant endocrine therapy among young women with breast cancer. J Natl Cancer Inst. 2015;107(10):djv245.

95. Land SR, Walcott FL, Liu Q, Wickerham DL, Costantino JP, Ganz PA. Symptoms and QOL as predictors of chemoprevention adherence in NRG Oncology/NSABP Trial P-1. J Natl Cancer Inst. 2016;108(4):djv365.

96. Murphy CC, Bartholomew LK, Carpentier MY, Bluethmann SM, Vernon SW. Adherence to adjuvant hormonal therapy among breast cancer survivors in clinical practice: a systematic review. Breast Cancer Res Treat. 2012;134(2):459–78.

97. Goodwin PJ, Ennis M, Pritchard KL, Trudeau M, Hood N. Risk of menopause during the first year after breast cancer diagnosis. J Clin Oncol. 1999;17(8):2365–70.

98. Petrek JA, Naughton MJ, Case LD, Paskett ED, Naftalis EZ, Singletary SE, et al. Incidence, time course, and determinants of menstrual bleeding after breast cancer treatment: a prospective study. J Clin Oncol. 2006;24(7):1045–51.

99. Sukumvanich P, Case LD, Van Zee K, Singletary SE, Paskett ED, Petrek JA, et al. Incidence and time course of bleeding after long-term amenorrhea after breast cancer treatment: a prospective study. Cancer. 2010;116(13):3102–11.

100. Ruddy KJ, Gelber SI, Tamimi RM, Ginsburg ES, Schapira L, Come SE, et al. Prospective study of fertility concerns and preservation strategies in young women with breast cancer. J Clin Oncol. 2014;32(11):1151–6.

101. Davies MC, Hall ML, Jacobs HS. Bone mineral loss in young women with amenorrhea. BMJ. 1990;301:790–3.

102. Colditz GA, Willett WC, Stampfer MJ, Rosner B, Speizer FE, Hennekens CH. Menopause and the risk of coronary artery disease in women. N Engl J Med. 1987;316(18):1105–10.

103. Rocca WA, Shuster LT, Grossardt BR, Maraganore DM, Gostout BS, Geda YE, et al. Long-term effects of bilateral oophorectomy on brain aging: unanswered questions from the Mayo Clinic Cohort Study of oophorectomy and aging. Womens Health (Lond). 2009;5(1):39–48.

104. Ganz PA, Greendale GA, Petersen L, Kahn B, Bower JE. Breast cancer in younger women: reproductive and late health effects of treatment. J Clin Oncol. 2003;21(22):4184–93.

105. Leining MG, Gelber S, Rosenberg R, Przypyszny M, Winer EP, Partridge AH. Menopausal-type symptoms in young breast cancer survivors. Ann Oncol. 2006;17(12):1777–82.

106. Crandall C, Petersen L, Ganz PA, Greendale GA. Association of breast cancer and its therapy with menopause-related symptoms. Menopause. 2004;11(5):519–30.

107. Webber K, Mok K, Bennett B, Lloyd AR, Friedlander M, Juraskova I, et al. If I am in the mood, I enjoy it: an exploration of cancer-related fatigue and sexual functioning in women with breast cancer. Oncologist. 2011;16(9):1333–44.

108. Kroenke CH, Chen WY, Rosner B, Holmes MD. Weight, weight gain, and survival after breast cancer diagnosis. J Clin Oncol. 2005;23(7):1370–8.
109. Avis NE, Crawford S, Manuel J. Quality of life among younger women with breast cancer. J Clin Oncol. 2005;23(15):3322–30.
110. Irwin ML, McTiernan A, Baumgartner RN, Baumgartner KB, Bernstein L, Gilliland FD, et al. Changes in body fat and weight after a breast cancer diagnosis: influence of demographic, prognostic, and lifestyle factors. J Clin Oncol. 2005;23(4):774–82.
111. Avis NE, Crawford S, Manuel J. Psychosocial problems among younger women with breast cancer. Psycho-Oncology. 2004;13(5):295–308.
112. Chan DS, Vieira AR, Aune D, Bandera EV, Greenwood DC, McTiernan A, et al. Body mass index and survival in women with breast cancer-systematic literature review and meta-analysis of 82 follow-up studies. Ann Oncol. 2014;25(10):1901–14.
113. Demark-Wahnefried W, Petersen BL, Winer EP, Marks L, Aziz N, Marcom K, et al. Changes in weight, body composition, and factors influencing energy balance among premenopausal breast cancer patients receiving adjuvant chemotherapy. J Clin Oncol. 2001;19(9):2381–9.
114. Holmes MD, Chen WY, Feskanich D, Kroenke CH, Colditz GA. Physical activity and survival after breast cancer diagnosis. JAMA. 2005;293(20):2479–86.
115. Kroenke CH, Rosner B, Chen WY, Kawachi I, Colditz GA, Holmes MD. Functional impact of breast cancer by age at diagnosis. J Clin Oncol. 2004;22(10):1849–56.
116. Howard-Anderson J, Ganz PA, Bower JE, Stanton AL. Quality of life, fertility concerns, and behavioral health outcomes in younger breast cancer survivors: a systematic review. J Natl Cancer Inst. 2012;104(5):386–405.
117. Wong-Kim EC, Bloom JR. Depression experienced by young women newly diagnosed with breast cancer. Psycho-Oncology. 2005;14(7):564–73.
118. Kendall AR, Mahue-Giangreco M, Carpenter CL, Ganz PA, Bernstein L. Influence of exercise activity on quality of life in long-term breast cancer survivors. Qual Life Res. 2005;14(2):361–71.
119. Harrison SA, Hayes SC, Newman B. Age-related differences in exercise and quality of life among breast cancer survivors. Med Sci Sports Exerc. 2010;42(1):67–74.
120. Partridge AH, Pagani O, Abulkhair O, Aebi S, Amant F, Azim HA, et al. First international consensus guidelines for breast cancer in young women (BCY1). Breast. 2014;23(3):209–20.

Young Age and Breast Cancer Biology

Hamdy A. Azim, Bastien Nguyen, and Hatem A. Azim Jr

2.1 Introduction

For the past three decades, it has been consistently shown that breast cancers arising in young women are associated with more aggressive clinicopathological features [1]. While the absence of screening programs in young women could partly explain the higher tendency of diagnosing tumors at a relatively advanced clinical stage, the association with aggressive pathological features remained hard to reconcile. This include more poorly differentiated and estrogen receptor-negative tumors [2–4]. While this would partly contribute to the poor prognosis observed in young breast cancer patients, interestingly several studies have found that young age remains a poor prognostic parameter independent of differences in tumor stage and pathological features [4–6]. This poor prognosis was observed more prominently in estrogen receptor-positive tumors or the luminal subtypes [4, 7]. This suggests that age is not just a surrogate for aggressive pathological features and that the biological makeup of these tumors is possibly more complex. It is plausible that the endocrine changes that take place during the reproductive age and changes occurring during pregnancy possibly influence the biology of these tumors, either directly or in a paracrine fashion via modulating the breast microenvironment. This would render these tumors rather biologically unique, as compared to their older counterparts.

Here we discuss key elements pertaining to the biology of tumors arising in young patients that could possibly open the door for defining tailored therapeutic interventions for these patients.

2.2 Gene Expression Profiling

Since the apparition of microarrays that allowed the evaluation of thousands of genes simultaneously to the high-throughput whole genome sequencing, the technological advances that have been made in the "omics" field have greatly improved our understanding of the biology of breast cancer in young women. This includes the characterization of breast cancer molecular subtypes but also key mRNA deregulations that were described in tumors arising at a young age.

H. A. Azim
Department of Clinical Oncology, Cairo University Hospital, Cairo, Egypt

B. Nguyen
Breast Cancer Translational Research Laboratory (BCTL), Institut Jules Bordet, UniversitéLibre de Bruxelles (ULB), Brussels, Belgium

H. A. Azim Jr (✉)
Division of Hematology/Oncology, Department of Internal Medicine, American University of Beirut (AUB), Beirut, Lebanon

© Springer Nature Switzerland AG 2020
O. Gentilini et al. (eds.), *Breast Cancer in Young Women*,
https://doi.org/10.1007/978-3-030-24762-1_2

2.2.1 Enrichment of Basal-Like Tumors in Young Women

In 2008, Anders et al. [8] published the first large-scale genomic analysis aiming to describe the biology of breast cancer in young women using gene expression profiling. This study included 411 patients with early-stage breast cancer from four publicly available datasets. They compared two groups: 200 patients classified as young ($\leq$45 years) versus 211 patients classified as older ($\geq$65 years). First, they focused the analysis on single genes that are routinely evaluated in standard practice and found that breast cancer in young patients is characterized by lower mRNA expression of estrogen receptor (ER) and progesterone receptor (PgR). This was in line with earlier studies that have reported a higher percentage of hormone receptor (HR)-negative disease in young women [9, 10]. In addition, they found a higher expression of human epidermal growth factor receptor 2 (HER-2) and epithelial growth factor receptor (EGFR) in breast cancer from young patients, an association not found consistently in prior studies [10, 11].

Subsequently, Azim Jr et al. [4] conducted the largest study so far to study the biology of breast cancer in young women by using gene expression data from 20 different datasets comprising a total of 3522 patients. They found that compared to patients 65 years or older, young breast cancer patients ($\leq$40 years) have nearly double the proportion of basal-like tumors (34.3% vs. 17.9%) but half the luminal A subtype (17.2% vs. 35.4%). Further work by the same group has highlighted that unlike postmenopausal breast cancer, ER-positive tumors arising in young women are predominantly the highly proliferative luminal B subtype and not the more indolent luminal A one [12].

Later on, Jenkins et al. [13] analyzed the discrepancy between the subtypes classified either by conventional immunohistochemistry or molecularly by PAM50 on around 4000 patients. One interesting finding is that in the younger group (<40 years), only 67% of the luminal patients by IHC (HR+/HER2−) were correctly classified as luminal A/B compared to 86% in the older group (>70 years). On the contrary, 80% of the triple-negative patients by IHC (HR−/HER2−) were correctly classified by PAM50 as basal-like compared to 57% in the older group (>70 years). This might indicate that in young patients, luminal breast cancer as defined by classical IHC could be enriched in more aggressive basal-like tumors and hence their poorer prognosis.

2.2.2 Unique Transcriptomic Alterations in Young Women

To further elucidate the biology of breast cancer diagnosed in young women, Azim Jr et al. evaluated the expression of more than 50 genes and gene signatures that are known to play a key role in breast cancer according to age [4]. Importantly, they tried to address if expression is related to age independent of differences in stage and molecular subtype. They found 12 genes and gene signatures significantly associated with age including higher expression of genes related to "stemness" like mammary stem cell signature, luminal progenitor signature, RANK-ligand (*RANKL*), and c-kit. The mammary stem cells are hormone receptor-negative cells known to give rise to mature epithelium of either the luminal or myoepithelial lineage via a series of lineage-restricted intermediates including luminal progenitors [14]. Other key molecular aberrations in tumors diagnosed in young women included deregulation of growth factor signaling like mitogen-activated protein kinase (MAPK) and phosphoinositide 3-kinase (PI3K) pathways. Moreover, breast cancer from young women was also enriched in a gene signature related to *BRCA1* mutation which is consistent with the relatively high prevalence of *BRCA1* mutations in younger patients [15, 16]. Further work by the same group has confirmed the enrichment of gene expression signatures related to endocrine resistance, proliferation, stem cells, and Notch signaling [11].

Several important messages and hypotheses could be derived from these findings. It is plausible that as women in their childbearing years have breast tissue enriched in stem cells to prepare for a potential pregnancy, this microenvironment, which is very sensitive to growth factor, could also promote tumor growth [17–19]. Increased number of luminal progenitors—the cell of origin of basal-like breast cancer—in young breast tissue could possibly explain the high expression of their regulating gene, *c-kit*, in tumors arising in young patients [14]. *BRCA1* and *RANKL* could also contribute to this phenomenon and this will be discussed later in more detail. Aberrations in PI3K and MAPK kinase pathways in addition to enrichment in endocrine resistance signature could all possibly explain, at least in part, the higher proportion of luminal B subtype (at the expense of luminal A) in younger women and the poorer outcome of ER-positive tumors in these patients.

2.3 Germline BRCA Mutation and the Interplay with PgR and RANKL Signaling

2.3.1 Germline BRCA Mutation in Young Breast Cancer Patients

Around 5–10% of breast cancers are secondary to germline mutations in either *BRCA1* or *BRCA2*, which are tumor suppression genes, dynamically involved in maintenance of genome integrity [20]. Both genes are considered key components of DNA homologous recombination repair pathway [21]; hence their loss leads to defective repair of damaged DNA, which increases cancer susceptibility.

Hence in *BRCA1* and *BRCA2* germline mutation carriers, the overall incidence of breast cancer rises dramatically compared to non *BRCA1/2* carriers [22]. Interestingly, such risk is more remarkable among young women, reaching 73- and 46-fold in women between 21–30 years and 31–40 years, respectively, for *BRCA1*, while in *BRCA2*, it is 60- and 20-fold in the two age groups, respectively [23]. Hence, diagnosis of breast cancer at a young age remains an absolute indication for germline *BRCA* testing [24], which currently has both preventive and therapeutic implications. In this context, Rosenberg et al.

have recently reported that in the USA, nearly all young breast cancer patients diagnosed in 2013 are subjected to *BRCA* testing compared to only 77% in 2006 [25].

Beyond the critical role of *BRCA1* in DNA repair [21], it is also implicated in the control of mammary cellular differentiation [14]. *BRCA1* deficiency was shown to disrupt the differentiation hierarchy present in the normal mammary gland and increases the proportion of the undifferentiated mammary stem cells [14]. Molecular analysis of benign breast tissues from women with *BRCA1* mutation revealed defects in progenitor cell lineage commitment even before cancer development. Furthermore, disrupting *BRCA1* in mice results in activation of epithelial-to-mesenchymal transition and induction of dedifferentiation of luminal progenitor cells, with accumulation of a luminal progenitor subset as a major cellular pool susceptible for neoplastic transformation [26]. Interestingly, the proportion of the hormone receptor-negative tumors in women with *BRCA1* mutations is highest among young women and gradually decreases with advanced age. These data runs in line with transcriptomic findings discussed earlier, highlighting how germline events impact the phenotype and molecular makeup of tumors diagnosed at a young age.

2.3.2 PgR and BRCA Crosstalk

On the other hand, *BRCA1* plays an important role in PgR degradation and was shown to inhibit progesterone-stimulated proliferation in breast cancer preclinical models [27]. Conversely, knockdown of endogenous *BRCA1* in in vitro models was shown to significantly enhance progesterone-stimulated activity of PgR[27]. In breast cancer patients, the expression of PgR was significantly higher in benign breast epithelium adjacent to invasive breast carcinoma in *BRCA1* mutation carriers compared to sporadic cases [27]. Furthermore, serum progesterone levels were shown to be higher in healthy and breast cancer patients harboring a *BRCA* mutation compared to controls [27]. These findings suggest that *BRCA1* regulates PgR expression, which—and via its paracrine signaling—can be also implicated in *BRCA1*-related mammary carcinogenesis.

These biological considerations may provide relevant therapeutic insights. The apparently inexplicable notion that, in *BRCA1* mutation carriers, prophylactic bilateral salpingo-oophorectomy is associated with reduced risk of developing breast cancer [28], despite the fact that *BRCA1*-associated tumors are mostly triple negative, could be possibly argued by the depletion of progesterone, given its important inference in the evolution of *BRCA1*-related breast cancer. Of note, the protective effect of salpingo-oophorectomy is more pronounced when performed before the age of 40.

2.3.3 *RANKL* Regulates PgR Signaling and Is Implicated in BRCA-Related Tumors

RANK and *RANKL* are principally recognized as the critical regulators of osteoclast maturation and activation and bone remodeling [29]. For many years now, targeting *RANKL* is recognized as an effective way to manage osteoporosis and reduce related skeletal events secondary to bone metastasis in patients with advanced cancers [29]. However, in recent years, there has been mounting evidence on the potential role of *RANKL* in breast carcinogenesis, particularly pertaining to the development of the disease at a young age.

The potential role of *RANKL* in breast cancer initiation and progression was initially elucidated in 2010 by two back-to-back studies, which showed that the pivotal role of progesterone in mammary carcinogenesis is mostly mediated by RANK/RANKL signaling [30, 31]. The PgR-positive luminal cells were found to upregulate *RANKL* expression that subsequently interacts with the RANK receptors present on the surface of mammary stem and luminal progenitor cells, which negatively express endocrine receptor suggesting a paracrine effect of *RANKL* in regulating mammary stem cells. Further evidence has also shown that administering *RANKL* inhibitor results in reducing mammary stem cell

pool [32] and in significant delay in developing progesterone-induced tumors [30, 31].

Two years later, Azim Jr et al. further showed that the expression of *RANKL* in primary breast cancer is much higher in younger patients compared to older counterparts [4]. In the same study, there was also high expression of signatures related to BRCA mutation and mammary stem cells. Further experiments by the same group showed that expression is also high on adjacent normal tissue, particularly in pregnant breast cancer patients [33], underscoring the potential impact of the breast microenvironment in altering tumor phenotype and possibly behavior.

Recently, two important studies shed light on the importance of RANK/RANKL signaling pathway in the context of BRCA1-related breast cancer [34, 35]. Sigl et al. found that RANKL/RANK signaling might have a role in the etiology of BRCA1/2 mutation-driven breast cancer. They found that *RANK* was highly expressed in human BRCA mutation carriers compared to wild-type malignant breast tumors. In a mouse model, they showed that genetic inactivation of *RANK* protected from *BRCA1* deletion-driven tumorigenesis. Nolan et al. have further demonstrated that *RANK* expression was highest in the luminal progenitor cells of BRCA1 mutation carriers compared to both wild-type and BRCA2 mutation carriers [35]. BRCA1 mutations were shown to induce RANK/RANKL-dependent expansion of mammary luminal progenitor cells, which as mentioned earlier are the major cellular subset responsible for the development of basal-like tumors [14]. The same group could also provide evidence that inhibition of RANKL has a substantial preventive effect on the development of mammary hyperplasia and tumors in BRCA1-deficient mice [35]. In addition, lower osteoprotegerin (*OPG*) levels—the endogenous antagonist receptor for *RANKL*—have been reported among BRCA1 mutation carriers [36]. Importantly, women with high plasma *OPG* had a significantly decreased risk of developing breast cancer, compared to women with low *OPG* [37]. These data suggest that RANK/RANKL signaling could represent a potential target for breast cancer prevention in BRCA1 mutation carriers.

Taken together, *RANKL* has been identified as a pivotal paracrine mediator of progesterone signaling, which is significantly deregulated during the process of *BRCA1*-associated oncogenesis (Fig. 2.1). The RANKL inhibitor, denosumab, is already indicated for postmenopausal, hormonal receptor-positive patients to reduce risk of osteoporosis and related skeletal events caused by endocrine therapy [38]. Currently, at least two studies are ongoing and expected to report soon. D-BEYOND is a window of opportunity study aiming to evaluate the impact of preoperative administration of denosumab on breast cancer biology in young breast cancer patients. Following the findings of Nolan et al., a pilot study (BRCA-D) has also been launched to evaluate if RANKL inhibition could represent a strategy for breast cancer prevention in BRCA1 and BRCA2 mutation carriers.

2.4 Copy Number Alterations According to Age

Somatic change in DNA copy number (copy number alterations (CNAs)) largely characterizes the architecture of breast cancer genomes [39]. It has been found that in breast cancer, CNAs account for 85% of the variation in expression [39]. Copy number gain of oncogenes and copy number loss of tumor suppressor genes drive breast cancer initiation and progression and influence disease outcomes [39]. Therefore, the study of these alterations could provide important insights on the biology of breast cancer in young women and might explain their relatively poor prognosis.

In 2007, Yau et al. [40] published the first study aiming to characterize breast cancer according to age using both transcriptomic and copy num-

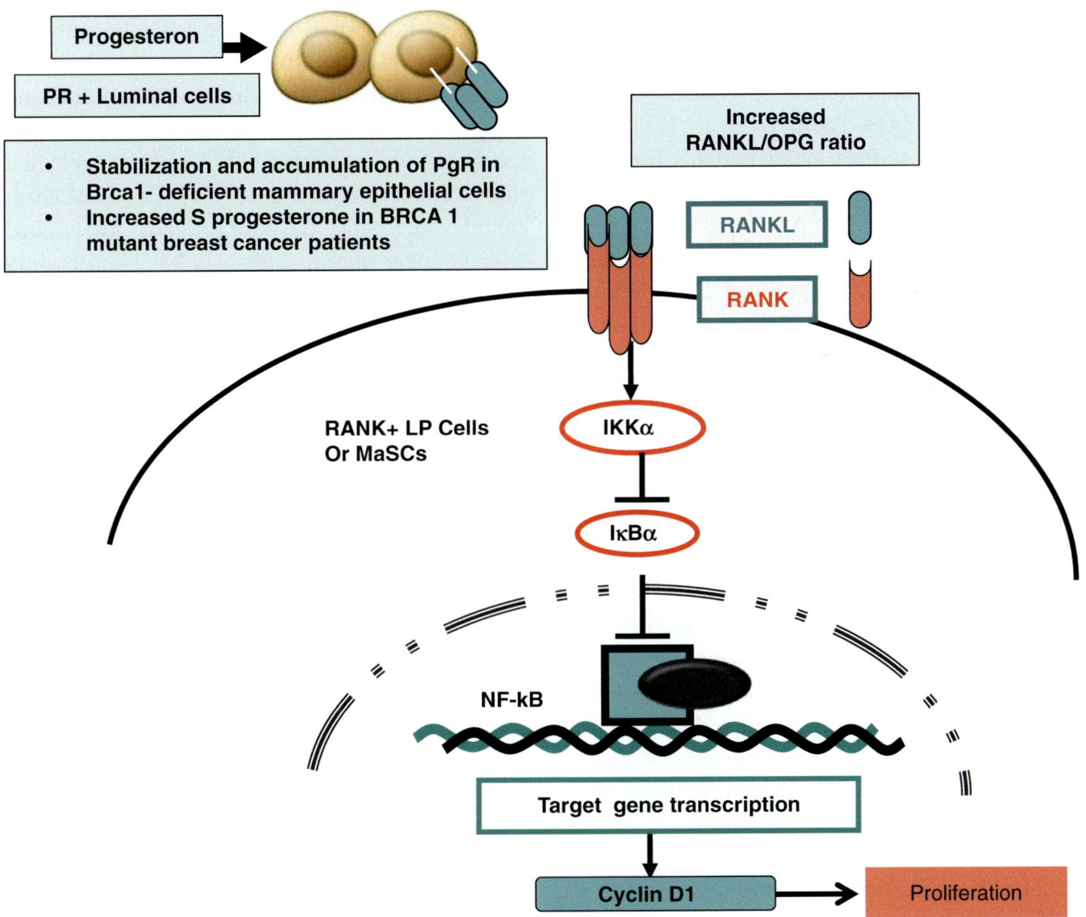

Fig. 2.1 Crosstalk of RANKL and progesterone signaling in BRCA mutant breast cancer

ber profiling. They retrospectively included 71 ER-positive breast cancer patients (27 diagnosed in young patients ($\leq$45 years) and 44 diagnosed in older patients ($\geq$70 years)). At the transcriptomic levels, they found some cancer-associated genes differentially expressed between the cohorts, with younger cases expressing more cell cycle genes and more than threefold higher levels of the growth factor amphiregulin and with older cases expressing higher levels of four different homeobox (HOX) genes in addition to ER (*ESR1*). They used comparative genomic hybridization array to compare the two age groups but did not find any significant differences in the fraction of genome altered nor in site-specific regions. However, this study had some limitations including the small sample size and the inclusion of ER-positive disease only. Moreover, the technology used to analyze copy number had low-density genomic arrays of only 2464 probes compared to the 900,000 probes used nowadays.

In a more recent in silico analysis using publicly available data from The Cancer Genome Atlas (TCGA) [41], Azim Jr et al. [11] found that breast cancer from older patients had globally more CNAs. This is likely due to the normal accumulation of CNAs in passenger genes as women age. Furthermore, they were able to identify a higher frequency of a focal deletion in chromosomal region 6q27 in young patients, a feature that has been previously associated with tumors of aggressive behavior [42].

2.5 Higher Frequency of GATA3 Mutations in Young Women with Breast Cancer

Recently, several groups have reported comprehensive analysis on the landscape of somatic mutations, copy number aberrations, and mutational signatures that are associated with different biological processes in large breast cancer cohorts [39, 41, 43, 44]. However, these studies had very poor representation of young breast cancer patients. In a secondary analysis of TCGA data, Azim Jr et al. [11] found 11 mutated genes that were independently associated with age at diagnosis. Among them *GATA3* was the only gene more frequently mutated in young women, in around 15% of cases, compared to 8% in older counterparts. The latter is known to regulate helper T-cell differentiation [45] and to have an important role in the development of the breast.

However, the contribution of *GATA3* mutations to cancer is poorly understood. Downregulation of *GATA3* results in epithelial-to-mesenchymal transition and basal-like tumors; thus *GATA3* has been considered as a tumor suppressor gene [46–48]. But a recent study by Mair et al. [49] had shed light on the fact that some frameshift mutation resulted in protein with an elongated C-terminus (namely *GATA*-ext) leading to a gain-of-function activity and hence could act as an oncogene. These specific mutations were associated with a worse DFS and resulted in differential drug sensitivity in cell line models. Further studies have shown that together with the estrogen receptor, *GATA3* controls the normal differentiation of the luminal epithelium in the terminal end buds in the mammary gland [50]. In addition, it has been suggested that *GATA3* plays a relevant role in endocrine resistance [51]. This is of clinical relevance, since the poor prognosis associated with younger age at diagnosis has been mainly observed in patients with luminal breast cancers [7]. Whether *GATA3* contributes to the poor prognosis of young ER-positive breast cancer patients and could act as a relevant therapeutic target remains to be explored.

2.6 Pregnancy Modulates Breast Cancer Biology

An important part of the development of the normal breast takes place during pregnancy. Several studies and meta-analyses have shown that women diagnosed with breast cancer during or shortly following pregnancy have poor prognosis compared to non-pregnancy-associated patients [52, 53]. In addition, women remain at an increased risk of developing breast cancer shortly after pregnancy [54]. This suggests that the physiological changes occurring during pregnancy possibly impact breast cancer initiation and progression, also via modulating the breast microenvironment.

Schedin et al. [55, 56] have published several experiments investigating the impact of post-pregnancy mammary changes on breast cancer initiation and progression. They showed that tumors developing in an involuting breast following pregnancy were highly proliferative, larger in size, and more in number compared to those developing in a nulliparous breast. Importantly, they found that biological changes that occur in the normal post-partum breast are well reflected on the tumors arising in these mice, particularly the deposition of collagen and expression of Cox-2, underscoring the impact of post-partum breast microenvironment on the nature of tumors developing in the same breast. In one of their experiments, they found that the inhibition of Cox-2 by a Cox-2 inhibitor resulted in reductions in the size of the tumors arising in the involuting breast. This work resulted in the initiation of a clinical trial that is expected to report soon investigating the role of Cox-2 inhibition on tumors arising in the post-partum phase.

Our group has worked on characterizing tumors diagnosed during pregnancy. These tumors are rare but could serve as a good model to understand impact of pregnancy on breast cancer biology. We found that RANKL, a gene that appears to play a key role in breast carcinogenesis in young women, is even more expressed in pregnant breast cancer patients, both on primary tumors and adjacent normal tissue, compared to non-pregnant young patients [33]. Using omics, pregnancy did not appear to impact considerably the distribution of breast cancer molecular subtypes using gene expression profiling [57]. However, by using an integrative analysis of gene expression, copy number alterations, and whole genome sequencing data, we found that tumors arising during pregnancy are enriched with non-silent mutations, a higher frequency of mutations in mucin gene family, and an enrichment of a mutational signature related to mismatch repair deficiency [58]. This suggests that these features may be implicated in promoting tumor

progression during pregnancy and may explain the aggressive behavior of BCP.

Taken together, pregnancy does appear to alter the molecular makeup of the already complex biology of cancers arising at young age.

2.7 Translating Biological Knowledge into Improving Patient Care

Accumulating evidence suggests that the biology of breast cancer in young women is rather unique. To date, treatments are tailored, irrespective of age, to the phenotypic subtype of the tumor as assessed by conventional factors, such as hormonal receptor and HER2 status as well as grade and proliferation rate [59–61]. In the current era of personalized medicine, it is of great importance to transfer the biological knowledge accumulated to improve breast cancer management in young women.

The upregulation of RANK/RANKL signaling pathway seen in young patients has led to a preoperative trial evaluating the impact of denosumab, a RANKL inhibitor, on the biology of breast cancer in young women (D-BEYOND; NCT01864798). This study could potentially define a role for denosumab in future management of young patients.

Younger breast cancer patients are enriched in *BRCA1/2* mutations, and the use of poly(ADP-ribose) polymerase (PARP) inhibitors to induce a synthetic lethality in those patients appears to be a very promising strategy [62]. Recent results in the metastatic setting have shown that the PARP inhibitor, olaparib, doubles the response rate and reduces the risk of disease progression by nearly 40% compared to standard of care chemotherapy [63], placing it as a novel standard of care option for metastatic breast cancer patients harboring a BRCA mutation. An even larger study is currently evaluating the value of the same agent in the adjuvant setting (NCT02032823), and a relatively large number of young patients will likely enroll.

Finally, better characterization of somatic mutations occurring in tumors arising in young women using next-generation sequencing could further identify key driver mutations that can be targeted in this challenging disease. Established in 2006, Helping Ourselves, Helping Others (HOHO): The Young Women's Breast Cancer Study has enrolled more than 1300 women who were 40 years or younger at the time of their diagnosis of breast cancer. This large study that included biobanking of tumor and blood samples represents a great opportunity to study the molecular characterization of young breast cancer. A lot of work is still required to expand our understanding of the biology of breast cancer diagnosed in young women while keeping in mind that the ultimate goal is to ensure optimal outcomes for these women.

References

1. Azim HA Jr, Partrdige AH. Biology of breast cancer in young women. Breast Cancer Res. 2014;16(4):427.
2. Gnerlich JL, Deshpande AD, Jeffe DB, Sweet A, White N, Margenthaler JA. Elevated breast cancer mortality in women younger than age 40 years compared with older women is attributed to poorer survival in early-stage disease. J Am CollSurg. 2009;208(3):341–7.
3. Han W, Kang SY, Korean Breast Cancer Society. Relationship between age at diagnosis and outcome of premenopausal breast cancer: age less than 35 years is a reasonable cut-off for defining young age-onset breast cancer. Breast Cancer Res Treat. 2010;119(1):193–200.
4. Azim HA Jr, Michiels S, Bedard PL, Singhal SK, Criscitiello C, Ignatiadis M, et al. Elucidating prognosis and biology of breast cancer arising in young women using gene expression profiling. Clin Cancer Res. 2012;18(5):1341–51.
5. Fredholm H, Eaker S, Frisell J, Holmberg L, Fredriksson I, Lindman H. Breast cancer in young women: poor survival despite intensive treatment. PLoS One. 2009;4(11):1–9.
6. Cancello G, Maisonneuve P, Rotmensz N, Viale G, Mastropasqua MG, Pruneri G, et al. Prognosis and adjuvant treatment effects in selected breast cancer subtypes of very young women (<35 years) with operable breast cancer. Ann Oncol. 2010;21(10):1974–81.
7. Partridge AH, Hughes ME, Warner ET, Ottesen RA, Wong YN, Edge SB, et al. Subtype-dependent relationship between young age at diagnosis and breast cancer survival. J ClinOncol. 2016;34(27):3308–14.
8. Anders CK, Hsu DS, Broadwater G, Acharya CR, Foekens JA, Zhang Y, et al. Young age at diagnosis correlates with worse prognosis and defines a subset of breast cancers with shared patterns of gene expression. J ClinOncol. 2008;26(20):3324–30.
9. Walker RA, Lees E, Webb MB, Dearing SJ. Breast carcinomas occurring in young women (< 35 years) are different. Br J Cancer. 1996;74(11):1796–800.
10. Colleoni M, Rotmensz N, Robertson C, Orlando L, Viale G, Renne G, et al. Very young women (<35 years) with operable breast cancer: features of disease at presentation. Ann Oncol. 2002;13(2):273–9.
11. Azim HA Jr, Nguyen B, Brohée S, Zoppoli G, Sotiriou C. Genomic aberrations in young and elderly breast cancer patients. BMC Med. 2015;13(1):266.
12. Azim HA Jr, Azim H. Breast cancer arising at a young age: do we need to define a cut-off? Breast. 2013;22(6):1007–8.
13. Jenkins EO, Deal AM, Anders CK, Prat A, Perou CM, Carey LA, et al. Age-specific changes in intrinsic breast cancer subtypes: afocus on older women. Oncologist. 2014;19(10):1076–83.
14. Lim E, Vaillant F, Wu D, Forrest NC, Pal B, Hart AH, et al. Aberrant luminal progenitors as the candidate target population for basal tumor development in BRCA1 mutation carriers. Nat Med. 2009;15(8):907–13.
15. Huzarski T, Byrski T, Gronwald J, Górski B, Domagala P, Cybulski C, et al. Ten-year survival in patients with BRCA1-negative and BRCA1-positive breast cancer. J ClinOncol. 2013;31(26):3191–6.
16. Young S, Pilarski RT, Donenberg T, Shapiro C, Hammond LS, Miller J, et al. The prevalence of BRCA1 mutations among young women with triple-negative breast cancer. BMC Cancer. 2009;9(1):86.
17. Kim JB, Stein R, O'Hare MJ. Tumour-stromal interactions in breast cancer: the role of stroma in tumourigenesis. Tumor Biol. 2005;26(4):173–85.
18. Bhowmick NA, Moses HL. Tumor–stroma interactions. CurrOpin Genet Dev. 2005;15(1):97–101.
19. McDaniel SM, Rumer KK, Biroc SL, Metz RP, Singh M, Porter W, et al. Remodeling of the mammary microenvironment after lactation promotes breast tumor cell metastasis. Am J Pathol. 2006;168(2):608–20.
20. Easton DF. How many more breast cancer predisposition genes are there? Breast Cancer Res. 1999;1(1):14–7.
21. Moynahan ME, Chiu JW, Koller BH, Jasin M. Brca1 controls homology-directed DNA repair. Mol Cell. 1999;4(4):511–8.
22. Burke W, Daly M, Garber J, Botkin J, Kahn MJ, Lynch P, et al. Recommendations for follow-up care of individuals with an inherited predisposition to cancer. II. BRCA1 and BRCA2. Cancer Genetics Studies Consortium. JAMA. 1997;277(12):997–1003.
23. Kuchenbaecker KB, Hopper JL, Barnes DR, Phillips K-A, Mooij TM, Roos-Blom M-J, et al. Risks of breast, ovarian, and contralateral breast cancer for *BRCA1* and *BRCA2*mutation carriers. JAMA. 2017;317(23):2402.
24. NCCN Guidelines Version 2.2017 Hereditary Breast and/or Ovarian Cancer Syndrome. [cited 2017 Nov 8].

http://www.nccn.org/professionals/physician_gls/pdf/genetics_screening.pdf

25. Rosenberg SM, Ruddy KJ, Tamimi RM, Gelber S, Schapira L, Come S, et al. *BRCA1* and *BRCA2* mutation testing in young women with breast cancer. JAMA Oncol. 2016;2(6):730.

26. Bai F, Chan HL, Scott A, Smith MD, Fan C, Herschkowitz JI, et al. BRCA1 suppresses epithelial-to-mesenchymal transition and stem cell dedifferentiation during mammary and tumor development. Cancer Res. 2014;74(21):6161–72.

27. Ma Y, Katiyar P, Jones LP, Fan S, Zhang Y, Furth PA, et al. The breast cancer susceptibility gene BRCA1 regulates progesterone receptor signaling in mammary epithelial cells. MolEndocrinol. 2006;20(1):14–34.

28. Metcalfe K, Lynch HT, Foulkes WD, Tung N, Kim-Sing C, Olopade OI, et al. Effect of oophorectomy on survival after breast cancer in *BRCA1* and *BRCA2* mutation carriers. JAMA Oncol. 2015;1(3):306.

29. Azim H, Azim HA Jr. Targeting RANKL in breast cancer: bone metastasis and beyond. Expert Rev Anticancer Ther. 2013;13(2):195–201.

30. Gonzalez-Suarez E, Jacob AP, Jones J, Miller R, Roudier-Meyer MP, Erwert R, et al. RANK ligand mediates progestin-induced mammary epithelial proliferation and carcinogenesis. Nature. 2010;468(7320):103–7.

31. Schramek D, Leibbrandt A, Sigl V, Kenner L, Pospisilik JA, Lee HJ, et al. Osteoclast differentiation factor RANKL controls development of progestin-driven mammary cancer. Nature. 2010;468(7320):98–102.

32. Asselin-Labat M-L, Vaillant F, Sheridan JM, Pal B, Wu D, Simpson ER, et al. Control of mammary stem cell function by steroid hormone signalling. Nature. 2010;465(7299):798–802.

33. Azim HA Jr, Peccatori FA, Brohée S, Branstetter D, Loi S, Viale G, et al. RANK-ligand (RANKL) expression in young breast cancer patients and during pregnancy. Breast Cancer Res. 2015;17(1):24.

34. Sigl V, Owusu-Boaitey K, Joshi PA, Kavirayani A, Wirnsberger G, Novatchkova M, et al. RANKL/RANK control Brca1 mutation-driven mammary tumors. Cell Res. 2016;26(7):761–74.

35. Nolan E, Vaillant F, Branstetter D, Pal B, Giner G, Whitehead L, et al. RANK ligand as a potential target for breast cancer prevention in BRCA1-mutation carriers. Nat Med. 2016;22(8):933–9.

36. Widschwendter M, Burnell M, Fraser L, Rosenthal AN, Philpott S, Reisel D, et al. Osteoprotegerin (OPG), the endogenous inhibitor of receptor activator of NF-κBligand (RANKL), is dysregulated in BRCA mutation carriers. EBioMedicine. 2015;2(10):1331–9.

37. Odén L, Akbari M, Zaman T, Singer CF, Sun P, Narod SA, et al. Plasma osteoprotegerin and breast cancer risk in BRCA1 and BRCA2 mutation carriers. Oncotarget. 2016;7(52):86687–94.

38. Gnant M, Pfeiler G, Dubsky PC, Hubalek M, Greil R, Jakesz R, et al. Adjuvant denosumab in breast cancer (ABCSG-18): a multicentre, randomised, double-blind, placebo-controlled trial. Lancet. 2015;386(9992):433–43.

39. Curtis C, Shah SP, Chin S-F, Turashvili G, Rueda OM, Dunning MJ, et al. The genomic and transcriptomic architecture of 2,000 breast tumours reveals novel subgroups. Nature. 2012;486(7403):346–52.

40. Yau C, Fedele V, Roydasgupta R, Fridlyand J, Hubbard A, Gray JW, et al. Aging impacts transcriptomes but not genomes of hormone-dependent breast cancers. Breast Cancer Res. 2007;9(5):R59.

41. TCGA. Comprehensive molecular portraits of human breast tumours. Nature. 2012;487(7407):61–70.

42. Noviello C, Courjal F, Theillet C. Loss of heterozygosity on the long arm of chromosome 6 in breast cancer: possibly four regions of deletion. Clin Cancer Res. 1996;2(9):1601–6.

43. Pereira B, Chin S-F, Rueda OM, Vollan H-KM, Provenzano E, Bardwell HA, et al. The somatic mutation profiles of 2,433 breast cancers refines their genomic and transcriptomic landscapes. Nat Commun. 2016;7(May):11479.

44. Nik-Zainal S, Davies H, Staaf J, Ramakrishna M, Glodzik D, Zou X, et al. Landscape of somatic mutations in 560 breast cancer whole-genome sequences. Nature. 2016;534(7605):1–20.

45. Tindemans I, Serafini N, Di Santo JP, Hendriks RW. GATA-3 function in innate and adaptive immunity. Immunity. 2014;41(2):191–206.

46. Asselin-Labat M-L, Sutherland KD, Barker H, Thomas R, Shackleton M, Forrest NC, et al. Gata-3 is an essential regulator of mammary-gland morphogenesis and luminal-cell differentiation. Nat Cell Biol. 2007;9(2):201–9.

47. Kouros-Mehr H, Kim J, Bechis SK, Werb Z. GATA-3 and the regulation of the mammary luminal cell fate. CurrOpin Cell Biol. 2008;20(2):164–70.

48. Kouros-Mehr H, Slorach EM, Sternlicht MD, Werb Z. GATA-3 maintains the differentiation of the luminal cell fate in the mammary gland. Cell. 2006;127(5):1041–55.

49. Mair B, Konopka T, Kerzendorfer C, Sleiman K, Salic S, Serra V, et al. Gain- and loss-of-function mutations in the breast cancer gene GATA3 result in differential drug sensitivity. PLoS Genet. 2016;12(9):1–26.

50. Chou J, Provot S, Werb Z. GATA3 in development and cancer differentiation: cells GATA have it! J Cell Physiol. 2010;222(1):42–9.

51. Yu-Rice Y, Jin Y, Han B, Qu Y, Johnson J, Watanabe T, et al. FOXC1 is involved in ERα silencing by counteracting GATA3 binding and is implicated in endocrine resistance. Oncogene. 2016;35(41):5400–11.

52. Azim HA Jr, Santoro L, Russell-Edu W, Pentheroudakis G, Pavlidis N, Peccatori FA. Prognosis of pregnancy-associated breast cancer: a meta-analysis of 30 studies. Cancer Treat Rev. 2012;38(7):834–42.

53. Hartman EK, Eslick GD. The prognosis of women diagnosed with breast cancer before, during and after pregnancy: a meta-analysis. Breast Cancer Res Treat. 2016;160(2):347–60.

54. Lambertini M, Santoro L, Del Mastro L, Nguyen B, Livraghi L, Ugolini D, et al. Reproductive behaviors and risk of developing breast cancer according to tumor subtype: a systematic review and meta-analysis of epidemiological studies. Cancer Treat Rev. 2016;49:65–76.

55. Lyons TR, O'Brien J, Borges VF, Conklin MW, Keely PJ, Eliceiri KW, et al. Postpartum mammary gland involution drives progression of ductal carcinoma in situ through collagen and COX-2. Nat Med. 2011;17(9):1109–15.

56. O'Brien J, Lyons T, Monks J, Lucia MS, Wilson RS, Hines L, et al. Alternatively activated macrophages and collagen remodeling characterize the postpartum involutingmammary gland across species. Am J Pathol. 2010;176(3):1241–55.

57. Azim HA Jr, Brohee S, Peccatori FA, Desmedt C, Loi S, Lambrechts D, et al. Biology of breast cancer during pregnancy using genomic profiling. EndocrRelat Cancer. 2014;21(4):545–54.

58. Nguyen B, Venet D, Azim HA Jr, Brown D, Desmedt C, Lambertini M, et al. Breast cancer diagnosed during pregnancy is associated with enrichment of non-silent mutations, mismatch repair deficiency signature and mucin mutations. NPJ Breast Cancer. 2018;4:23.

59. Paluch-Shimon S, Pagani O, Partridge AH, Abulkhair O, Cardoso MJ, Dent RA, et al. ESO-ESMO 3rd international consensus guidelines for breast cancer in young women (BCY3). Breast. 2017;35:203–17.

60. Rosenberg SM, Partridge AH. Management of breast cancer in very young women. Breast. 2015;24:S154–8.

61. Partridge AH. Chemotherapy in premenopausal breast cancer patients. Breast Care. 2015;10(5):307–10.

62. Balmaña J, Domchek SM, Tutt A, Garber JE. Stumbling blocks on the path to personalized medicine in breast cancer: the case of PARP inhibitors for *BRCA1/2* -associated cancers. Cancer Discov. 2011;1(1):29–34.

63. Robson M, Im SA, Senkus E, Xu B, Domchek SM, Masuda M, et al. Olaparib for metastatic breast cancer in patients with a germline BRCA mutation. N Engl J Med. 2017;377(6):523–33.

Tanja Gagliardi

3.1   Introduction

Breast cancer is a disease, which does not stop with young age. Although uncommon in young women under the age of 40, young women are not unusual visitors in symptomatic breast clinics. Early diagnosis is crucial, since breast cancer in young women is more likely to display aggressive biological features paired with often indeterminate morphological imaging characteristics. This makes it a dangerous mixture, which likely is underestimated in routine clinical settings and might fall short of appropriate clinical attention. Many signs and symptoms of young women are dismissed as cysts, nodular breast tissue, and fibroadenomas. Women are discouraged to refer to specialist breast units unless symptoms continue longer than one menstrual cycle. In the vast majority of women, this is a sensible approach, while for the few dealing with breast cancer, this is valuable time lost. By the time a lump has grown to a size it is clinically palpable, the chances of survival might have reduced, particularly given the aggressive nature of most cancers affecting young women.

For young mutation carriers and young women at high risk of breast cancer, well-established guidelines facilitating early diagnosis exist and are introduced in most countries of the developed world. For the rest, breast cancer comes with the same disadvantages as any other rare cancer. It is often overlooked, likely dismissed, delayed in diagnosis, and hence likely to be more advanced than in older women.

3.2   Specific Imaging Characteristics in Young Women with Breast Cancer

The American College of Radiology developed a structured reporting system to facilitate a common language among radiologists when reporting various imaging modalities [1]. A lesion is assessed by its shape, margin, density, associated calcifications and architectural distortion on mammography, and degree of echogenicity on ultrasound. It categorizes imaging features to allow an estimate of suspicion, ranging from benign categories I and II to indeterminate category III and suspicious/malignant categories IV and V. A typical malignant lesion presents as an ill-defined, spiculated, dense lesion sometimes with associated architectural distortion on mammography and associated microcalcifications. When reviewing MRI images of young breast cancer patients according to their morphological features, various groups [2, 3] described differences compared with their older counterparts. Young women's cancers appear more likely to

T. Gagliardi (✉)
University of Aberdeen, Aberdeen, UK
e-mail: t.gagliardi@nhs.net

© Springer Nature Switzerland AG 2020
O. Gentilini et al. (eds.), *Breast Cancer in Young Women*,
https://doi.org/10.1007/978-3-030-24762-1_3

display round, oval, or lobular mass shapes and smooth margins. They are more likely to have high signal intensity on T2-weighted images, a finding often seen in fibroadenomas. Those features can be regarded as benign or indeterminate according to the BI-RADS classification, with a follow-up in 6 months being one of the assessment options. The expected spectrum of abnormalities in young, symptomatic women ranges from simple to inspissated cysts, fibroadenomas, phyllodes tumors and galactoceles, and lactating adenomas in breastfeeding women, with breast cancer being the least likely of all (Figs. 3.1, 3.2, 3.3, and 3.4).

The rather indeterminate to benign-looking imaging characteristics of young women's cancers paired with the low incidence in this age group impose a challenge in the diagnosis of breast cancer in symptomatic women, let alone in the asymptomatic, high-risk group.

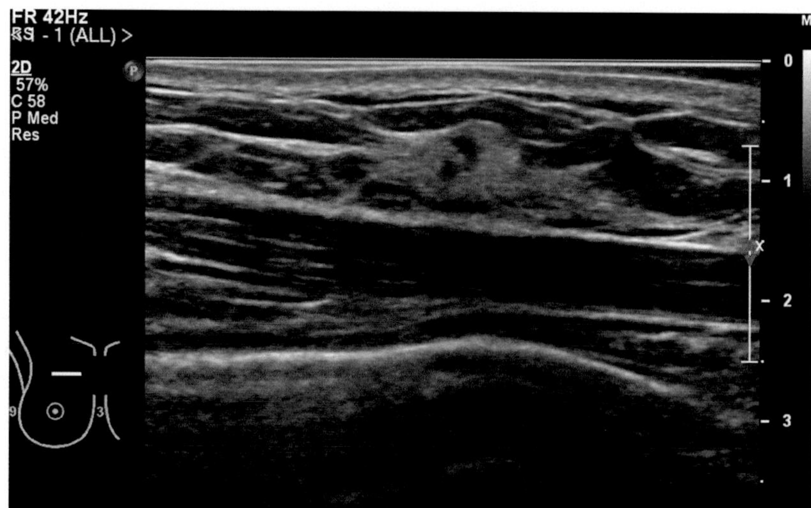

Fig. 3.1 30-year-old woman, palpable lump in upper, inner aspect of the right breast. Well-defined, hyperechoic with central hypoechoic features. No infiltration of Cooper ligaments. Histology: invasive ductal cancer, triple negative

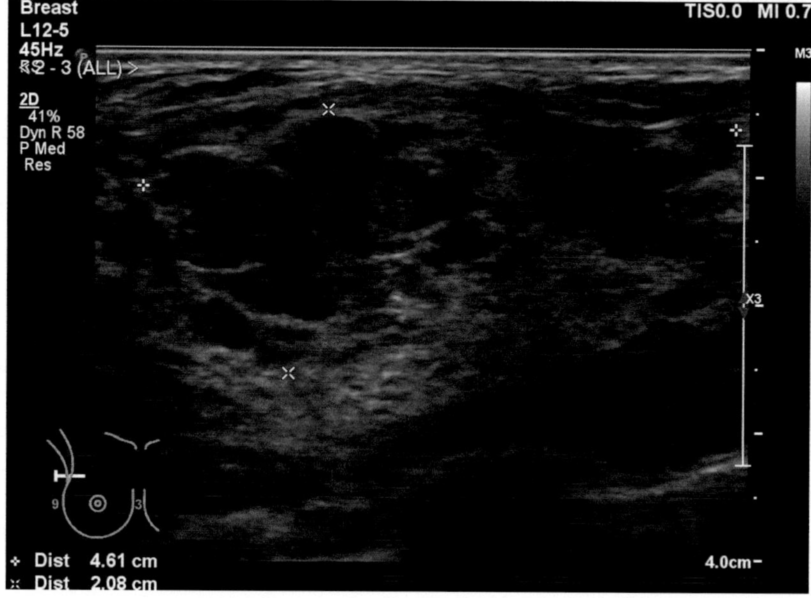

Fig. 3.2 26-year-old woman, presented with palpable lump in the upper outer quadrant of the right breast. Polylobulated, heterogeneous mass lesion with internal septations, partly irregular margins. Histology: malignant phyllodes tumor

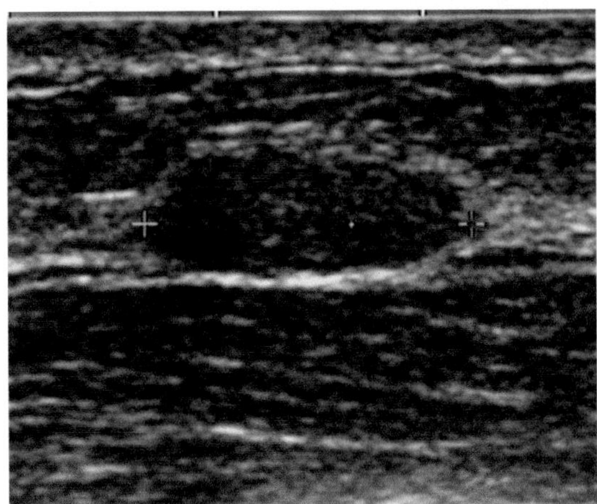

Fig. 3.3 28-year-old woman, presented with palpable lump. Oval-shaped, well-defined mass lesion, wider-than-tall orientation without interruption of Cooper ligaments. Histology: fibroadenoma

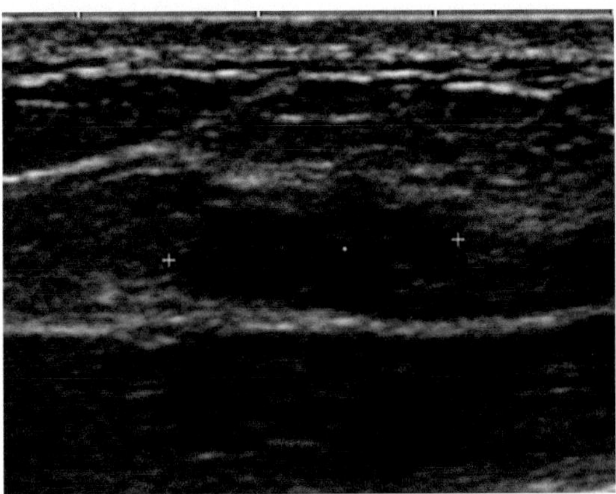

Fig. 3.4 34-year-old woman, palpable abnormality left inner aspect of the breast, 7 o'clock position. Hypoechoic lesion with irregular margins. Histology: high-grade invasive ductal cancer

3.3 Breast Density

The breast is composed of 15–20 breast lobules on a background of fatty tissue mixed in with fibro-connective tissue. During a woman's lifetime, breast lobules are likely to be replaced with fatty tissue. Breast lobules appear as "white" matter on a background of fatty tissue, which is featured as "black" material on mammography. Young women are much more likely to have plenty of breast lobules, which makes them feel firmer, and much less fatty tissue, depending on patients' body habitus. The so-called "density" of the breast relates to these incremental findings and developmental changes. A classical cancer will appear as a white mass on mammography. In dense breast tissue, it can be a tall order to detect a small white mass on a background of dense, white breast tissue. Similar problems can occur with MRI, where the density itself is not a problem as such, but the presence of moderate or strong "background enhancement" resulting in multiple, usually bilateral enhancing foci. This lowers the sensitivity of the examination and can be a challenge [4]. In an attempt to minimize this effect, premenopausal women should be scanned between day 7 and day 10 of their menstrual cycle, and the same should apply to mammography, since this is the time when performing a mammogram is less painful.

There appears to be a significant inverse relation between age and breast density according to a study of Checka et al. with 81% of women under the age of 40 having dense breast tissue [5]. On top of this, breast density is an independent risk factor associated with a four to six times increase in a woman's risk of developing a breast cancer [6]. In order to quantify the density, the American College of Radiology has addressed this issue and included density in their standardized reporting system [1]. This gives referring clinicians an overall idea of how well the reporting radiologist was able to make an assessment, since the density affects the sensitivity of all imaging modalities (Figs. 3.5 and 3.6).

3.4 Sonography

Sonography is deemed to be the first-line examination in symptomatic young women below the age of 35 years. Its value as a screening tool is limited due to its high false-positive rate, the variability between operators, and the considerable physician time for image acquisition. However, when compared to mammography and MRI, it lacks disadvantages such as X-ray dose, unavailability, and expense which are drawbacks in real-life scenarios.

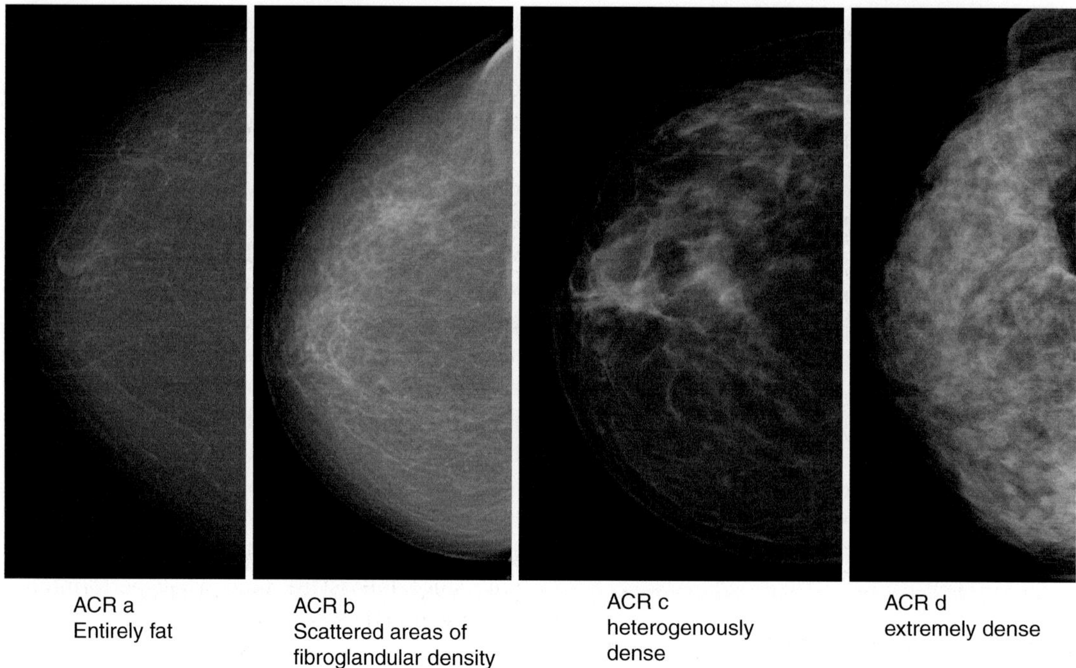

Fig. 3.5 Breast density categories according to the American College of Radiology

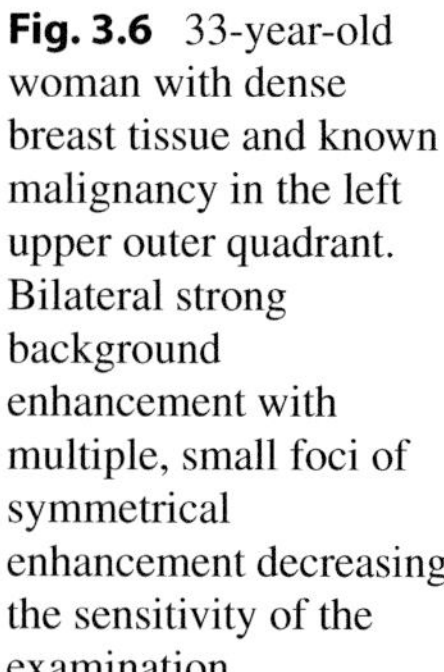

Fig. 3.6 33-year-old woman with dense breast tissue and known malignancy in the left upper outer quadrant. Bilateral strong background enhancement with multiple, small foci of symmetrical enhancement decreasing the sensitivity of the examination

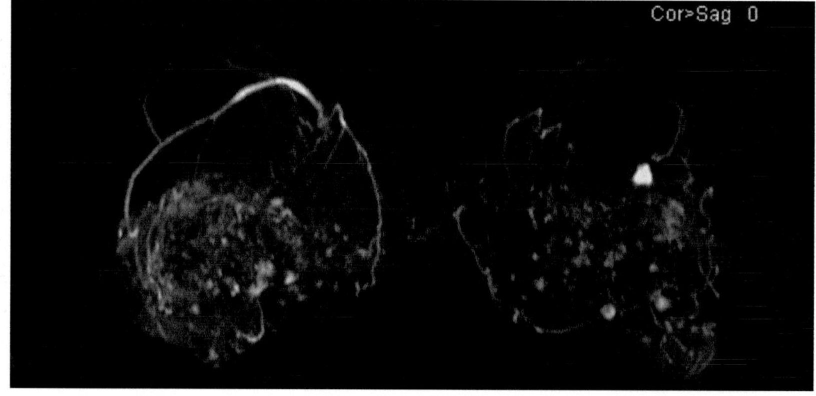

Sonography is a relatively cheap, mostly widely available imaging technique, not confined to exclusive use of radiologists and hence most suitable in the evaluation of symptomatic patients. It is an interactive, dynamic, and real-time modality. Ultrasound-guided biopsy is the primary biopsy method used to achieve a tissue diagnosis. In a landmark study, Stavros et al. [7] showed in 1995 that solid breast lesions could be differentiated between benign and malignant by using high-resolution gray-scale ultrasound imaging. Benign findings include a few gentle lobulations, ellipsoid shape, thin capsule, as well as a homogeneously echogenic texture. Malignant lesions have similar characteristics as described on mammography, with spiculation, taller-than-wide orientation, angular margins, microcalcifications, and posterior acoustic shadowing being the main features [8]. However, there is considerable overlap between benign and malignant ultrasound features. Specifically in the young women patient group, some benign features appear to be more often present in malignant lesions (Fig. 3.7).

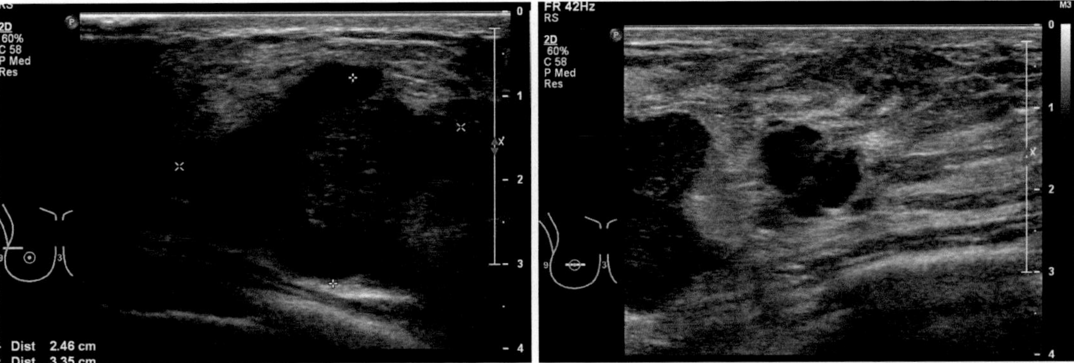

Figs. 3.7 and 3.8 26-year-old woman with palpable lump right breast. Ultrasound image shows a multilobulated, in part irregular mass lesions without posterior shadowing

Correlation with clinical findings, ideally linked with mammography, is essential. Sonography is commonly used as an adjunct to MRI, used as a second-look targeted imaging modality to evaluate findings detected on MRI.

Recent developments like Doppler imaging, elastography, and three-dimensional ultrasound are deemed to improve specificity and avoid unnecessary biopsies. The most promising development might be the introduction of three-dimensional automated breast ultrasound (3D ABUS). This offers the opportunity to standardize the examination by scanning the entirety of the breast in sections, using automated high-frequency transducers with an examination time of approximately 15 min for each breast. Images are than reconstructed and can be reviewed at a dedicated workstation allowing reproducibility to a level so far only seen with mammography and MRI. The actual interpretation time is deemed to be 5 min. Early studies using 3D automated ultrasound with mammography in dense breasts in asymptomatic women revealed promising results [9]. Adding 3D automated breast ultrasound to mammography added 1.9 additional cancers per 1000 women screened with 30 among the 82 cancers detected being seen with ABUS only. However, in this particular study, the recall rate almost doubled when ABUS was implemented leading to an increased number of false-positive results. A more recent study in Sweden with a lower volume of women screened in a similar setting described more

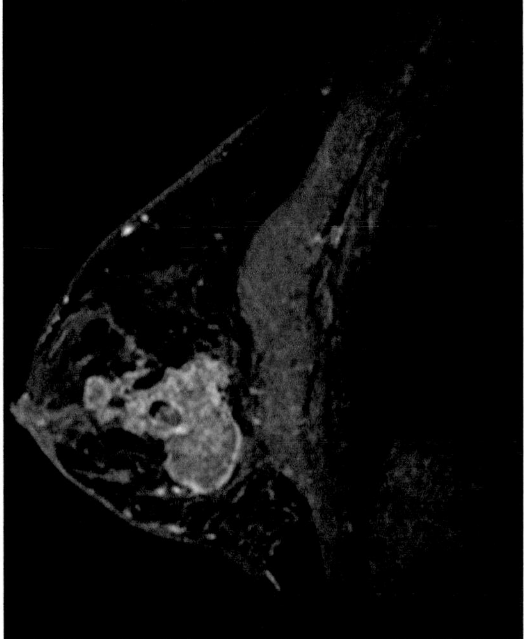

Fig. 3.9 Corresponding MRI images (T1 fat-saturated post-gadolinium image) show a multifocal tumor with features of peripheral enhancement. Histology: invasive ductal cancer, triple negative, BRCA 2 mutation carrier

promising results with a similar cancer detection rate and a much lower recall rate of only 9 women per 1000 screened [10]. So far this approach has not been studied in young symptomatic women. The benefits of standardization and lack of radiation remain appealing, and studies are needed to prove whether this might be a step forward to improve cancer detection rate in young women (Figs. 3.8 and 3.9).

3.5   Mammography

Mammography is the working horse of breast examination for the majority of women. It falls short to achieving its potential in dense breast tissue in young women, with a reported sensitivity in those under 45 years of as low as 72% [11] while compared to an estimated sensitivity for detection in the general population of 83% [12]. In BRCA mutation carriers, in which young women are often well represented, the sensitivity is estimated with 30% [13]. The sensitivity of ultrasound in those under 45 years instead appears to be 85% [11]. The specificity of both examinations is comparable.

Given the weak performance of mammography in young women, in addition to the negative impact related to the X-ray dose applied, common recommendations suggest ultrasound to be the first-line diagnostic method for young women. The Royal College of Radiologists stated in their "Guidance on Screening and Symptomatic Breast Imaging" in 2013 [14]: "There is no evidence of a mortality benefit from mammographic screening of women under the age of 35 years. There is also a greater risk of induced breast cancer from the use of diagnostic X-ray mammography in young women. Routine screening in the absence of significant breast cancer risk factors is not recommended."

The next step to improve the performance of digital mammography is digital tomosynthesis. Digital tomosynthesis is the creation of a 3D image of the breast by digital processing of multiple X-ray projection images. A series of usually seven to nine low-dose images are recorded as the mammographic unit moves gradually in a small arc over the compressed breast. These images can be reconstructed into a series of high-resolution slices of 1 mm allowing images to be reviewed in slices, labs, or cinemode. While tomosynthesis promises to improve cancer detection rate and decrease the recall rate in a general screening setting, the hopes to increase detection rate in dense breast tissue have so far failed to gain momentum, although recent publications point strongly in this direction [15]. When compared to ultrasound as adjunct to mammography, tomosynthesis did at least not show inferiority, but failed to perform in very dense breast tissue [16]. The issue of applying X-ray dose in young women, carrying at least a minimal risk of radiation-induced breast cancer, remains and should be taken into consideration.

3.6   MRI

Without doubt MRI is the most sensitive examination available throughout the spectrum of breast imaging with earlier and more recent studies constantly confirming this statement [17–19]. Most of the data stems from screening trials in genetic carriers and women being at high risk of developing a breast cancer. Kuhl compared the diagnostic accuracies of ultrasound, mammography, and MRI alone and in combination. Mammography alone reached 33% sensitivity, ultrasound 40%, and MRI 91%. Even when mammography and ultrasound were combined, the two modalities together did not reach the same sensitivity as MRI alone. This comes with the cost of decreased specificity and increased false-positive rate. In 2010, the European Society of Breast Cancer Specialists gathered and reviewed all available information published regarding diagnostic performance and indications for MRI [20]. Based on their findings, they recommended that annual MRI should be available for the high-risk patient group starting at the age of 30. Since the benefit of MRI for in situ disease is less consistent, annual mammography should also be applied in this patient group.

More recent published papers point to an even more tailored approach in the mutation carrier group. Obdeijn [21] and colleagues investigated the diagnostic performance of mammography as an adjunct to screening MRI in the high-risk group. Their study demonstrated that digital mammography added only 2% to the breast cancer detection in BRCA1 patients, with no additional benefit of mammography in women below age 40. A review of six high-risk screening trials confirmed those findings; however, it saw a screening benefit with mammography in BRCA2 mutation carriers, especially below the age of 40 years [22].

Yet, MRI has its drawbacks with MRI displaying a lower specificity than radiologists wish for. Especially in young women, hormonal influences may limit the sensitivity of the examination, and scanning within the 7th–10th day of the menstrual cycle is recommended to limit this effect. This might delay diagnosis and treatment. If MRI reveals unexpected findings, not previously seen on ultrasound and mammography, second-look ultrasound is the next recommended step. An abnormality seen only on MRI requires MRI-guided biopsy to establish a diagnosis. This is costly and time consuming and might only be available in specific centers, with patients being asked to travel to complete the work-up with delays being the consequences. Furthermore, thus far the evidence whether preoperative MRI can fulfill the promises made is not there. It was hypothesized that detection and removal of pre-

viously unrecognized cancer deposits would lead to improved outcomes with regard to surgical planning and decreased re-excision rates (Figs. 3.10 and 3.11).

This should lead to fewer local recurrences and even fewer distant metastases and death. Houssami and colleagues reviewed a meta-analysis pooling data from 3169 women and looked at the impact of performing a preoperative MRI on re-excision rates, mastectomy rates, local recurrence, and disease-free survival [23, 24]. Weak evidence was found that MRI reduces re-excision surgery in patients with invasive lobular carcinoma, at the expense of increased mastectomy rates with no reduction of local recurrence or disease-free survival. Those findings led to the recommendation stipulated by an expert forum which led to the Second International Consensus Guidelines for Breast Cancer in Young Women

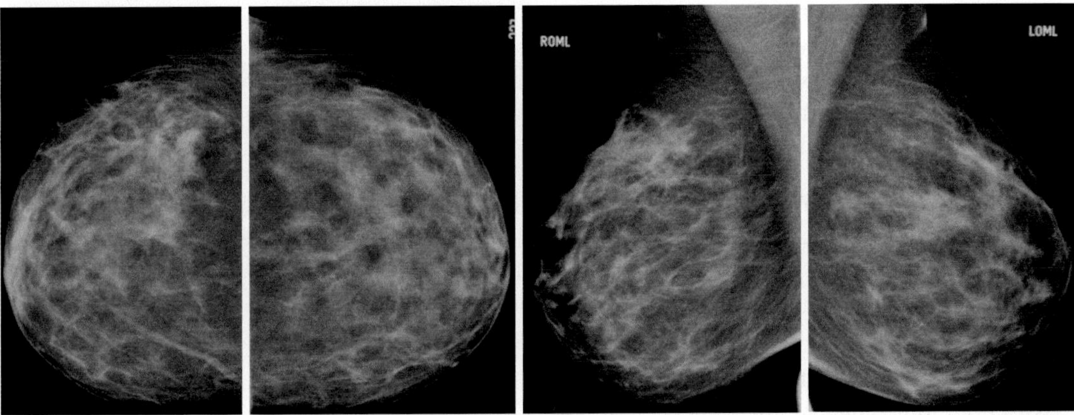

Fig. 3.10 34-year-old woman, palpable asymmetry in the upper aspect of the right breast. Dense breast tissue with very subtle asymmetry on mammography

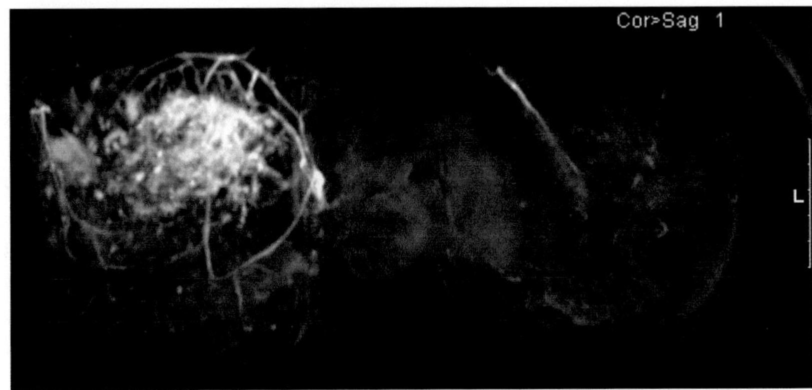

Fig. 3.11 Histology confirmed a high-grade DCIS extending over the entire aspect of the right breast on MRI examination (3D MIP reconstruction of dynamic series)

(BCY2), which are also endorsed by the European Society of Breast Cancer Specialists (EUSOMA) [25]. They recommend the use of screening breast MRI in the high-risk group. If MRI is to be used in the symptomatic setting, this should be done by nationally/regionally approved and audited services with appropriate expertise and knowledge present. MRI-guided biopsies and bracketing should be available to execute the highest standard possible and avoid unnecessary mastectomies.

3.7 Pregnant and Lactating Women

Pregnancy and breastfeeding reduces a woman's lifetime risk of developing a breast cancer especially in young women [26]. Yet the breast remains susceptible during this time in life to all disorders that affect the breast in non-pregnant, non-lactating women. There are further pathologies like lactating adenoma, galactocele, and mastitis complicated with abscesses, which are specific to this particular patient group [27] (Figs. 3.12 and 3.13).

During pregnancy, proliferative changes occur, with lobular hyperplasia, hyperemia, and fluid retention being present. Lactogenesis occurs in the second half of the pregnancy. These are dramatic changes leading to a further increase in breast density, making the diagnosis of breast masses even more challenging. In general, ultrasound is used as a first-line imaging modality often combined with biopsies to confirm the diagnosis. The risk of milk fistulas is small although reports in the literature exist [28]. The hormonal changes lead to an increased hypoechogenicity of the breast parenchyma with breast-feeding women's breast tissue displaying hyperechoic features on ultrasound. Both findings may hamper the visibility of a palpable lump, the cardinal finding in women presenting to symptomatic breast clinics [29]. The sensitivity of ultrasound is described as 100% with mammography resulting in an ability to pick up a cancer of up to 86%.

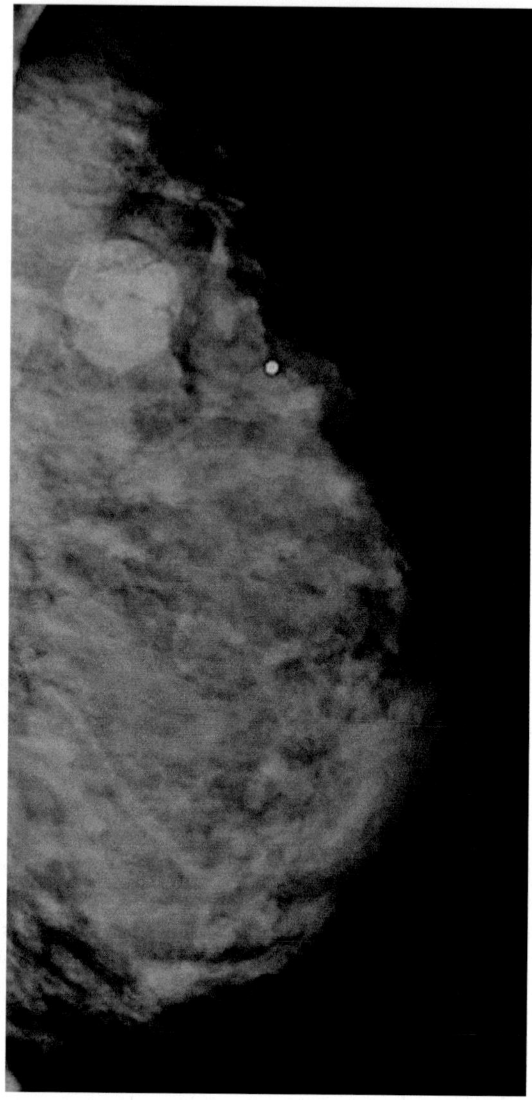

Fig. 3.12 Left medio-lateral oblique image in a lactating breast with a palpable lump in the upper outer quadrant. Dense, multilobulated, well-defined mass on mammography representing a galactocele

If ultrasound reveals a suspicious finding or malignancy is confirmed on biopsy, mammography can be safely performed even in pregnant women. Shielding of the abdomen is advised reducing the risk to the fetus to a non-significant amount [30]. Women are encouraged to express milk immediately prior to imaging in an attempt to decrease the density lowering the diagnostic value of the examination (Figs. 3.14, 3.15, and 3.16).

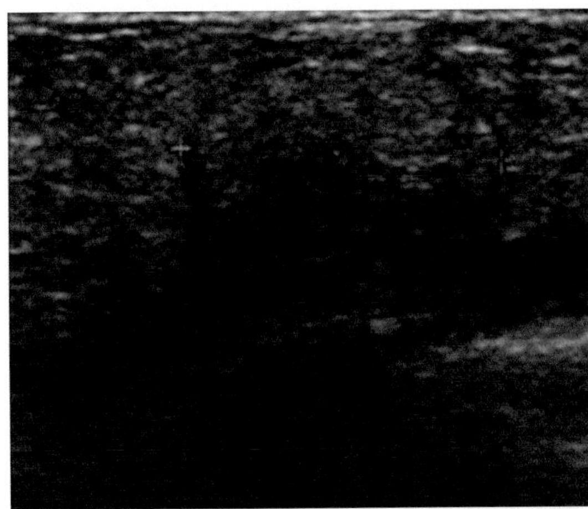

Fig. 3.13 Corresponding ultrasound image displaying heterogeneous, hyperechoic parenchyma with a well-defined, equally heterogeneous mass lesion

There is a limited role for breast MRI in pregnant women as gadolinium crosses the blood/placenta barrier and the risk-benefit ratio should be clear. A possible scenario is to establish the full extent of disease. MRI can be performed in breastfeeding women, with the infant being abstained from breastfeeding for 24 h and the milk discarded. However, strong background enhancement related to breastfeeding may cause an overlap of enhancement characteristics of invasive cancers with lactating breast tissue [31].

In addition to the underlying difficulties in imaging, common fibroadenomas in young women can appear with atypical characteristics like cystic changes, increased vascularity, microlobulations, irregular margins, and posterior acoustic shadowing: findings mimicking features

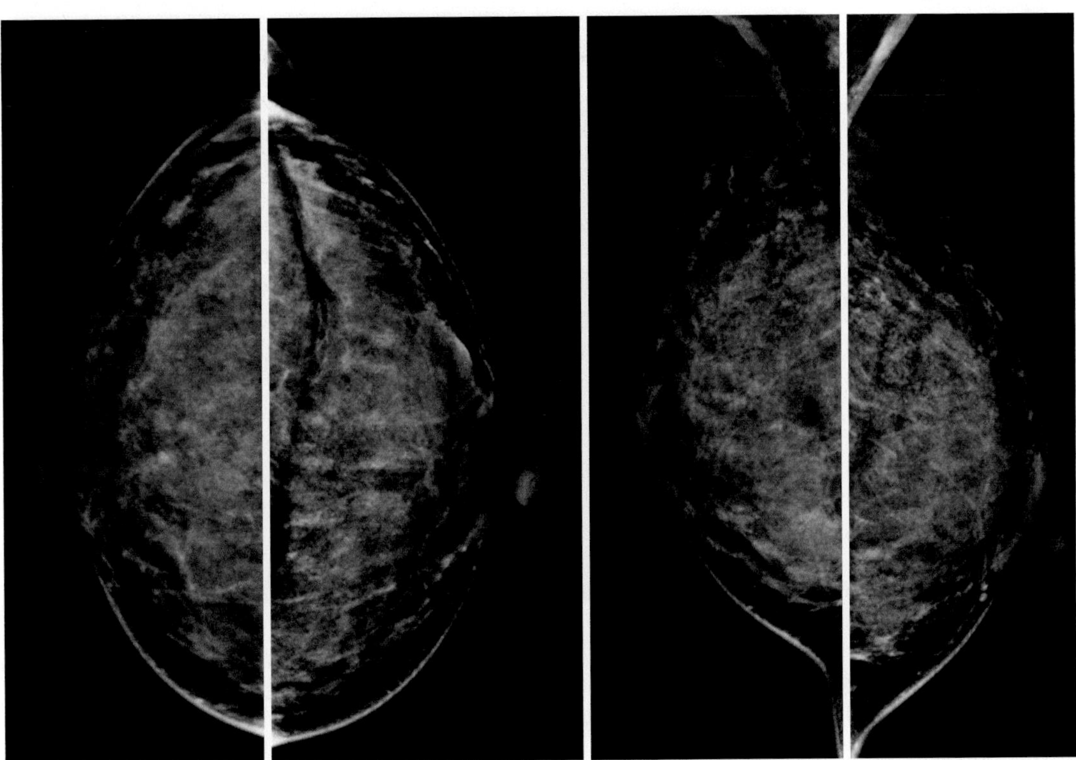

Fig. 3.14 37-year-old, pregnant woman with palpable lump at 6 o'clock position of the right breast. Dense breast without abnormality in CC views and only a very subtle asymmetry in the inferior aspect of the right breast, when compared to the left breast. Histology: grade 3 invasive ductal cancer, triple negative

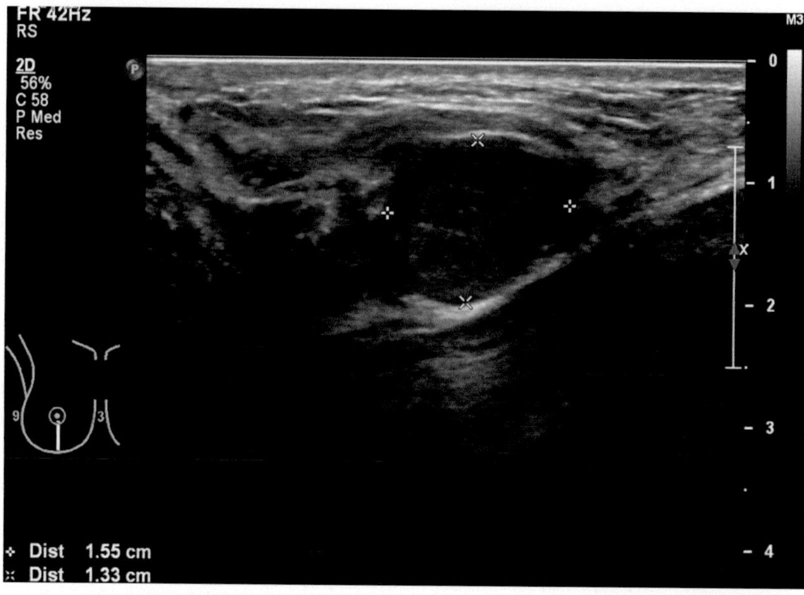

Fig. 3.15 Ultrasound of the palpable lump shows a hypoechoic, well-defined mass with areas of irregular extension without posterior acoustic shadowing

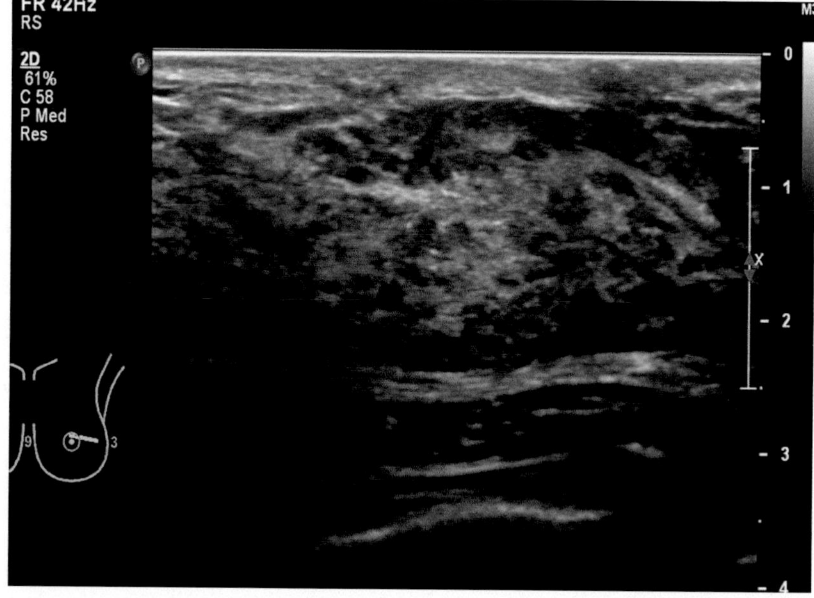

Fig. 3.16 Generalized hyperechoic, heterogeneous breast tissue on ultrasound reflecting the changes in pregnancy

of a breast cancer. Granulomatous mastitis is another entity usually seen in young women following pregnancy. Patients can present with clinical and imaging features of a malignancy with treatment being challenging [32].

All these factors make dealing with pregnant or breastfeeding women a challenge, highlighting the need for experienced and knowledgeable clinicians and radiologists being a prerequisite to deliver excellent patient care.

3.8 Conclusion

Breast cancer in young women is uncommon. The perception of clinicians and radiologists that cancers hardly occur in young women might lead to delays in diagnosis. The majority of young women present with a palpable lump in symptomatic breast services. A malignancy in young women often does not display the typical morphological features of a cancer on imaging, which might lead to misinterpretation. Young women tend to have dense breast tissue decreasing the sensitivity of clinical and radiological examinations. To facilitate early diagnosis, we need to have an imaging tool on hand, which is readily available, affordable, radiation-free and of diagnostic value in dense breast tissue, and operator independent as a standardized examination, with low false-positive rate and recall rates. Thus far such an all-in-one imaging tool is not available; hence there is no role for routine screening by any imaging. For the high-risk group, screening with MRI should be offered according to national guidelines in experienced centers.

References

1. American College of Radiology. Breast imaging reporting and data system (BI-RADS™). 5th ed. Reston, VA: American College of Radiology; 2013.
2. Kim JY, Lee SH, Lee JW, et al. Magnetic resonance imaging characteristics of invasive breast cancer in women aged less than 35 years. ActaRadiol. 2015;56(8):924–32.
3. Veltman J, Mann R, Kok T. Breast tumor characteristics of BRCA1 and BRCA2 gene mutation carriers on MRI. EurRadiol. 2008;18:931–8.
4. Giess C, Yeh E, Raza S, et al. Background parenchymal enhancement at breast MR imaging: normal patterns, diagnostic challenges, and potential for false-positive and false-negative interpretation. Radiographics. 2014;34(1):234–47.
5. Checka CM, et al. The relationship of mammographic density and age: implications for breast cancer screening. AJR Am J Roentgenol. 2012;198(3):W292–5.
6. Boyd NF, Guo H, Martin LJ. Mammographic density and the risk and detection of breast cancer. NEnglJMed. 2007;356(3):227–36.
7. Stavros AT, Thickman D, Rapp CL, et al. Solid breast nodules: use of sonography to distinguish between benign and malignant lesions. Radiology. 1995;196(1):123–34.
8. Holley RJ, Scoutt LM, Philpotts LE. Breast ultrasonography: state of the art. Radiology. 2013;268(3):642–59.
9. Brem RF, Tabar L, Duffy S, et al. Assessing improvement in detection of breast cancer with three-dimensional automated breast ultrasound in women with dense breast tissue: the SomoInsightstudy. Radiology. 2015;274(3):663–73.
10. Wilczek B, Wilczek H, Rasouliyan L, Leifland K. Adding 3D automated breast ultrasound to mammography screening in women with heterogeneously and extremely dense breasts: report from a hospital-based, high-volume, single-center breast cancer screening program. Eur J Radiol. 2016;85(9):1554–63.
11. Houssami N, Simpson IL, et al. Sydney breast imaging study accuracy study: comparative sensitivity and specificity of mammography and sonography in young women with symptoms. AJR Am J Roentgenol. 2003;180(4):935–40.
12. Kemp Jacobsen K, O'Meara ES, Key D, et al. Comparing sensitivity and specificity of screening mammography in the United States and Denmark. Int J Cancer. 2015;137(9):2198–207.
13. Warner E, Plewes DB, Hill KA, et al. Surveillance of BRCA1 and BRCA2 mutation carriers with magnetic resonance imaging, ultrasound, mammography and clinical breast examination. JAMA. 2004;292(11):1317–25.
14. The Royal College of Radiologists. Guidance on screening and symptomatic breast imaging,3rd edition.2013.
15. Houssami N, Turner RM. Rapid review: estimates of incremental breast cancer detection from tomosynthesis (3D-mammography) screening in women with dense breasts. Breast. 2016;30:141–5.
16. Kim WH, Chang JM, Lee J. Diagnostic performance of tomosynthesis and breast ultrasonography in women with dense breasts: a prospective comparison study. Breast Cancer Res Treat. 2017;162(1):85–94.
17. Berg WA, Gutierrez L, Ness Aiver MS. Diagnostic accuracy of mammography, clinical examination, US and MR imaging in preoperative assessment of breast cancer. Radiology. 2004;233(3):830–49.
18. Warner E, Hill K, Causer P, et al. Prospective study of breast cancer incidence in women with a BRCA1 or BRCA2 mutation under surveillance with and without magnetic resonance imaging. J ClinOncol. 2011;29(13):1664–9.
19. Kriege M, Brekelmanns CT, Boetes C, et al. Efficacy of MRI and mammography for breast cancer screening in women with a familial and genetic predisposition. N Engl J Med. 2004;351(5):427–37.
20. Sardanelli F, Boetes C, Borisch B, et al. Magnetic resonance imaging of the breast: recommendations from the EUSOMA working group. Eur J Cancer. 2010;46:1296–316.
21. Obdeijn IM, Winter-Warnars GA, Mann RM, et al. Should we screen BRCA1 mutation carriers only with MRI? A multicenter study. Breast Cancer Res Treat. 2014;144(3):577–82.
22. Phi X, Saadatmand S, De Bock G, et al. Contribution of mammography to MRI screening in BRCA mutation carriers by BRCA status and age: individual patient data meta-analysis. Br J Cancer. 2016;114(6):631–7.
23. Houssami N, Turner R, Macaskill P, et al. An individual person data meta-analysis of preoperative magnetic resonance imaging and breast cancer recurrence. J Clin Oncol. 2014;32(5):392–401.
24. Houssami N, Turner R, Morrow M. Preoperative magnetic resonance imaging in breast cancer: meta-analysis of surgical outcomes. Ann Surg. 2013;257(2):249–55.

25. Paluch-Shimon S, Pagani O, Partridge A, et al. Second International Consensus guidelines for breast cancer in young women (BCY2). Breast. 2016;26:87–99.
26. Russo J, Moral R, Balogh GA, et al. The protective role of pregnancy in breast cancer. Breast Cancer Res. 2005;7(3):131–42.
27. Faguy K. Breast disorders in pregnant and lactating women. Radiol Technol. 2015;86(4):419–38.
28. Schackmuth EM, Harlow CL, Norton LW. Milk fistula: a complication after breast core biopsy. AJR. 1993;161:961–2.
29. Robbins J, Jeffries D, Roubidoux M, et al. Accuracy of diagnostic mammography and breast ultrasound during pregnancy and lactation. AJR Am J Roentgenol. 2011;196(3):716–22.
30. Magno S, Terribile D, Franceschini G, et al. Early onset lactating adenoma and the role of breast MRI: a case report. J Med Case Rep. 2009;3:43.
31. Talele AC, SLanetz PJ, Edmister WB, et al. The lactating breast: MRI findings an literature review. Breast J. 2003;9:237–40.
32. Joshi S, Dialani V, Marotti J, et al. Breast disease in the pregnant and lactating patient: radiological-pathological correlation. Insights Imaging. 2013;4:527–38.

Establishing a Program for Young Women at High Risk for Breast Cancer

Soley Bayraktar and Banu Arun

4.1 Defining the "High-Risk Patient": Risk Factors and Risk Categories

The American Cancer Society [1] defines high risk as a lifetime risk of 20% or more, moderate risk as a lifetime risk of 15–20%, and normal risk as a lifetime risk of less than 15%. Knowledge of risk factors will help clinicians develop risk levels and make clinical decisions. A system to select the patients who require further evaluation should be created to optimize resources and acceptability.

4.1.1 Non-genetic Risk Factors for Breast Cancer

4.1.1.1 Age

The risk of developing breast cancer increases with age. According to the Surveillance, Epidemiology, and End Results (SEER) database, the probability of a woman in the United States developing breast cancer is 1 in 8 over a lifetime, 1 in 202 from birth to age 39 years of age, 1 in 26 from 40 to 59 years, and 1 in 28 from 60 to 69 years [2]. Young women who develop breast cancer appear to have worse disease-free survival (DFS) and overall survival (OS) and present with more aggressive-appearing biological characteristics than older women [3].

4.1.1.2 Environmental and Lifestyle Risk Factors

Most breast cancers are related to female hormones, and therefore any factor that increases exposure to these hormones is a potential risk factor. In particular, reproductive factors associated with increased exposure to endogenous estrogens produced by the ovaries, such as earlier menarche, late menopause, low parity, and late age at first birth, are recognized breast cancer risk factors [4–6]. Similarly, women exposed to exogenous hormones (e.g., through menopausal hormone therapy (MHT) or oral contraceptives) are often at increased risk [7–9].

Lifestyle factors are also associated with breast cancer. There is an estimated 10% increase in risk per 10 g of ethanol consumed every day [10]. Being overweight or obese is also associated with breast cancer risk, but only in postmenopausal women, with a gain of 5 kg/m² in body mass index (BMI) resulting in an 8% increase in disease risk. On the contrary, excess weight is associated with a decrease in risk in premenopausal women. Again, these associations can be explained by

S. Bayraktar
Biruni Univeristy School of Medicine, Protokol Yolu, Istanbul, Turkey

B. Arun (✉)
Department of Breast Medical Oncology and Clinical Cancer Genetics Program, The University of Texas MD Anderson Cancer Center, Houston, TX, USA
e-mail: barun@mdanderson.org

© Springer Nature Switzerland AG 2020
O. Gentilini et al. (eds.), *Breast Cancer in Young Women*,
https://doi.org/10.1007/978-3-030-24762-1_4

hormonal factors: alcohol consumption and postmenopausal obesity are related to higher circulating estrogen levels [11]. In postmenopause, elevated estrogen levels are most probably due to extraglandular production in the adipose tissue, whereas in premenopause, the decrease in female hormone synthesis associated with anovulatory cycles in obese women likely explains the inverse association with breast cancer [11].

Radiation exposure from various sources, including medical treatment and nuclear explosion, increases the risk of breast cancer. Radiation to the chest wall for treatment of childhood cancer increases the risk of breast cancer linearly with chest radiation dose [12]. Survivors of childhood cancers who received therapeutic radiation are at a dose-dependent risk for the development of breast cancer, and those treated for Hodgkin's disease are at highest risk (RR = 7) [13]. Radiation effects on the development of female breast cancer were also demonstrated in Japan after the nuclear attacks on Hiroshima and Nagasaki [14] and positively correlated with age younger than 35 years at time of exposure. The incidence of breast cancer has also increased in areas of Belarus and Ukraine. A significant twofold increase was observed in the most contaminated areas around Chernobyl following the nuclear accident and manifested in women who were younger at the time of the exposure [15].

4.1.1.3 Mammographic Breast Density

Mammographic breast density (MBD), alone or in combination with other risk factors, is associated with an increased risk of breast cancer [16–18]. Percentage dense area (PDA) is the most common measurement of mammographic density. A four- to sixfold greater risk of breast cancer has been reported in women for whom more than 75% of the total area on mammogram is occupied by dense area [19]. In addition to PDA, the absolute dense area of the breast obtained during an assessment of PDA is an independent risk factor for breast cancer, and its inclusion in risk-assessment tools has been proposed [20].

4.1.1.4 Breast Pathology

Proliferative breast disease is associated with an increased risk of breast cancer. Proliferative breast lesions without atypia, including usual ductal hyperplasia, intraductal papillomas, sclerosing adenosis, and fibroadenomas, confer only a small increased risk of breast cancer development, approximately 1.5–2 times that of the general population [21, 22]. Atypical hyperplasia, including both ductal and lobular, which are usually incidentally found during screening mammography, confers a substantial increased risk of breast cancer. Women with lobular atypia have an approximately four to five times increased lifetime risk of developing breast cancer in either the ipsilateral or contralateral breast compared with the general population [23].

In lobular carcinoma in situ (LCIS), premalignant cells are growing in the lobules, but not growing through the wall of the lobules. LCIS is a risk factor and a nonobligate precursor of breast carcinoma. The relative risk of invasive carcinoma after classic LCIS diagnosis is approximately nine to ten times that of the general population.

Previously uncommon, ductal carcinoma in situ (DCIS) now comprises ~20% of all breast carcinoma diagnoses [24]. DCIS shares many of the epidemiological risk factors as invasive breast cancer (IBC) including age, family history, parity, and some other hormonal factors and high mammographic density [25]. Because of its nature as a potential precursor for IBC, excision of DCIS is recommended; however, most DCIS would never progress to invasive disease nor give rise to any morbidity. Indeed, autopsy studies indicate that occult DCIS exists in ~9% of women (range 0–15%) [26]. In the few studies with small numbers of DCIS where misdiagnosis led to omission of surgery, 14–53% of women developed IBC over 30 years [27–29]. A recent meta-analysis placed the 15-year invasive recurrence rate after surgery alone for DCIS at 28% and breast cancer-specific mortality at 18% [30].

4.1.2 Genetic Risk Factors for Breast Cancer

4.1.2.1 Personal History of Breast Cancer

A personal history of breast cancer is a significant risk factor for the development of a second ipsilateral or contralateral breast cancer. In fact, the most common cancer among breast cancer survivors is metachronous contralateral breast cancer (CBC) with a mean annual incidence rate of 0.13% [31]. Factors associated with an increased risk of a second breast cancer include an initial diagnosis of DCIS, stage IIB, hormone receptor-negative cancers, and young age [32].

4.1.2.2 Family History of Breast Cancer

A woman's risk of breast cancer is increased if she has a family history of the disease. In the Nurses' Health Study follow-up, women with a mother diagnosed before age 50 had an adjusted relative risk (RR) of 1.69, and women with a mother diagnosed at 50 or older had an RR of 1.37 compared with women without a family history of breast cancer. A history of a sister with breast cancer was associated with an increased RR of 1.66 if the diagnosis was made prior to age 50 and an RR of 1.52 if diagnosed after age 50 compared with patients without a family history [33]. The highest risk is associated with an increasing number of first-degree relatives diagnosed with breast cancer at a young age (younger than 50). Compared with women who had no affected relative, women who had one, two, or three or more affected first-degree relatives had risk ratios of 1.80, 2.93, and 3.90, respectively [34].

4.1.2.3 Genetic Predisposition

Approximately 20–25% of breast cancer patients have a positive family history, but only 5–10% of breast cancer cases demonstrate autosomal dominant inheritance [35, 36]. Genetic predisposition alleles have been described in terms of clinical significance [37]. High-risk predisposition alleles conferring a 40–85% lifetime risk of developing breast cancer include BRCA1 and BRCA2 mutations and mutations in TP53 resulting in Li-Fraumeni syndrome, PTEN resulting in Cowden syndrome, STK11 causing Peutz-Jeghers syndrome, NF1 resulting in neurofibromatosis, and CDH-1 resulting in E-cadherin impairment [38]. Half of the breast cancer predisposition syndromes are associated with mutations in BRCA1 and BRCA2. Women with BRCA1 or BRCA2 deleterious mutations have a significantly higher risk of developing breast cancer than the general population, and they develop breast cancer at a younger age. In a large study by the Consortium of Investigators of Modifiers of BRCA1/2 (CIMBA), the median age of breast cancer diagnosis was 40 years among BRCA1 and 43 years among BRCA2 mutation carriers [39]. Lifetime breast cancer risk ranges from 65% to 81% for BRCA1 mutation carriers and 45% to 85% for BRCA2 carriers [40–42]. BRCA1 and BRCA2 mutation carriers develop DCIS more frequently and at an earlier age than the general population [43] and are significantly more likely to have occult DCIS in prophylactic mastectomies than age-matched non-carriers from autopsy studies [17]. Women carrying a BRCA1 or BRCA2 germline mutation also have increased risk of other cancer types, such as ovarian cancer and fallopian tube cancer, male breast cancer, prostate cancer, pancreas cancer, gastrointestinal cancers (e.g., gallbladder, bile duct, and stomach), and melanoma [44–46].

Moderate-risk genes, including homozygous ataxia-telangiectasia mutations (ATM) [47], somatic mutations in tumor suppressor gene CHEK2, and the BRCA1 and BRCA2 modifier genes BRIP1 [48] and PALB2 [49], confer a 20–40% lifetime risk of breast cancer. A study suggested an association between germline TP53 mutations and early-onset HER2-positive breast cancer [50]. Numerous low-risk common alleles have been identified, largely through genome-wide association studies [37], and the clinical implications of these mutations have not been determined.

Families carrying genetic mutations in the abovementioned genes exhibit an apparently dominant inheritance pattern and are often characterized by early age of onset and overrepresentation of ovarian, bilateral breast, and male breast cancers [51]. In a large study by the Consortium of Investigators of Modifiers of BRCA1/2 (CIMBA), the median age of breast cancer diagnosis was 40 years among BRCA1 and 43 years among BRCA2 mutation carriers [39].

4.2   Genetic Counseling and Breast Cancer Risk Assessment Models

The National Comprehensive Cancer Network (NCCN) has guidelines regarding who should be offered genetic testing on the basis of personal and family history [52]. In the presence of predictive factors for a hereditary cancer syndrome, it would be appropriate to refer an individual for genetic counseling even if they do not have a personal history of invasive breast cancer.

For patients with risk factors based on personal or family history, different models are available for assessing and quantifying risk [53–55]. The Gail, Claus, and Tyrer-Cuzick models are some of the more commonly used models that estimate breast cancer risk. Of note, these models are different than models such as BRCAPRO or BOADICEA, which are more commonly used to estimate the likelihood of a BRCA1 or BRCA2 mutation. Additionally, these models are not appropriate for use in women with a known deleterious gene mutation associated with a hereditary breast cancer syndrome, as the models will likely underestimate the woman's breast cancer risk.

The accuracy of any breast cancer risk assessment model is dependent on the accuracy of the reported family history. In general, breast cancer is often accurately reported in families, whereas abdominal cancers, such as gynecologic cancers, are often misreported. The cancer genetics professional will work with the patient to try to obtain the most accurate family history possible, either through the use of medical or death records or by asking follow-up questions regarding how the cancer was diagnosed or treated. Finally, the cancer genetics professional will choose the model(s) that best account for the patient's personal and family history risk factors for breast cancer. If genetic testing is deemed unnecessary, or once genetic testing is complete, and if an inconclusive negative result or a VUS is identified, breast cancer risk assessment models can be used to estimate a woman's breast cancer risk and make appropriate recommendations about risk management.

Assignment of risk levels permits tailored screening and risk reduction strategies. The genetics counselor will review her family medical history, talk about the role of genetics in cancer, and perform a hereditary cancer risk assessment. This assessment should cover:

- Patient's chances of having a genetic mutation
- Personalized genetic testing recommendations
- A general estimate of personal cancer risks
- Individualized cancer screening and prevention recommendations

Since 2013, because of changes in patent law, BRCA1/BRCA2 genetic testing is now offered at a variety of laboratories, and an increasing number of laboratories are utilizing next-generation sequencing (NGS) to offer extensive hereditary cancer panel testing, which includes analysis of many genes simultaneously.

4.3   Cancer Genetic Risk Assessment

Despite advances in genetic testing, assessment of cancer family history and pedigree structure remains central to accurate risk assessment. The pedigree allows for a visual assessment of patterns of cancer as well as the informativeness of the family structure as a whole. In some cases, appreciation of many unaffected relatives can reduce concern for a hereditary condition, while in others, small family size or individuals with early deaths or interventions that reduce cancer risk (such as oophorectomy) can limit the ability to recognize a hereditary syndrome if one were present in the family. The risk assessment should also assess physical features, for example, skin hyperpigmentation, mucocutaneous tumors, and macrocephaly, which can aid in the identification of Peutz-Jeghers syndrome, and non-genetic risk factors, such as reproductive history and exposure to radiation or endogenous estrogens or progestins, which might explain breast cancer in a family. The possibility of non-paternity and undisclosed adoption as well as the accuracy of the reported information should also be considered when deciding whether genetic testing should be offered.

Genetic testing recommendations not only include which test(s) are indicated but also who in the family is the best genetic testing candidate. Genetic testing is most informative when an affected family member is tested first. Thus, patients who are referred for cancer genetic risk assessment may need to prepare themselves to discuss genetic testing with family members. However, there are circumstances in which an unaffected person in the family may be the first person to undergo genetic testing, such as when affected family members are deceased. In any case, the benefits, risks, limitations, testing process, and possible results of genetic testing should be discussed. The goal of this discussion is to allow the patient to make an informed decision regarding genetic testing and to understand how genetic testing may influence her breast cancer risk management.

4.4 Genetic Test Results

Patients who undergo genetic testing can receive three possible test results: positive, negative, or variant of uncertain significance (VUS). A positive result means that a mutation that is known to be deleterious was identified and the patient is at increased risk for certain types of cancer. The increased cancer risks may include breast cancer, as well as a variety of other cancers, depending on in which gene the mutation was identified. A positive result does not guarantee that a patient will develop breast or other cancers, nor does it predict at what age a cancer might develop. A positive result does allow the patient and her phy-

sician to consider more aggressive screening or risk reduction options, which will be discussed in greater detail later in this review.

The next possible genetic test result is a negative result. There are actually two types of negative results: true negative and inconclusive negative. A true-negative result can only occur when a positive result has previously been identified in a patient's family member. In the case of a true-negative result, the patient undergoes testing for the mutation that was identified in her relative, and the patient is found not to have the same mutation. In contrast, an inconclusive negative result occurs when a patient undergoes genetic testing and no deleterious mutations are identified. Inconclusive negative results require an individualized breast cancer risk management plan based on the patient's personal and family history.

The last possible genetic test result is a VUS. A VUS is a mutation whose effect on the function of the gene is unknown. A VUS could be a deleterious mutation that is associated with an increased risk of cancer, or it could be a harmless change in the gene that is not at all associated with an increased risk of cancer. Variants of uncertain significance also require an individualized breast cancer risk management plan based on the patient's personal and family history.

4.5 Why Is Genetic Testing Important?

Once we identify young women carrying a breast cancer predisposition gene, it is important to apply proper steps as part of a multidisciplinary approach at a high-risk clinic. Based on the current evidence, high-risk individuals require different screening and risk reduction strategies from those deployed for the population at large. Importantly, taking appropriate steps as part of a multidisciplinary approach would ensure that these women are treated with appropriate chemotherapy as they have a differential sensitivity to chemotherapeutic agents. For example, it could lead to offering a patient neoadjuvant chemotherapy with PARP inhibitors, or platinums, or enrolling her in specific clinical trials.

Genetic evaluation before surgical decision making is also important as knowledge of mutation status may influence immediate treatment recommendations including the performance of concomitant contralateral risk-reducing mastectomy and RRSO in a patient who would otherwise undergo only lumpectomy or unilateral mastectomy [56]. Genetic testing could get lost in the shuffle of complicated medical care and other immediate decisions that need to be made. The optimum window of opportunity for genetic testing to influence surgical decisions would be during neoadjuvant chemotherapy if it is prescribed; then the definitive decision occurs after chemotherapy is completed and before the surgery or initiation of radiotherapy. If the patient is not a candidate for neoadjuvant chemotherapy, then expedited genetic testing may play a role in order to avoid a delay in surgical procedures. However, the timing of genetic counseling and testing must balance the necessity for immediate testing with the stress patients feel as they cope with the diagnosis of cancer, treatment plans, and prognosis.

4.5.1 Implications for the Affected Individuals

4.5.1.1 Implications on the Systemic Therapy Options

Traditionally, for those who develop breast or ovarian cancer, systemic therapy has been selected similarly to those with sporadic cancers, and the choice of chemotherapy (adjuvant or neoadjuvant as appropriate), endocrine therapy, and radiation has been based on ER/PR/HER2 status, lymph node involvement, and the size of the tumor. However, the approach to treatment is changing based on the recent data suggesting that BRCA1-defective cell lines are sensitive to DNA-damaging agents, such as platinum, and are relatively resistant to taxanes compared with BRCA-competent cell lines [57–60].

An important recent advance is that the FDA has approved the first molecularly targeted therapy olaparib, a poly(ADP-ribose) polymerase (PARP) inhibitor, for the treatment of patients with deleterious or suspected deleterious germ-line BRCA-mutated, HER2-negative metastatic breast cancer who have been treated with chemotherapy either in the neoadjuvant, adjuvant, or metastatic setting [61]. Because BRCA1 and BRCA2 proteins are critical in double-strand DNA repair, combining PARP inhibition with tumors that have defective BRCA1 or BRCA2 proteins exerts a synergistic lethal effect [62].

When it comes to endocrine therapy recommendations, some studies have reported that tamoxifen reduces the risk of contralateral breast cancer (CBC) by 50–70% in BRCA mutation carriers; other studies have not reported a significant reduction [63, 64]. However, overall, studies suggested that tamoxifen was associated with a risk reduction in patients with BRCA mutation-associated ER-positive breast cancer with or without oophorectomy. Currently, the role of aromatase inhibitors (AI) after RRSO or as an adjuvant endocrine therapy in BRCA mutation-associated breast cancer is unknown. The IBIS-II study is evaluating anastrozole versus placebo in high-risk women. In addition, there is an ongoing French study evaluating letrozole versus placebo in women with BRCA mutations [ClinicalTrials.gov identifier: NCT00673335].

4.5.1.2 Implications on the Surgical Interventions

In addition to the risk of ipsilateral recurrence (IPR), breast cancer patients with a deleterious BRCA1 mutation have up to a 43.4% 10-year risk of contralateral breast cancer (CBC), while BRCA2 mutation carriers have up to a 34.6% 10-year risk. The risk increases exponentially in women diagnosed at a younger age [65]. Most studies have reported that oophorectomy reduces the risk of CBC in BRCA mutation carriers by 50–70%, with the greatest benefit observed if the surgery is performed before the age of 50 [66]. Despite the significant reduction in the risk of CBC associated with prophylactic contralateral mastectomy in BRCA mutation carriers, the procedure has not currently been found to improve survival, although studies have been limited by short follow-up [67]. In this multicenter, prospective cohort study by Domchek et al., salpingo-oophorectomy was associated with a reduction of ovarian cancer and ovarian cancer mortality, a reduction of subsequent breast cancer and breast cancer mortality, and a reduction of overall mortality. The above findings justify the practice of offering the option for risk-reducing surgeries to women with BRCA mutations; however, a detailed discussion with the patient regarding the surgical risk-reducing intervention and its long-term side effects is central to the management of mutation carriers.

4.5.2 Implications for the Unaffected Individuals

There is general agreement that women with a higher lifetime risk of breast cancer, such as that conferred by a BRCA mutation, should undergo earlier and more frequent screening, with additional imaging modalities considered. A consolidated summary of breast cancer screening recommendations published by the National Comprehensive Cancer Network (NCCN), American Cancer Society (ACS), American College of Radiology (ACR), and other national organizations for the asymptomatic, female, BRCA mutation carrier includes the following [52]:

- Monthly breast self-exam (BSE) beginning at the age of 18 years
- Semiannual clinical breast exam (CBE) beginning at the age of 25 years
- Alternating annual mammograms with annual breast magnetic resonance imaging (MRI) beginning at the age of 25–30 years or individualized based on the earliest age of cancer onset in the family [68]

Women with mutations in genes of uncertain clinical validity for breast cancer assessment (such as BARD1, BRIP1, MRE11A, RAD50/51, RAD51B/C/D, and certain missense mutations in CHEK2) are not recommended to undergo MRI screening based on the presence of the mutation alone. For these women, however, a family-history-based model might predict sufficient risk to warrant MRI screening [69].

While risk-reducing salpingo-oophorectomy (RRSO) is more effective in preventing ovarian cancer in these women compared to general population, some may not opt to pursue this intervention until after their childbearing years. In the absence of more effective screening methods, transvaginal ultrasound (TVU) and CA-125 levels continue to be recommended and endorsed by national organizations for women who are at high risk for hereditary breast and ovarian cancer syndromes (HBOC). Current NCCN screening guidelines for BRCA mutation carriers who are not undergoing RRSO include the following [52]:

- Semiannual concurrent pelvic exam, TVU, and CA-125 antigen determination beginning at the age of 30–35 years or 5–10 years earlier than the youngest age at which any family member was diagnosed with ovarian cancer.
- RRSO between 35 and 40 years of age appears appropriate for BRCA1 mutation carriers, while delaying RRSO until the early 40s for the BRCA2 mutation carrier appears safe[42, 70].

Mutations in the tumor suppressor genes BRCA1 and BRCA2 place male and female carriers at increased risk for a number of other cancers, notably pancreatic, melanoma, colorectal, and other gastrointestinal tumors. No expert consensus or evidence-based guidelines exist regarding screening for these cancers. Some literature and investigational studies support considering the following additional surveillance modalities [71, 72]:

- Pancreatic: annual endoscopic ultrasound, beginning at the age of 50 years or 10 years prior to the earliest pancreatic cancer diagnosis in the family
- Melanoma: annual full body skin and ocular exam
- Colorectal: population screening guidelines, beginning at the age of 50 years and continuing until 75 years old
- Annual fecal occult blood testing
- Sigmoidoscopy every 5 years or colonoscopy every 10 years

4.5.3 Implications for the Family Members

The abovementioned risk-reducing surgeries, chemoprevention, and surveillance strategies are not only for mutation carriers but also for unaffected women who carry the cancer-predisposing genes. Family members of a woman who carry a germline genetic mutation should be referred to a high-risk breast cancer clinic and undergo predictive genetic testing and if found positive discuss risk management options. In fact a study showed that, with appropriate risk management, breast and ovarian cancer risk could be reduced by 23% and 41%, respectively, in first-degree family members with BRCA mutations (Kwon and Arun JCO 2010).

4.6 How to Establish a Program for Young Women at High Risk for Breast Cancer

A program for patients at high risk for breast cancer needs to be developed according to the current legislation and healthcare conditions in the country where the program will be located and local decisions regarding what is wanted or needed. Regardless of where the program is developed, it may be useful to consider the list of goals outlined by MacDonald [73] (Table 4.1).

Table 4.1 Goals of a cancer genetics service

– Identify individuals at high risk for cancer and genetic mutation carriage
– Stratify patients according to risk and tailor screening and management according to risk
– Promote a healthy lifestyle as a primary preventive intervention
– Provide genetic counseling regarding cancer risk
– Protect patient privacy and confidentiality
– Provide education about factors that confer a high risk of breast cancer to clinicians and the community
– Establish research collaborations
– Publish your actions and the results of your interventions
– Promote your initiative and encourage the development of new programs for patients at high risk
– Create a cost-effective breast program

The staff should include genetic counselors, nurses, physicians, psychologists, social workers, secretaries, and a data manager. A medical director is needed to assist with development and monitor achievements and opportunities for improving the program.

Since high-risk evaluation, especially genetic counseling and genetic testing, is a part of a multidisciplinary evaluation of the affected patient with breast cancer, it would be ideal to have several "stakeholders" involved in the multidisciplinary physician team. These would include surgeons, medical oncologists, radiologists, gynecologists, and gynecology oncologists. Periodic high-risk and genetic patient care boards/meetings are encouraged to establish and maintain a productive process and clinic flow. With recent improvements in technology (e.g., multipanel gene testing), genetic testing and management guidelines change rapidly; hence regular meetings enable a platform to discuss current guidelines and their implementation in the clinics. These meetings would also serve as an important infrastructure to ask clinically relevant research questions. We stress also the importance of building a prospective high-risk and genetics database that would allow to prospectively collect data, blood, and tissue samples for research.

Along with a promotional plan, a simple referral guide should be created for distribution to physicians. Ideally, the guide should be kept visible in the clinics that may refer patients. Having health insurance support may encourage other institutional staff to participate and allow easy referral process. To get health insurance companies to cover the services provided in the high-risk program, it should be explained that an economic benefit is expected from promoting prevention, screening, chemoprevention, and prophylactic surgeries, allowing resources to be focused where they are needed the most [74].

While the importance of identifying individuals for high-risk and/or genetic testing is widely recognized, unfortunately studies have shown that only 22% of eligible individuals are actually referred to genetic evaluation and testing [75, 76]. As discussed previously, among patients newly diagnosed with cancer, a positive test result will often prompt more aggressive surgical treatment (e.g., bilateral salpingo-oophorectomy or prophylactic contralateral mastectomy) with the goal of minimizing the potential for second primary cancers or prompt consideration of new systemic therapies such as PARP inhibitors for ovarian cancer. A positive test result may also prompt consideration of BRCA1/2 testing among at-risk relatives of the cancer patient so that those testing positive can benefit from more aggressive prevention and screening.

Studies are trying to address the reasons behind low genetics referral practices; it is thought to be related to decreased awareness among healthcare providers, not having a referral system, not having a specialized high-risk and genetics clinic in place, as well as patient-related factors (anxiety about genetic risk, stigmata, and insurance concerns, among others). A well-diverse multidisciplinary high-risk team and clinic can address some of these issues and increase awareness and access to these services with the ultimate aim of not missing any patient that would benefit from risk assessment and genetic testing.

The ideal location of high-risk clinics is as follows: In some high-risk programs, breast cancer screening and prevention services for high-risk individuals are offered in a centralized high-risk clinic located in a different area from the breast cancer unit. Other high-risk programs offer their services in the clinic where breast cancer patients are treated. In this arrangement, the high-risk team interacts with the oncology team, sharing examination rooms and clinics, allowing continuous feedback. This approach allows for multidisciplinary management and ongoing communication between the patients and multiple healthcare providers.

Legal issues must be addressed by every high-risk program. Depending on the country, there may be important issues related to the lack of laws about genetic syndromes and risk assessment. The information that is going to be generated must be managed confidentially; disclosure of such information to insurance companies and healthcare providers may be threatening for patients if there is no legislation that protects patients. High-risk programs should obtain approval from patients and institutions to share very sensitive information and should create an information-sharing system that protects patient privacy. Such a system is particularly important in the case of referral or assessment of patients who live outside the city or country where the high-risk program is located.

References

1. https://cancerstatisticscenter.cancer.org.
2. Siegel RL, Miller KD, Jemal A. Cancer statistics, 2018. CA Cancer J Clin. 2018;68(1):7–30.
3. Litton JK, Eralp Y, Gonzalez-Angulo AM, Broglio K, Uyei A, Hortobagyi GN, et al. Multifocal breast cancer in women < or =35 years old. Cancer. 2007;110(7):1445–50.
4. Clamp A, Danson S, Clemons M. Hormonal risk factors for breast cancer: identification, chemoprevention, and other intervention strategies. Lancet Oncol. 2002;3(10):611–9.
5. Collaborative Group on Hormonal Factors in Breast Cancer. Menarche m, and breast cancer risk: individual participant meta-analysis, including 118 964 women with breast cancer from 117 epidemiological studies. Lancet Oncol. 2012;13(11):1141–51.
6. Cadeau C, Fournier A, Mesrine S, et al. Postmenopausal breast cancer risk and interactions between body mass index, menopausal hormone therapy use, and vitamin D supplementation: Evidence from the E3N cohort. Int J Cancer. 2016;139(10):2193–200.
7. Rossouw JE, Anderson GL, Prentice RL, LaCroix AZ, Kooperberg C, Stefanick ML, et al. Risks and benefits of estrogen plus progestin in healthy postmenopausal women: principal results From the Women's Health Initiative randomized controlled trial. JAMA. 2002;288(3):321–33.
8. Travis R, Key T. Oestrogen exposure and breast cancer risk. Breast Cancer Res. 2003;5(5):239–247.
9. Hilakivi-Clarke L, de Assis S, Warri A. Exposures to synthetic estrogens at different times during the life, and their effect on breast cancer risk. J Mammary Gland Biol Neoplasia. 2013;18:25–42.
10. World Cancer Research Fund/American Institute for Cancer Research. Food, nutrition, physical activity, and the prevention of cancer: a global perspective. Washington, DC: AICR; 2007. http://www.wcrf.org/int/research-we-fund/continuous-update-project-cup/second-expert-report
11. Travis RC, Key TJ. Oestrogen exposure and breast cancer risk. Breast Cancer Res. 2003;5(5):239–47.

12. Henderson TO, Amsterdam A, Bhatia S, Hudson MM, Meadows AT, Neglia JP, et al. Systematic review: surveillance for breast cancer in women treated with chest radiation for childhood, adolescent, or young adult cancer. Ann Intern Med. 2010;152(7):444–55. W144–54

13. Guibout C, Adjadj E, Rubino C, Shamsaldin A, Grimaud E, Hawkins M, et al. Malignant breast tumors after radiotherapy for a first cancer during childhood. J ClinOncol. 2005;23(1):197–204.

14. Preston DL, Cullings H, Suyama A, et al. Solid cancer incidence in atomic bomb survivors exposed in utero or as young children. J Natl Cancer Inst. 2008;100:428–36.

15. Pukkala E, Kesminiene A, Poliakov S, et al. Breast cancer in Belarus and Ukraine after the Chernobyl accident. Int J Cancer. 2006;119:651–8.

16. Barlow WE, White E, Ballard-Barbash R, Vacek PM, Titus-Ernstoff L, Carney PA, et al. Prospective breast cancer risk prediction model for women undergoing screening mammography. J Natl Cancer Inst. 2006;98(17):1204–14.

17. Boyd NF, Guo H, Martin LJ, Sun L, Stone J, Fishell E, et al. Mammographic density and the risk and detection of breast cancer. N Engl J Med. 2007;356(3):227–36.

18. McCormack VA, dos Santos Silva I. Breast density and parenchymal patterns as markers of breast cancer risk: a meta-analysis. Cancer EpidemiolBiomarkPrev. 2006;15:1159–69.

19. Pettersson A, Hankinson SE, Willett WC, Lagiou P, Trichopoulos D, Tamimi RM. Nondense mammographic area and risk of breast cancer. Breast Cancer Res. 2011;13(5):R100.

20. Rauh C, Hack CC, Häberle L, Hein A, Engel A, Schrauder MG, et al. Percent mammographic density and dense area as risk factors for breast cancer. GeburtshilfeFrauenheilkd. 2012;72:727–33.

21. Cote ML, Ruterbusch JJ, Alosh B, Bandyopadhyay S, Kim E, Albashiti B, et al. Benign breast disease and the risk of subsequent breast cancer in African American women. Cancer Prev Res (Phila). 2012;5(12):1375–80.

22. Hartmann LC, Sellers TA, Frost MH, Lingle WL, Degnim AC, Ghosh K, et al. Benign breast disease and the risk of breast cancer. N Engl J Med. 2005;353(3):229–37.

23. Dupont WD, Parl FF, Hartmann WH, Brinton LA, Winfield AC, Worrell JA, et al. Breast cancer risk associated with proliferative breast disease and atypical hyperplasia. Cancer. 1993;71(4):1258–65.

24. Ward EM, De Santis CE, Lin CC, Kramer JL, Jemal A, Kohler B, et al. Cancer statistics: Breast cancer in situ. CA Cancer J Clin. 2015;65(6):481–95.

25. Kerlikowske K. Epidemiology of ductal carcinoma in situ. J Natl Cancer Inst Monogr. 2010;2010(41):139–41.

26. Welch HG, Black WC. Using autopsy series to estimate the disease "reservoir" for ductal carcinoma in situ of the breast: how much more breast cancer can we find? Ann Intern Med. 1997;127:1023–8.

27. Collins LC, Tamimi RM, Baer HJ, Connolly JL, Colditz GA, Schnitt SJ. Outcome of patients with ductal carcinoma in situ untreated after diagnostic biopsy: results from the Nurses' Health Study. Cancer. 2005;103(9):1778–84.

28. Erbas B, Provenzano E, Armes J, Gertig D. The natural history of ductal carcinoma in situ of the breast: a review. Breast Cancer Res Treat. 2006;97(2):135–44.

29. Sanders ME, Schuyler PA, Simpson JF, Page DL, Dupont WD. Continued observation of the natural history of low-grade ductal carcinoma in situ reaffirms proclivity for local recurrence even after more than 30 years of follow-up. Mod Pathol. 2015;28(5):662–9.

30. Stuart KE, Houssami N, Taylor R, Hayen A, Boyages J. Long-term outcomes of ductal carcinoma in situ of the breast: a systematic review, meta-analysis and meta-regression analysis. BMC Cancer. 2015;15:890.

31. Inskip PD, Curtis RE. New malignancies following childhood cancer in the United States, 1973–2002. Int J Cancer. 2007;121(10):2233–40.

32. Buist DS, Abraham LA, Barlow WE, Krishnaraj A, Holdridge RC, Sickles EA, et al. Diagnosis of second breast cancer events after initial diagnosis of early stage breast cancer. Breast Cancer Res Treat. 2010;124(3):863–73.

33. Colditz GA, Kaphingst KA, Hankinson SE, Rosner B. Family history and risk of breast cancer: nurses' health study. Breast Cancer Res Treat. 2012;133(3):1097–104.

34. Collaborative Group on Hormonal Factors in Breast Cancer. Familial breast cancer: collaborative reanalysis of individual data from 52 epidemiological studies including 58,209 women with breast cancer and 101,986 women without the disease. Lancet. 2001;358(9291):1389–99.

35. Lynch HT, Lynch JF. Breast cancer genetics in an oncology clinic: 328 consecutive patients. Cancer Genet Cytogenet. 1986;22(4):369–71.

36. Margolin S, Johansson H, Rutqvist LE, Lindblom A, Fornander T. Family history, and impact on clinical presentation and prognosis, in a population-based breast cancer cohort from the Stockholm County. Familial Cancer. 2006;5(4):309–21.

37. Lalloo F, Evans DG. Familial breast cancer. Clin Genet. 2012;82(2):105–14.

38. Sharif S, Moran A, Huson SM, Iddenden R, Shenton A, Howard E, et al. Women with neurofibromatosis 1 are at a moderately increased risk of developing breast cancer and should be considered for early screening. J Med Genet. 2007;44(8):481–4.

39. Mavaddat N, Barrowdale D, Andrulis IL, et al. Pathology of breast and ovarian cancers among BRCA1 and BRCA2 mutation carriers: results from the Consortium of Investigators of Modifiers of BRCA1/2 (CIMBA). Cancer EpidemiolBiomark Prev. 2012;21:134–47.

40. Ford D, Easton DF, Stratton M, Narod S, Goldgar D, Devilee P, et al. Genetic heterogeneity and penetrance analysis of the BRCA1 and BRCA2 genes in breast cancer families. The Breast Cancer Linkage Consortium. Am J Hum Genet. 1998;62(3):676–89.

41. Antoniou A, Pharoah PD, Narod S, Risch HA, Eyfjord JE, Hopper JL, et al. Average risks of breast and ovarian cancer associated with BRCA1 or BRCA2 mutations detected in case Series unselected for family history: a combined analysis of 22 studies. Am J Hum Genet. 2003;72(5):1117–30.

42. King MC, Marks JH, Mandell JB, New York Breast Cancer Study G. Breast and ovarian cancer risks due to inherited mutations in BRCA1 and BRCA2. Science. 2003;302:643–6.

43. Ziegler RG, Hoover RN, Pike MC, Hildesheim A, Nomura AM, West DW, et al. Migration patterns and breast cancer risk in Asian-American women. J Natl Cancer Inst. 1993;85(22):1819–27.

44. Thompson D, Easton D. The genetic epidemiology of breast cancer genes. J Mammary Gland Biol Neoplasia. 2004;9(3):221–36.

45. Diez O, Osorio A, Duran M, Martinez-Ferrandis JI, de la Hoya M, Salazar R, et al. Analysis of BRCA1 and BRCA2 genes in Spanish breast/ovarian cancer patients: a high proportion of mutations unique to Spain and evidence of founder effects. Hum Mutat. 2003;22(4):301–12.

46. Mersch J, Jackson MA, Park M, Nebgen D, Peterson SK, Singletary C, et al. Cancers associated with BRCA1 and BRCA2 mutations other than breast and ovarian. Cancer. 2015;121(2):269–75.

47. Thompson D, Duedal S, Kirner J, McGuffog L, Last J, Reiman A, et al. Cancer risks and mortality in heterozygous ATM mutation carriers. J Natl Cancer Inst. 2005;97(11):813–22.

48. Seal S, Thompson D, Renwick A, Elliott A, Kelly P, Barfoot R, et al. Truncating mutations in the Fanconi anemia J gene BRIP1 are low-penetrance breast cancer susceptibility alleles. Nat Genet. 2006;38(11):1239–41.

49. Wong MW, Nordfors C, Mossman D, Pecenpetelovska G, Avery-Kiejda KA, Talseth-Palmer B, et al. BRIP1, PALB2, and RAD51C mutation analysis reveals their relative importance as genetic susceptibility factors for breast cancer. Breast Cancer Res Treat. 2011;127(3):853–9.

50. Melhem-Bertrandt A, Bojadzieva J, Ready KJ, Obeid E, Liu DD, Gutierrez-Barrera AM, et al. Early onset HER2-positive breast cancer is associated with germline TP53 mutations. Cancer. 2012;118(4):908–13.

51. Honrado E, Benitez J, Palacios J. The molecular pathology of hereditary breast cancer: genetic testing and therapeutic implications. Mod Pathol. 2005;18(10):1305–20.

52. NCCN Guidelines version 1.2018. BRCA-related breast and/or ovarian cancer syndrome. http://www.nccn.org/professionals/physician_gls/pdf/

53. Tyrer J, Duffy SW, Cuzick J. A breast cancer prediction model incorporating familial and personal risk factors. Stat Med. 2004;23(7):1111–30.

54. Antoniou AC, Cunningham AP, Peto J, Evans DG, Lalloo F, Narod SA, et al. The BOADICEA model of genetic susceptibility to breast and ovarian cancers: updates and extensions. Br J Cancer. 2008;98(8):1457–66.

55. Powell M, Jamshidian F, Cheyne K, Nititham J, Prebil LA, Ereman R. Assessing breast cancer risk models in Marin County, a population with high rates of delayed childbirth. Clin Breast Cancer. 2014;14(3):212–20.e1.

56. Armstrong J, Toscano M, Kotchko N, Friedman S, Schwartz MD, Virgo KS, et al. Utilization and outcomes of BRCA genetic testing and counseling in a National Commercially Insured Population: The ABOUT Study. JAMA Oncol. 2015;1(9):1251–60.

57. Domagala P, Hybiak J, Rys J, Byrski T, Cybulski C, Lubinski J. Pathological complete response after cisplatin neoadjuvant therapy is associated with the downregulation of DNA repair genes in BRCA1-associated triple-negative breast cancers. Oncotarget. 2016;7(42):68662–73.

58. Byrski T, Huzarski T, Dent R, Gronwald J, Zuziak D, Cybulski C, et al. Response to neoadjuvant therapy with cisplatin in BRCA1-positive breast cancer patients. Breast Cancer Res Treat. 2009;115(2):359–63.

59. Arun B, Bayraktar S, Liu DD, Gutierrez Barrera AM, Atchley D, Pusztai L, et al. Response to neoadjuvant systemic therapy for breast cancer in BRCA mutation carriers and noncarriers: a single-institution experience. J ClinOncol. 2011;29(28):3739–46.

60. Tutt A, Paul E, Kilburn L, Gilett C, Pinder S, Abraham J, et al. The TNT trial: a randomized phase III trial of carboplatin compared with docetaxel for patients with metastatic or recurrent locally advanced triple negative or BRCA 1/2 breast cancer. Cancer Res. 2014;75:S3–01.

61. Robson M, Goessl C, Domchek S. Olaparib for metastatic germline BRCA-mutated breast cancer. N Engl J Med. 2017;377(18):1792–3.

62. Ame JC, Spenlehauer C, de Murcia G. The PARP superfamily. BioEssays. 2004;26(8):882–93.

63. Gronwald J, Robidoux A, Kim-Sing C, Tung N, Lynch HT, Foulkes WD, et al. Duration of tamoxifen use and the risk of contralateral breast cancer in BRCA1 and BRCA2 mutation carriers. Breast Cancer Res Treat. 2014;146(2):421–7.

64. Narod SA, Brunet JS, Ghadirian P, Robson M, Heimdal K, Neuhausen SL, et al. Tamoxifen and risk of contralateral breast cancer in BRCA1 and BRCA2 mutation carriers: a case-control study. Hereditary Breast Cancer Clinical Study Group. Lancet. 2000;356(9245):1876–81.

65. Metcalfe K, Lynch HT, Ghadirian P, Tung N, Kim-Sing C, Olopade OI, et al. Risk of ipsilateral breast cancer in BRCA1 and BRCA2 mutation carriers. Breast Cancer Res Treat. 2011;127(1):287–96.

66. Metcalfe K, Lynch HT, Ghadirian P, Tung N, Olivotto I, Warner E, et al. Contralateral breast cancer in BRCA1 and BRCA2 mutation carriers. J ClinOncol. 2004;22(12):2328–35.

67. Domchek SM, Friebel TM, Singer CF, Evans DG, Lynch HT, Isaacs C, et al. Association of risk-reducing surgery in BRCA1 or BRCA2 mutation carriers with cancer risk and mortality. JAMA. 2010;304(9):967–75.

68. Le-Petross HT, Whitman GJ, Atchley DP, Yuan Y, Gutierrez-Barrera A, Hortobagyi GN, et al. Effectiveness of alternating mammography and magnetic resonance imaging for screening women with deleterious BRCA mutations at high risk of breast cancer. Cancer. 2011;117(17):3900–7.

69. Tung N, Domchek SM, Stadler Z, Nathanson KL, Couch F, Garber JE, et al. Counselling framework for moderate-penetrance cancer-susceptibility mutations. Nat Rev ClinOncol. 2016;13(9):581–8.

70. Ramus SJ, Antoniou AC, Kuchenbaecker KB, Soucy P, Beesley J, Chen X, et al. Ovarian cancer susceptibility alleles and risk of ovarian cancer in BRCA1 and BRCA2 mutation carriers. Hum Mutat. 2012;33(4):690–702.

71. Brentnall TA. Cancer surveillance of patients from familial pancreatic cancer kindreds. Med Clin North Am. 2000;84(3):707–18.

72. Canto MI, Goggins M, Hruban RH, Petersen GM, Giardiello FM, Yeo C, et al. Screening for early pancreatic neoplasia in high-risk individuals: a prospective controlled study. ClinGastroenterolHepatol. 2006;4(6):766–81. quiz 665

73. Kuerer H. Establishing a cancer genetics service. In: Kuerer's breast surgical oncology. New York: McGraw-Hill Professional, Inc.; 2010.

74. MacDonald DJ, Blazer KR, Weitzel JN. Extending comprehensive cancer center expertise in clinical cancer genetics and genomics to diverse communities: the power of partnership. J Natl Compr Cancer Netw. 2010;8(5):615–24.

75. Febbraro T, Robison K, Wilbur JS, Laprise J, Bregar A, Lopes V, et al. Adherence patterns to National Comprehensive Cancer Network (NCCN) guidelines for referral to cancer genetic professionals. GynecolOncol. 2015;138(1):109–14.

76. Levy DE, Garber JE, Shields AE. Guidelines for genetic risk assessment of hereditary breast and ovarian cancer: early disagreements and low utilization. J Gen Intern Med. 2009;24(7):822–8.

Maria João Cardoso

5.1 Introduction

Breast cancer is the most frequent cancer in high-income countries, and although survival is one of the highest, it is still the most common cause of cancer-related death in women.

Although the majority of breast cancers are sporadic, approximately 10% of breast cancers develop in the setting of hereditary gene mutations.

The risk of developing a breast cancer in women who carry a germline mutation depends on gene penetrance. Gene penetrance is defined as the probability of the effect (phenotype) of a mutation (genotype) will become clinically detected.

The majority of hereditary breast cancers are attributed to mutations in the BRCA1 and BRCA2 genes. Together BRCA1 and BRCA2 mutations account for around 30% of inheritable breast cancers. BRCA mutations increase also the risk of cancer in the ovaries, fallopian tubes, peritoneum, breast cancer in males, prostate cancer in younger men, pancreatic cancer and melanoma constituting what is known as Hereditary Breast and Ovarian Cancer Syndrome [1].

Other gene mutations with varying penetrance and frequencies that are less common than BRCA mutations have also been associated with heredi-

tary breast cancer (Table 5.1). Women who test negative for BRCA mutations and have a strong family history suggesting an hereditary cancer syndrome may be advised to undergo multigene test assessment. However, a word of caution is fundamental in this setting because the amount of evidence-based knowledge related to other genes, especially the moderate and low penetrance genes, is still very scarce.

The current chapter will focus mainly on the locoregional treatment of breast cancer in the setting of BRCA1 and BRCA2 mutations.

BRCA mutation carriers have a high lifetime risk of breast cancer that ranges from 30 to 85%.

Breast cancers that arise in the context of a deleterious BRCA1 or BRCA2 gene mutation have unique biologic features that directly affect surgical decisions, radiation therapy options and the choice of systemic agents.

For women without a mutation, facing a new breast cancer diagnosis, breast conserving treatment (BCT), if possible, is the preferred option, conferring a superior breast cancer-specific survival to mastectomy (M) particularly in early stages of disease [2]. However, in the presence of a confirmed or suspicious mutation carrier status, local management decisions need to be balanced taking into account the risk of ipsilateral breast recurrence (IBR), the risk of contralateral breast cancer (CBC), the potential survival benefit of prophylactic mastectomy and the modifying factors that could either increase or decrease the risk for IBR or CBC [3].

M. J. Cardoso (✉)
Breast Unit, Champalimaud Clinical Center/
Champalimaud Foundation, Lisbon, Portugal
e-mail: maria.joao.cardoso@fundacaochampalimaud.pt

© Springer Nature Switzerland AG 2020
O. Gentilini et al. (eds.), *Breast Cancer in Young Women*,
https://doi.org/10.1007/978-3-030-24762-1_5

Table 5.1 Genes, associated syndromes and lifetime risk of breast cancer

Gene	Hereditary syndrome; associated cancers	Lifetime risk of breast cancer
Frequent mutations—highly penetrant genes		
BRCA1	Hereditary Breast and Ovarian Cancer Syndrome; early-onset breast cancer, ovarian cancer, modest increase in male breast cancer risk	65–81%
BRCA2	Hereditary Breast and Ovarian Cancer Syndrome; early-onset/late-onset breast cancer, ovarian cancer, melanoma, pancreatic cancer, male breast cancer	45–85%
Rare mutations—highly penetrant genes		
TP53	Li-Fraumeni syndrome; very-early-onset breast cancer, sarcoma, adrenocortical carcinoma, brain tumours, phyllodes tumour, others (many), ER-positive, PR-positive, human epidermal growth factor receptor 2-positive breast cancer	50–80%
PTEN	Cowden syndrome; breast cancer, benign and malignant thyroid disease, endometrial cancer, colorectal cancer, macrocephaly, trichilemmomas, palmar-plantar keratoses, oral mucosal papillomatosis, benign breast disease; de novo mutations 11–48%	50–85%
SKT-11	Peutz-Jeghers syndrome; very-early-onset breast cancer, gastrointestinal cancer, pancreatic cancer, ovarian cancer, hamartomatous polyps of the gastrointestinal tract, oral-labial pigmentation; de novo mutation rate may be as high as 50%	35–50%
CDH1	Invasive lobular cancer, diffuse gastric cancer with signet ring cells	39–52%
Frequent mutations—moderately penetrant genes		
CHEK2	Similar cancer spectrum as Li-Fraumeni syndrome but lower penetrance; male breast cancer	15–25%
ATM	Ataxia-telangiectasia; leukaemia, lymphoma and breast cancer	15–20%
PALB2	Later-onset breast cancer, male breast cancer, pancreatic cancer	20–30%

5.2 Breast Cancer Diagnosis and Testing for BRCA Mutation Status: Clinical Scenarios

In the clinical setting, there are three main scenarios that can modify the locoregional treatment approach. The first scenario is a diagnosis of a breast cancer in a known mutation carrier; the second one is a detection of a mutation carrier status after the completion of a breast cancer treatment; the third one, and possibly the most challenging, is the hypothesis of harbouring a mutation at the time of diagnosis of breast cancer.

Genetic testing is becoming more frequent and can influence treatment decision making. Testing for BRCA1 and BRCA2 has been available for the last 20 years, but new sequencing technologies and easier patent laws have made multipanel testing widely available at lower costs. However, clinical needs for genetic testing may not be adequately recognized due to physician's lack of training in identifying high-risk patients. Although several guidelines are available to guide in the detection of patients with a high probability of harbouring a mutation, it is important to have a simple and reproducible methodology to lessen the possibility of missing BRCA mutation carriers in the first approach of a newly diagnosed breast cancer patient.

In breast cancer diagnosed at young age, in triple negative breast cancer, in bilateral breast cancer and with a strong family history of breast and ovarian cancer, BRCA1 and BRCA2 are the most commonly assessed mutations. Identification of carriers will allow an informed discussion of treatment options.

In highly organized centres, the presence of a geneticist can be a facilitator to make the screening of those patients that can harbour a germline mutation and can be proposed for a genetic testing. Usually the threshold for carrying on with a genetic test is the possibility of $\geq 10\%$ of harbouring a mutation. Various models have been developed to determine the probability of BRCA1 and BRCA2 mutations, the Myriad models, BRCAPRO and BOADICEA. However, they are not easy to use in a medical appointment as a screening tool.

Being aware of major family risk factors and, more recently, also histology-related factors can help clinicians to stratify risk and more accurately propose patients to genetic testing in the setting of a recently diagnosed or previous breast cancer. The Manchester Scoring System 3 (MSS) is an easy-to-use, clinic-friendly, paper-based model that compares well with other computer-based models and takes into account several pathology adjustments that further refined the system's previous versions (Table 5.2) [4].

Table 5.2 The Manchester Scoring System—MSS3 (pathology adjustment)

Type of cancer, age at diagnosis	BRCA1	BRCA2
Female breast cancer (FBC), <30	6	5
Female breast cancer (FBC), 30–39	4	4
Female breast cancer (FBC), 40–49	3	3
Female breast cancer (FBC), 50–59	2	2
Female breast cancer (FBC), >59	1	1
Male breast cancer (MBC), <60	5	8
Male breast cancer (MBC), ≥60	5	5
Ovarian cancer, <60	8	5
Ovarian cancer, ≥60	5	5
Pancreatic cancer	0	1
Prostate cancer, <60	0	2
Prostate cancer, ≥60	0	1
Breast cancer pathology adjustment in index case		
Grade 3	2	0
Grade 1	−2	0
ER positive	−1	0
ER negative	1	0
Triple negative	4	0
HER 2 positive (3+ or ISH)	−6	0
Ductal carcinoma in situ	−2	0
Lobular invasive		
Ovarian cancer pathology adjustment—any case in family		
Mucinous germ cell or borderline tumours	0	0
High-grade serous, <60	2	0
Adopted no known status in blood relatives	2	2

MSS3 is based on empirical data from the Manchester mutation-screening programme

Each individual and family characteristic (from one side of the family only) is given a numerical weight, and these are added to give a score for each of the two genes—BRCA1/2
The combined score of 15–19 correlates to the 10% probability of carrying a mutation and a score of 20 points to 20% in BRCA1 or 2 (sequential screening). If analysed separately, 10 points in each gene correlate with a 10% probability for either gene

5.2.1 Diagnosis of a Breast Cancer in a Known Mutation Carrier

In this particular scenario, breast cancer diagnosis is usually made in a carrier that initially opted for surveillance. Those patients are usually well aware of the associated risks, and the attitude in terms of locoregional treatment is frequently towards a more radical surgery, comprising both breasts.

5.2.2 Detection of a Mutation Carrier Status After Completion of Breast Cancer Treatment

After a previous breast cancer treatment, the confirmation of a carrier status raises the question of further surgery in the operated breast in case of a unilateral cancer, previously treated with breast conservation, considering the possibility of a ipsilateral breast recurrence (IBR) and also the risk of a contralateral breast cancer (CBC) and the possibility of a prophylactic mastectomy.

5.2.3 Suspicion of a Mutation Carrier Status at the Time of Diagnosis of a New Breast Cancer

This is by far the most challenging of the three scenarios. Patients are confronted at the same time with two frightening news: the breast cancer diagnosis and the possibility of being a mutation carrier. Some authors argue that this particular moment is not the time to confront the patient with the possibility of being a mutation carrier. However, this knowledge can influence not only surgical decision but also systemic treatment.

Recently, several studies have demonstrated that genetic testing at diagnosis and before starting treatment is considered positively by the majority of patients and does not have a negative psychological impact [5].

A recent report by Kurian and colleagues reports that the major reason for not performing genetic test in high-risk patients is not the fear patients have of harbouring a mutation and have to deal with the result but that the clinical need for testing may not be recognized by physicians [6].

The vast majority of women, who are aware of their mutation status before surgery, use this knowledge in their decision process, meaning more bilateral mastectomies as opposite to those who are not aware of their mutation and opt for a conservative approach [7].

One important factor to consider is the interval from sample collection to the reception of results. It is not clear if the wait delays surgery, and there are not many publications confirming or denying this factor. However, genetic counselling and testing is evolving, and results can usually be obtained in 2–3 weeks, although this median time can vary between countries [8].

Usually BRCA-associated breast cancers have a more aggressive nature [9], and as a consequence more patients will be submitted to chemotherapy, either adjuvant or neo-adjuvant. When neo-adjuvant chemotherapy is decided, genetic test results are usually available before surgery, allowing for a more informed decision.

5.3 Ipsilateral and Contralateral Breast Cancer Risk and Modifying Factors

Independently of the clinical scenario at stake, it is important to accurately explain to BRCA patients the expected risks, when compared to sporadic breast cancer situations. It is also essential to be aware of the possible risk-modifying factors that can help in the choice of the optimal locoregional treatment.

5.3.1 Risk of Ipsilateral Breast Cancer Recurrence (IBR)

Although BCT in sporadic breast cancer is the treatment of choice, when feasible, in early breast cancer, it is debatable if it is also an option for BRCA mutation carriers. There were also concerns about the harmful effect of radiotherapy after breast conservation in mutation carriers that turned out to be unconfirmed, and several studies support the approach of breast conservation surgery with radiotherapy as a possible approach in this particular group of patients [10]. However, the fear of a higher rate of IBR is still the main question arising in BRCA carriers that consider BCT as a possible strategy.

An IBR can be either a true local recurrence or a new primary cancer. Most studies have not been able to differentiate between those, and both are denominated IBR. The rate of true local recurrences after BCT is probably similar between mutation carriers and non-carriers. However, the rate of new primary cancers is probably higher. Such a difference is expected to be more evident after longer follow-up intervals because the remaining breast tissue is still susceptible to the mutation effect [3].

Valachis and colleagues, in a meta-analysis of retrospective studies, investigated the risk of IBR after BCT in BRCA carriers versus non-carriers, including 6 cohort and 4 case-control studies with a total of 526 carriers and 2320 controls. The rate of IBR was 17.3% (95% CI 11.4–24.2%) for BRCA carriers and 11% (95% CI 6.5–15.4%) for controls without a significant difference between both groups (RR 1.45, 95% CI 0.98–2.14, p value = 0.07). The rate of IBR was no different between BRCA1 and BRCA2 carriers. However, if follow-up time was considered in the analysis, a significant higher risk for IBR in BRCA carriers was confirmed in studies with a follow-up of more than 7 years (23.7% for BRCA mutation carriers with 95% CI 12.1–37.8 and 15.9% for controls with 95% CI 8.7–24.8%, RR 1.51, 95% CI 1.15–1.98, p value = 0.003) [3].

This difference in results according to duration of follow-up seems to be explained by a higher risk of new primaries in BRCA carriers due to the continuous risk in the remaining breast tissue. These new cancers will arrive later than true recurrences that are more frequent in the first years after treatment. However, no overall survival difference was observed between carriers and controls who opted for breast conservation treatment.

Few data are available comparing IBR in BCT with M in BRCA carriers. Published results show a significantly increased risk of local failure in BRCA1/2 mutation carriers treated with BCT compared to carriers treated with M; however, breast cancer-specific and overall survivals are similar.

In the study by Pierce and colleagues published in 2010, no significant difference in breast cancer-specific or overall survivals was observed by local treatment type. Breast cancer-specific survivals with BCT were 93.6% and 91.7% at 10 and 15 years vs. 93.5% and 92.8% with M (p = 0.85). Overall survivals with BCT group were 92.1% and 87.3% at 10 and 15 years and 91.8% and 89.8% with M (p = 0.73) [10].

The modifying risk factors for IBR after BCT in BRCA carriers have been thoroughly investigated, and until today two factors stand out as protectors as demonstrated in the Valachis meta-analysis: adjuvant chemotherapy (RR 0.51, 95% CI 0.31–0.84) and ovariectomy (RR 0.42, 95% CI 0.22–0.81) [3]. Tamoxifen was not associated with a reduced risk of IBR in the meta-analysis although there the evidence is still conflicting and some authors claim that Tamoxifen is a protector independently of the mutation carrier status [10].

5.3.2 Risk of Contralateral Breast Cancer (CBC)

A BRCA mutation carrier who had breast cancer is at higher risk for a new primary breast cancer in the contralateral breast. The annual risk of contralateral breast cancer for a mutation carrier is around 3%, compared with 0.5% in the sporadic breast cancer population.

In the meta-analysis by Valachis, 11 studies (7 cohort and 4 case–control studies) presented data on the risk for CBC between BRCA-mutation carriers and non-carriers (807 carriers and 3163 non-carriers). The rates of CBC for BRCA-mutation and controls were 23.7% (95% CI 17.6–30.5%) and 6.8% (95% CI 4.2–10%), respectively. Patients with BRCA mutation had a higher risk for CBC compared with non-carriers (RR 3.56, 95% CI 2.50–5.08, p value <0.001) [3].

Regarding the risk of CBC in BRCA1-mutation versus BRCA2- mutation carriers, several studies investigated this difference. In the beforementioned publication, 1532 BRCA1-mutation carriers were compared to 950 BRCA2-mutation carriers. BRCA1-mutation carriers had an increased risk for CBC compared to BRCA2-mutation carriers (21.1% for BRCA1-mutation carriers with 95% CI 15–28.2% and 15.1% for controls with 95% CI 10–21%, RR 1.42, 95% CI 1.01–1.99, p value = 0.04) [3].

It is estimated that BRCA1- and BRCA2-mutation carriers have a 3.5-fold higher relative risk of CBC compared to non-carriers and that CBC risk increases up to 42% in BRCA1 compared to BRCA2 carriers.

The 10-year cumulative risk of CBC in BRCA-mutation carriers with breast cancer varies between 20 and 35% and may even further differ by age or menopausal status at diagnosis of the first breast cancer, type of treatment and other clinical and pathological factors of the first tumour in the breast.

Although it is clear that the risk of CBC is higher in BRCA-mutation carriers, it is not equally obvious if contralateral prophylactic mastectomy (CPM) has an impact in breast cancer-specific survival and overall survival. CPM aims at preventing CBC in carriers. However, until now there is no proof that it improves survival. Studies were small, and retrospective in the majority of cases and follow-up is rather short [3]. More recently, there has been a growing body of evidence of an improvement in survival demonstrated in longer follow-ups. Metcalfe et al. showed a 20-year survival rate of 88% for women submitted to CPM versus 66% for those who did not even after controlling for associated factors [11].

There are two ***risk-modifying factors*** generally considered to be associated with a lower risk of CBC in BRCA mutation carriers: ovariectomy and older age at diagnosis (>50 years). According to the study by Metcalfe et al., the cumulative risk of CBC at 5, 10 and 15 years was 14.2%, 23.9% and 37.6% for women <50 at diagnosis and 8.6%, 14.7% and 16.8% for women >50 at diagnosis [12]. Tamoxifen can also have a protective effect mostly in women not previously submitted to ovariectomy [10].

5.4 Type of Locoregional Treatment in BRCA Mutation Carriers

5.4.1 Breast Conservation Surgery and Radiotherapy

There are no specific indications other than those applied to non-carriers regarding surgery in BRCA patients.

The type of breast-conserving treatment, the use of oncoplastic techniques and margin width all should be according to the rules used in the treatment of sporadic breast cancer.

In case of known carriers that choose to undergo breast conservation, it is important to be aware of the need of further surgery.

If neo-adjuvant chemotherapy is the primary treatment, the choice between BCT or mastectomy will be dependent of tumour response and also patient preference.

All patients submitted to breast conservation have a clear indication to undergo adjuvant radiotherapy.

If patients have an absolute contraindication for radiotherapy, they should be advised to choose a mastectomy to allow a better local control of the disease.

All BRCA carriers are excluded from partial breast irradiation techniques as per ASTRO and ESTRO guidelines.

5.4.2 Mastectomy

When mastectomy is considered for the treatment of the primary cancer in a BRCA mutation carrier, rules should follow the general indications for non-carriers.

The choice between the type of mastectomy—total mastectomy, skin-sparing or even nipple-sparing mastectomy—will depend on the safety regarding size and location of the tumour

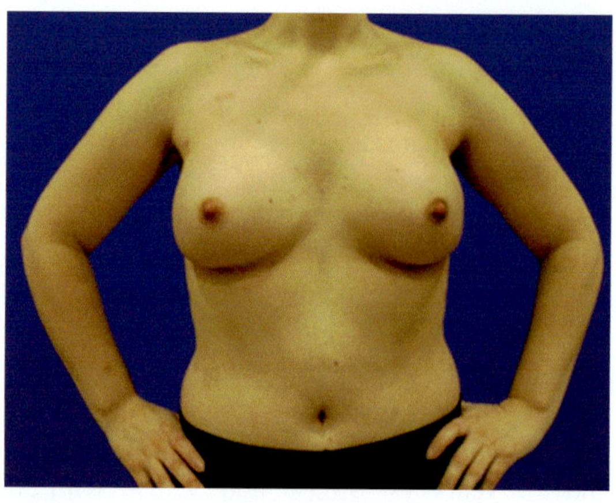

Fig. 5.1 Bilateral Skin-Sparing Mastectomy. Therapeutic mastectomy with sentinel lymph node and radiotherapy (left) and contralateral prophylactic mastectomy (right). Immediate breast reconstruction with implants and ADM. Post-operative adjuvant radiotherapy

to the skin. Nipple-sparing mastectomy, due to the preservation of the complete envelope, is usually associated with a better aesthetic outcome (Fig. 5.1) [13].

Several studies have demonstrated that preservation of the nipple areolar complex, in nipple-sparing mastectomy, is safe and with no additional risk of local recurrence compared to sporadic cases. Locoregional recurrences are low with reported values of 2% at 5 years follow-up [13].

There is no impediment to any type of reconstruction, and the decision should be entirely dependent on patient's choice after a proper discussion of pros and cons with the surgeon. Decision to undergo immediate reconstruction will depend on institutional indications and patients desire. In many institutions around the globe, adjuvant radiotherapy is still a contraindication to undergo immediate reconstruction.

Regarding CPM, the most common choice is nipple-sparing mastectomy with immediate reconstruction if the patient desires to do so. Again in this situation the risk of leaving mammary tissue behind the nipple is very small, and there are no studies showing, until now, that the risk of CBC is higher with this type of surgery.

5.4.3 Axillary Approach

Axillary staging and treatment in the presence of a breast cancer in a mutation carrier should follow the same principles as in sporadic early breast cancer.

All clinically negative axilla should be treated with sentinel node biopsy.

Special care should be given to recent guidelines in case of axillae with a low burden of disease, like the Z011 protocol bearing in mind that the published study did not include BRCA-mutated patients [14].

If considering a CPM, there is no clear evidence that sentinel lymph node biopsy will be of benefit [14]. Considering that the risk of associated lymphedema exists, although low, and that it's around 3–4% in sentinel node biopsy, and the possibility of having a positive lymph node in a CPM is around 1%, due to a non-detected breast cancer at imaging, surgeons should not consider proposing, as routine, the sentinel node biopsy without a discussion of the associated risks and benefits [15].

5.5 Locoregional Treatment Options Considering Different Scenarios and Different Risk-Modifying Factors in BRCA-1 and BRCA2-Mutation Carriers

As discussed before, there are three different situations regarding mutation status that can impact the choices of patients regarding locoregional treatment. In any of these situations, additional risk for IBR, CBC and possible impact in survival should be carefully discussed with patients and compared with identical risks in non-carriers (Table 5.3).

In case of a previously known mutation carrier status, when the breast cancer is diagnosed, usually patient's choice is towards a more radical surgery, usually bilateral [7].

On the contrary, when the mutation status is known only after breast cancer treatment, patients

Table 5.3 Differences in IBR and CBC between sporadic breast cancer and breast cancer in BRCA1 and BRCA2 mutation carriers

	BRCA positive (%/year)	BRCA negative (%/year)
IBR	1–2% (2–4% >7 years)	1–2%
CBC	3% (BRCA1) 2% (BRCA2)	0.5%

Similar breast cancer-specific survival and overall survival

are usually more cautious and try to understand better the risks and benefits of further surgery.

When breast cancer is diagnosed and at the same time there is a high possibility of being a mutation carrier, the situation is a little more stressful. In case of neo-adjuvant chemotherapy, genetic test can be done at the beginning of treatment, and results are usually available for discussion before surgery. In case of surgery as the first treatment, a complete discussion should have place with the patient to understand if the test should be undertaken before the operation with the consequent waiting time or if the decision of locoregional treatment should be done without knowing the result accepting the consequences of a positive test result after treatment.

For each of these situations, there are higher risk groups of BRCA-mutated patients where a more aggressive surgical approach may be preferable always respecting individual patient's preferences (Table 5.4). Discussion in a multidisciplinary team is mandatory, and a case by case approach will lead to a more balanced choice using the published available evidence.

Age is by far the most important risk-modifying factor in IBR as there is more time to the development of new cancers. Younger patients have a higher risk of IBR and also CBC. Adjuvant and neo-adjuvant chemotherapy are associated with a 50% reduction of IBR as is ovariectomy.

Regarding CBC, there are also three factors associated with a decreased risk: age again with younger patients having higher risk of CBC, ovariectomy and also adjuvant Tamoxifen.

When BRCA1 patients are compared to BRCA2, the former ones have a higher risk of CBC.

Table 5.4 Proposed locoregional approach according to modifying risk factors

More aggressive approach	More conservative approach
Younger patients (<50 years)	Older patients
No oophorectomy	Oophorectomy
No adjuvant Tamoxifen	Adjuvant Tamoxifen
BRCA1	BRCA2

Younger BRCA1 carriers with hormonal receptor-negative breast cancer would benefit more of a more aggressive approach possibly bilateral. By contrast, older patients with a BRCA2 mutation with an hormonal receptor-positive breast cancer could consider a more conservative approach and accept the smaller CBC risk that would be further reduced by the use of anti-oestrogen treatment. Prophylactic ovariectomy should always be considered and adapted in each case according to risk and to childbearing plans.

References

1. Valencia OM, Samuel SE, Viscusi RK, Riall TS, Neumayer LA, Aziz H. The role of genetic testing in patients with breast cancer: a review. JAMA Surg. 2017;152(6):589–94.
2. Gentilini OD, Cardoso MJ, Poortmans P. Less is more. Breast conservation might be even better than mastectomy in early breast cancer patients. Breast. 2017;35:32–3.
3. Valachis A, Nearchou AD, Lind P. Surgical management of breast cancer in BRCA-mutation carriers: a systematic review and meta-analysis. Breast Cancer Res Treat. 2014;144(3):443–55.
4. Evans DG, Harkness EF, Plaskocinska I, Wallace AJ, Clancy T, Woodward ER, et al. Pathology update to the Manchester Scoring System based on testing in over 4000 families. J Med Genet. 2017;54(10):674–81.
5. Wevers MR, Ausems MG, Verhoef S, Bleiker EM, Hahn DE, Brouwer T, et al. Does rapid genetic counseling and testing in newly diagnosed breast cancer patients cause additional psychosocial distress? Results from a randomized clinical trial. Genet Med. 2016;18(2):137–44.
6. Kurian AW, Griffith KA, Hamilton AS, Ward KC, Morrow M, Katz SJ, et al. Genetic testing and counseling among patients with newly diagnosed breast cancer. JAMA. 2017;317(5):531–4.
7. Yadav S, Reeves A, Campian S, Sufka A, Zakalik D. Preoperative genetic testing impacts surgical decision making in BRCA mutation carriers with breast cancer: a retrospective cohort analysis. Hered Cancer Clin Pract. 2017;15:11.
8. Wevers MR, Aaronson NK, Bleiker EMA, Hahn DEE, Brouwer T, van Dalen T, et al. Rapid genetic counseling and testing in newly diagnosed breast cancer: patients' and health professionals' attitudes, experiences, and evaluation of effects on treatment decision making. J Surg Oncol. 2017;116(8):1029–39.
9. Shah PD, Patil S, Dickler MN, Offit K, Hudis CA, Robson ME. Twenty-one-gene recurrence score assay in BRCA-associated versus sporadic breast cancers: differences based on germline mutation status. Cancer. 2016;122(8):1178–84.
10. Pierce LJ, Phillips KA, Griffith KA, Buys S, Gaffney DK, Moran MS, et al. Local therapy in BRCA1 and BRCA2 mutation carriers with operable breast cancer: comparison of breast conservation and mastectomy. Breast Cancer Res Treat. 2010;121(2):389–98.
11. Metcalfe K, Gershman S, Ghadirian P, Lynch HT, Snyder C, Tung N, et al. Contralateral mastectomy and survival after breast cancer in carriers of BRCA1 and BRCA2 mutations: retrospective analysis. BMJ. 2014;348:g226.
12. Metcalfe K, Gershman S, Lynch HT, Ghadirian P, Tung N, Kim-Sing C, et al. Predictors of contralateral breast cancer in BRCA1 and BRCA2 mutation carriers. Br J Cancer. 2011;104(9):1384–92.
13. Peled AW, Irwin CS, Hwang ES, Ewing CA, Alvarado M, Esserman LJ. Total skin-sparing mastectomy in BRCA mutation carriers. Ann Surg Oncol. 2014;21(1):37–41.
14. Lyman GH, Temin S, Edge SB, Newman LA, Turner RR, Weaver DL, et al. Sentinel lymph node biopsy for patients with early-stage breast cancer: American Society of Clinical Oncology clinical practice guideline update. J Clin Oncol. 2014;32(13):1365–83.
15. Burger A, Thurtle D, Owen S, Mannu G, Pilgrim S, Vinayagam R, et al. Sentinel lymph node biopsy for risk-reducing mastectomy. Breast J. 2013;19(5):529–32.

Systemic Therapies of Young Breast Cancer Patients at High Genetic Risk

6

Shani Paluch-Shimon, Bella Kaufman, and Ella Evron

6.1 Background

More than 90% of hereditary cases of breast and ovarian cancer are thought to be a result of a mutation in *BRCA1/2* [1]. The estimated prevalence of *BRCA1* and *BRCA2* mutations is dependent on the population and can vary between 1 in 300 and 1 in 800, respectively. More than 2000 different mutations have been identified in *BRCA1/2* genes. Founder mutations are prevalent in 2.5% of the general Ashkenazi Jewish population, specifically, mutations in *BRCA1* (185delAG [= c.68_69delAG], 5382InsC [=c.5266dupC]) or *BRCA2* (6174delT [=c.5946delT]) [2], and have also been described in Northern, Western, and Eastern Europe. A germline mutation in *BRCA1* or *BRCA2* results in a significantly elevated lifetime risk of developing breast and ovarian cancer, estimated at up to 7 and 25 times (respectively) that of the average-risk population [3–6], depending on the population studied, while a mutation in *BRCA2* has been demonstrated in multiple studies to be associated with an increased risk in prostate cancer, melanoma, and pancreatic cancer [7]. Women with a germline mutation in *BRCA1* and *BRCA2* typically present with breast cancer at a younger age, particularly those harboring a *BRCA1* mutation [6]. In a contemporary cohort, the cumulative risk by age 40 for developing breast cancer was 24% for *BRCA1* carriers and 13% for *BRCA2* carriers [6].

Genetic susceptibility to breast cancer has also been associated with mutations in other genes, some of which are associated with known hereditary cancer syndromes, such as *p53*, *PTEN*, *CDH1*, *STK11*, *PALB2*, *CHEK2*, *ATM*, *NBN*, and *NF-1* [8].

A recent study demonstrated that 87% of young women ($\leq$40) will have completed genetic testing by 1 year from their breast cancer diagnosis, and the percentage of those who had been tested within a year of diagnosis was highest in the most contemporary cohorts [9]. In this study 81% of women had in fact received their results within 3 months of diagnosis, and while many reported that the results impacted their surgical choices, the results of the genetic testing did not have a significant impact on these women's choices of systemic therapies. Undoubtedly, as research in the field of systemic therapies for women with hereditary breast cancer evolves, the therapeutic impact of genetic testing will grow.

S. Paluch-Shimon (✉)
Breast Oncology Unit, Shaare Zedek Medical Centre, Jerusalem, Israel
e-mail: shanips@szmc.org.il

B. Kaufman
Breast Oncology Institute, Sheba Medical Centre, Ramat Gan, Israel

E. Evron
Sackler School of Medicine, Tel Aviv University, Tel Aviv, Israel

© Springer Nature Switzerland AG 2020
O. Gentilini et al. (eds.), *Breast Cancer in Young Women*,
https://doi.org/10.1007/978-3-030-24762-1_6

6.2   BRCA-Associated Breast Cancer

6.2.1   Role of BRCA1 and BRCA2 in DNA Repair

BRCA1 and *BRCA2* are tumor suppressor genes that encode very large nuclear proteins and are widely expressed in proliferating cells of various normal tissues. The two genes reside on different chromosomes and have no homology in nucleotide sequence or in protein functional domains. However, both play an essential role in preserving genomic stability during cell division as it was shown earlier that *BRCA1* [10] and *BRCA2* [11] deficiency leads to accumulation of chromosomal aberrations which may result in carcinogenesis. Genome integrity is repeatedly interfered throughout the cell's life span, either during DNA replication and cell division or in response to endogenous or exogenous genotoxic stress. Consequently, cellular mechanisms of DNA damage response (DDR) are activated to allow DNA repair and prevent transmission of genetic errors to the daughter cells. Both *BRCA1* and *BRCA2* are involved in DDR [12], primarily by taking part in homologous recombination (HR), an error-free DNA repair mechanism of double-strand breaks in DNA [13–15]. Whereas *BRCA2* binds directly to DNA breaks and recruits the recombinase RAD51 [16, 17], *BRCA1* forms complexes with other key components of the HR machinery including PALB2 (partner and localizer of BRCA2), BRCA2, and RAD51 [18–20]. Consequently, lack of either of these genes leads to loss of DNA damage-induced formation of RAD51 foci and impaired HR, which further activates alternative error-prone repair mechanisms, resulting in aberrations in chromosomal structure and number and genomic instability [21–23]. In addition to HR, *BRCA1* is involved in multiple DDR protein complexes that activate cell cycle checkpoints and attenuate S phase or mitosis entry, thus extending the time window for DNA repair.

While germline heterozygosity for *BRCA* mutations is enough for relative tissue-specific cancer predisposition, cancers that arise in mutation carriers usually lose the second *BRCA* allele during tumor progression. Loss of heterozygosity (LOH) is the most common second hit for inactivation of the *BRCA* tumor suppressor genes and more than 90% of *BRCA1* and *BRCA2* carcinomas have LOH of the non-mutated allele [24]. Moreover, LOH of the wild-type *BRCA* allele has been found in peri-tumoral non-neoplastic tissues and in situ lesions, suggesting that LOH is an early event in *BRCA*-associated carcinogenesis [25]. The way in which germline heterozygous mutations in *BRCA* predispose humans to cancer remains poorly understood. Although heterozygosity of *BRCA* may engender a low but significant rate of chromosomal instability [26], it is the loss of the second allele that appears to trigger an inflection in the rate of genetic alteration. Nevertheless, the presence of broken or aneuploid chromosomes usually triggers cell cycle arrest and apoptosis. Hence, knockout of both *BRCA* alleles caused early embryonal lethality in mice [27, 28], and in humans no individuals were described that carry homozygous biallelic deleterious mutations in these genes, although compound germline heterozygosity for concomitant *BRCA1* and *BRCA2* has been reported [29, 30]. Clearly, on top of *BRCA* deficiency, additional alterations in cell cycle checkpoints or apoptotic pathways are required to escape death signals and promote carcinogenesis [22]. In accordance with this hypothesis is the high frequency of p53 mutations detected in *BRCA*-deficient cancers [31, 32]. Another unanswered question is that of tissue specificity, why germline mutations in *BRCA* predispose to cancer primarily in the breast and ovary rather than in other organs [12, 14, 33]. It is possible that tissue-specific epigenetic and genetic alterations as well as local factors such as hormones may synergize with *BRCA* deficiency to support carcinogenesis [34]. For example, *BRCA*-deficient tumors may arise in tissues that support the prolonged survival of cells that have inactivated both *BRCA* alleles, providing a window in which additional mutations necessary for outgrowth can occur [35]. Interestingly, recent data suggest that increased genomic instability and impaired DNA damage repair may be observed in *BRCA1*-haplo-insufficient human mammary epithelial cells but not in human mammary fibroblasts prior to the loss of the second *BRCA1* allele [36].

6.2.2 Phenotype of BRCA-Associated Breast Cancer

Hereditary breast cancers in carriers of *BRCA1* and *BRCA2* mutations have distinct clinicopathological features as compared to sporadic breast cancers [22, 37, 38]. *BRCA1*-related cancers are usually high-grade, invasive ductal carcinomas with a higher incidence of medullary carcinoma histological subtype, lymphocytic infiltration, foci of necrosis, and pushing margins. Between 60% and 90% of *BRCA1* tumors are estrogen receptor negative and fall into the "basal-like" subgroup of breast cancers [38–41], although it was suggested that they actually arise from luminal progenitors rather than from basal progenitor cells [42–44]. In addition, *BRCA1*-associated breast cancers have higher incidence of p53 mutations [31, 32], lack of PTEN expression [45], c-myc amplification, and EGFR expression [22]. In contrast, tumors arising in BRCA2 mutation carriers do not differ from sporadic tumors with regard to ER and PR expression, and ER positivity was reported in the majority of these tumors [38, 39]. It has been suggested that HER2 over-expression is uncommon in *BRCA1* and *BRCA2* carcinomas, with reported frequencies ranging from 0 to 3.7% [39, 46]. However, in their comprehensive report of 3797 BRCA1-associated and 2392 BRCA2-associated breast cancers, Her2 positivity was reported in 10% and 13%, respectively [38]. Both BRCA1- and BRCA2-associated tumors tend to be of high grade. Thus 77% and 50% of the tumors, respectively, were classified grade III in the CIMBA report [38]. Accordingly, it has been reported that ER-positive tumors of *BRCA1* and *BRCA2* mutation carriers score significantly higher Oncotype Dx RS as compared to ER-positive tumors in non-carriers, suggesting more aggressive phenotype [47, 48].

6.2.3 Prognosis of BRCA-Associated Breast Cancer

Several studies have focused on prognosis and outcome of *BRCA*-associated breast cancers as compared with sporadic tumors. Most recent larger studies where patients were subjected to modern chemotherapy and hormonal therapies found similar disease outcome in *BRCA* mutation carriers and non-carriers. Goodwin et al. compared breast cancer recurrence and death of 94 patients with *BRCA1* mutations, 72 with *BRCA2* mutations, and 1550 with sporadic breast cancer. The outcome of *BRCA1* mutation carriers did not differ significantly from the outcome of the sporadic tumors group or from the outcome of sporadic TNBC. For *BRCA2* mutation carriers, worse outcome was suggested by univariate analysis. However, this difference disappeared after adjustment for patient and tumor characteristics and for the administration of adjuvant chemotherapy. Interestingly, worse outcome was observed in *BRCA2* mutation carriers when adjuvant hormonal therapy was administered, likely reflecting more aggressive characteristics of *BRCA2*-mutated tumors [49]. A retrospective study by Rennert et al. reported no adverse effect on outcome by the presence of *BRCA1/2* mutations in 128 mutation carriers compared with 1189 non-carriers [50]. A number of studies reported similar results [51–56]. However, few studies reported worse breast cancer outcome in *BRCA* mutation carriers, especially with mutations in *BRCA1* [57–59], and differential response of *BRCA*-mutated tumors to certain chemotherapy drugs had been proposed [60, 61]. Several meta-analyses have been published regarding breast cancer survival of *BRCA1/2* mutation carriers [62–65]. Zhong et al. found that *BRCA1* mutation carriers had worse OS (HR 1.50, 95%CI 1.11–2.04) but not PFS compared to non-carriers. In their analysis a *BRCA2* mutation was not associated with breast cancer prognosis. Van den Broek et al. concluded that current evidence does not support worse breast cancer survival of *BRCA1/2* mutation carriers in the adjuvant setting and that any differences if at all are likely to be small. The largest and most recent meta-analysis that involved 105,220 breast cancer patients, including 3588 (3.4%) carriers of *BRCA* mutations, concluded that *BRCA1* carriers had worse OS compared to sporadic non-carrier breast cancer patients. However, when carrier patients with triple-negative breast cancers were compared to non-carriers with triple-negative cancers only, the difference in OS was no longer apparent. This meta-analysis also found that *BRCA1* carriers with early-stage non-metastatic breast cancer had worse OS and breast cancer-specific survival (BCSS) as compared to non-carrier patients and that *BRCA2* carriers also had worse BCSS than non-carrier breast cancer patients [65].

Given these data we conclude that when adjusted for tumor phenotype and treatment, the current evidence does not support significant differences in the outcome of breast cancers in *BRCA* mutation carriers compared to non-carriers.

6.3 Systemic Therapies and Treatment Response for *BRCA*-Associated Breast Cancer

6.3.1 Chemotherapy

Preclinical models demonstrated that *BRCA* mutant cells were more sensitive to chemotherapeutic agents that cause double-strand breaks in DNA, such as platinum compounds, anthracyclines, and alkylators [66–69]. Numerous retrospective studies suggested differing clinical responses of *BRCA1/2*-mutated breast cancers to different chemotherapy drugs [60, 61, 70], specifically, that *BRCA1*-deficient tumors may be more responsive to platinum compounds [71, 72] and less responsive to taxanes and CMF (cyclophosphamide/methotrexate/fluorouracil) [70, 73–75].

Numerous retrospective studies of neo-adjuvant therapy have demonstrated that *BRCA1/2*-associated breast cancers have higher pathological complete response (pCR) rates to neo-adjuvant therapy compared with non-carriers. Byrski et al. reported pCR rate as high

as 83% (10/12) in *BRCA1* carriers who received neo-adjuvant cis-platinum [71, 74]. In addition, lower response rates to neo-adjuvant CMF or AT (doxorubicin/docetaxel) were noted in *BRCA1* mutation carriers in these studies [71]. Another neo-adjuvant study from MD Anderson reported superiority of anthracycline- and taxane-containing regimens in *BRCA1*-mutated breast cancers. Thus, 26 of 57 *BRCA1* carriers (46%) achieved a pCR, compared to 3 of 23 *BRCA2* carriers (13%) and 53 of 237 *BRCA* non-carriers (22%) ($P = 0.0008$). Interestingly, *BRCA1* status predicted pCR independent of ER negativity, suggesting that it is not simply the association of *BRCA1* mutations with a particular intrinsic subtype that explains the sensitivity of these cancers to chemotherapy [55]. One study reported low pCR rate in only 3 of 29 (10%) *BRCA2*-mutated breast cancer patients compared to 13 of 67 (19%) sporadic ER-positive patients and suggested that these patients are less responsive to neo-adjuvant chemotherapy [76]. Notably these studies included diverse molecular subtypes and treatment regimens, and the number of *BRCA* mutation carriers was limited, $n = 44$ [74], $n = 102$ [71], and $n = 80$ [55]. A study on TNBC in which all patients received dose-dense AC-T demonstrated a significantly higher pCR among *BRCA1* carriers; however, unlike the non-BRCA cases who had an excellent outcome if a pCR was achieved, those with a *BRCA1* mutation and a pCR did not have superior outcome to those with residual disease and a *BRCA1* mutation, suggesting that, despite greater chemo-sensitivity among *BRCA1* carriers, this did not necessarily translate into a survival benefit [77].

In some of the clinical studies, *BRCA1*-mutated cancers were grouped with sporadic TNBC. In addition to the phenotypic similarities between them, it was shown that TNBC have reduced function of *BRCA* proteins (often termed "BRCAness") [22]. Several mechanisms were reported to inhibit *BRCA1* in TNBC, including methylation of the *BRCA1* promoter [78], low *BRCA1* mRNA expression, and high levels of ID4, a negative regulator of *BRCA1* [79]. It was also shown that TNBC were associated with defective DNA repair pathways [80, 81].

Whether sporadic tumors with reduced *BRCA1* expression behave in the same way as *BRCA1*-mutated tumors remains unresolved. Numerous studies have demonstrated that the presence of a germline *BRCA* mutation, somatic *BRCA* deficiency, or tumors with significant homologous recombination deficiency (HRD) or genomic instability have greater sensitivity to platinum agents [82–85].

The favorable response of *BRCA*-mutated and triple-negative breast cancers to platinum was demonstrated in the prospective neo-adjuvant study by Silver et al. [86]. The CALGB 40603 (Alliance) trial was a phase II study that randomized patients with stage II–III TNBC in a 2 × 2 factorial design to test the addition of either carboplatin or bevacizumab or both to standard neo-adjuvant chemotherapy of weekly paclitaxel ×12 followed by four cycles of dose-dense AC. In this study 23% of the patients were<40 years. The addition of carboplatin to weekly paclitaxel increased pCR in the breast and axilla to 54% as compared to 41%, *P* = 0.0029. A further update presented at SABCS in 2015 failed to demonstrate a survival advantage for the addition of carboplatin but the trial was underpowered to do so. However, no data was presented as to the proportion of patients harboring *BRCA1/2* mutations. The GeparSixto was also a phase II study that randomized patients with stage II–III TNBC to receive neo-adjuvant therapy with paclitaxel and non-pegylated liposomal doxorubicin with or without carboplatin or bevacizumab or both. In this study 23% of the patients were<40 years and 17.2% harbored a *BRCA1/2* mutation. The pCR in the non-carboplatin arm for those with a BRCA1/2 mutation was 66.7% compared with 36.4% in the non-*BRCA* patients. The addition of carboplatin increased the pCR in the non-*BRCA* patients to 55% but did not increase the pCR in the *BRCA*-mutated patients. The addition of carboplatin only improved the DFS in the patients that did not have a *BRCA* mutation [87, 88]. It is worth noting that in this study the chemotherapy protocol did not include an alkylating agent.

Notably, definitive evidence for survival advantage from adding platinum to standard treatment is still lacking [60, 89].

In the metastatic setting, the TNT study, presented by Tutt et al., demonstrated superior response rate for women with metastatic TNBC and a *BRCA1/2* mutation compared to those without a mutation and an improved progression-free survival among the *BRCA* carriers that received carboplatin compared to the non-carriers. Of note, in this study the Myriad HRD score did not predict for platinum sensitivity.

A retrospective French study evaluated outcome for women with MBC and a *BRCA* mutation who received high-dose chemotherapy and autologous stem cell transplantation between 2003 and 2012. The study included 235 patients of whom only 15 (6.4%) had a *BRCA* mutation. On multivariate analysis patients without a *BRCA* mutation had a worse prognosis with an HR of 3.08 (96%CI 1.1–8.6) compared to those with a *BRCA* mutation [90].

6.3.2 Hormonal Therapy

One study demonstrated that androgen receptor (AR) expression was present overall in 30% of *BRCA1*-associated tumors and 78% of *BRCA2*-associated tumors (as compared with 76% of non-*BRCA*-associated tumors). Specifically, in the case of triple-negative tumors, 16% of *BRCA1*-associated tumors had AR expression as compared to 50% of *BRCA2*-associated tumors (and as compared to 0% of non-BRCA-associated tumors) [91]. This would suggest that further study of anti-androgen therapies is warranted in this group of patients.

6.3.3 PARP Inhibitors

Poly(ADP-ribose) polymerase-1 (PARP-1) plays a key role in the repair of DNA single-strand breaks through base excision repair. The inhibition of PARP-1 leads to the accumulation of single-strand breaks in DNA and consequently to double-strand breaks at the replication forks. Normally, these double-strand breaks are repaired by homologous recombination (HR). However, when cancer cells deficient of HR due to absent

BRCA are exposed to PARP-1 inhibitors, they accumulate unrepaired double-strand breaks that result in collapse of the replication forks and cell death. Such synergistic cell death resulting from concomitant inhibition of molecular pathways that are each dispensable when inactivated solely is a concept known as "synthetic lethality." Since the normal cells of *BRCA*-mutated carriers contain one functional allele of *BRCA*, they can still use HR and repair DSB, and therefore they are resistant to PARP inhibition. Thus, PARP inhibitors selectively target only the cancer cells and are associated with relatively minor damage to the normal tissues [92]. Long-term effects of PARP inhibitors are not yet known, and concern exists about future risk of second malignancies, such as leukemia, induced by PARP inhibitors.

6.3.3.1 Olaparib

Olaparib is an orally available PARP inhibitor and was the first FDA-approved PARP inhibitor both for germline *BRCA*-mutated advanced ovarian cancer and advanced breast cancer. The pivotal trial assessing PARP inhibitors in a study population enriched for *BRCA* mutation carriers was published by Fong et al. [93]. This phase I trial of 60 patients, 22 of whom harbored known *BRCA* mutations, established the maximum tolerated dose (MTD) of olaparib at 400 mg twice daily. The most common reported side effects were grade 1–2 fatigue and mild gastrointestinal complaints and there was minimal hematological toxicity. Evidence of sustained antitumor activity was limited to patients with *BRCA*-associated cancers, of whom 63% experienced clinical benefit. A proof-of-concept study evaluating olaparib in *BRCA*-associated advanced breast cancer was next published by Tutt et al. [94]. This was a phase II multicenter, multi-national study assessing two dosing schedules of olaparib: 100 mg or 400 mg twice daily. The study included 54 women who had received a median of three previous chemotherapy regimens. The objective response rate (ORR) was 41% (11/27) in the cohort receiving 400 mg twice daily and 22% (6/27) in the cohort on the lower dosing schedule. Stable disease was achieved in 44% of both cohorts. Most toxicities were low grade, the most common being fatigue, nausea, vomiting, and anemia. Further phase

II studies supported activity of olaparib among women with advanced breast cancer and a germline *BRCA* mutation [95, 96]. The first phase III study of olaparib for advanced breast cancer was published in 2017. In the study by Robson et al., women were randomized 2:1 to receive either olaparib 300 mg twice daily or treatment of physician's choice (eribulin, capecitabine, or vinorelbine); in this study patients had received prior anthracycline and taxane, those that were HR+ had progressed on at least one line of endocrine therapy, and patients had not relapsed within 12 months of neo-adjuvant platinum therapy or progressed during platinum therapy in the advanced setting. Two hundred and five women received olaparib and 97 received standard therapy. Median age was 44 years (range 22–76). The olaparib arm had superior response rate, progression-free survival, and toxicity profile to the standard therapy arm, with a response rate of 59.9% compared with 28.8% and a median PFS of 7 months compared to 4.2 months (HR 0.58, 96%CI 0.43–0.8). Subgroup analyses suggested benefit was most significant among those with triple-negative disease and those with no previous platinum exposure.

Phase I studies combining olaparib with other chemotherapeutic agents (paclitaxel, cisplatin, and carboplatin) [97–99] have been published with promising results and are being further explored in a phase II setting. Results have also been published for a phase I study of olaparib with the PI3K inhibitor, BKM120 [100]. There are ongoing phase II studies evaluating these combinations and ongoing studies evaluating the combination with the anti-programmed death ligand-1 antibody durvalumab, pembrolizumab, the oral PI3kinase inhibitor BYL719, the oral mTORC1/2 inhibitor AZD2014 or the oral AKT inhibitor AZD5363, and the VEGF inhibitor, cediranib.

Olaparib is being evaluated in the neo-adjuvant setting in combination with chemotherapy. OLYMPIA is an international phase III randomized, placebo blinded study evaluating adjuvant olaparib in *BRCA1/2* mutation carriers with triple-negative breast cancer or high-risk endocrine-responsive breast cancer after completion of standard adjuvant chemotherapy and radiotherapy, aiming to recruit 1320 patients.

6.3.3.2 Veliparib

Veliparib (ABT-888) is a potent orally available inhibitor of PARP-1 and PARP-2. The common side effects include nausea, fatigue, and pancytopenia.

In a phase I study combining veliparib with doxorubicin and cyclophosphamide, partial responses were seen exclusively in the 3/5 included *BRCA1/2* carriers, with no partial responses in the non-carriers [101]. In a trial combining veliparib with carboplatin in 22 patients with *BRCA*-associated metastatic breast cancer, overall response rate was demonstrated in 67% of patients [102]. In a phase II trial assessing veliparib and temozolomide in 41 patients with metastatic breast cancer by Isakoff et al. [103], clinical activity was seen exclusively among the eight *BRCA1/2* mutation carriers.

Phase I/II studies have been published or are ongoing evaluating combinations of veliparib with different chemotherapeutic agents including irinotecan, mitomycin, vinorelbine, metronomic cyclophosphamide, cisplatin, gemcitabine, eribulin, liposomal doxorubicin, carboplatin, and paclitaxel. Specifically, the results of the phase II BROCADE study were presented at the San Antonio Breast Cancer Symposium (2016)—the study randomized patients to taxol and carboplatin with or without veliparib. The study initially had a study arm combining temozolomide and veliparib but this arm was ceased following a futility evaluation. The overall response rate was 77.8% compared to 61.3% ($p = 0.027$) favoring the veliparib-containing arm. There was a trend to improved PFS and OS that did not reach statistical significance favoring the veliparib-containing arm. The addition of veliparib did not increase the toxicity of the chemotherapy. The combination is being further evaluated in the phase III BROCADE 3 study.

Veliparib is being evaluated in combination with carboplatin in the I-SPY 2 neo-adjuvant trial, an adaptive phase II study. In this study *BRCA1/2* mutation carriers with TN subtype were significantly more likely to achieve a pCR than non-*BRCA* TN, with a predicted pCR of 75% compared with 29% [104], and gene expression-like signature profiling that distinguished between *BRCA1*ness and non-*BRCA1*-like signatures indicated greater response to the combination for the *BRCA1*ness [105].

Veliparib is also being evaluated in combination with the anti-programmed death ligand-1 antibody atezolizumab.

6.3.3.3 Rucaparib

Rucaparib is a potent PARP inhibitor available in both intravenous (IV) and oral formulation. Most common side effects include hematogical toxicity, nausea, vomiting, fatigue, and diarrhea. A phase II study evaluating rucaparib in *BRCA* mutation carriers with advanced ovarian and breast cancer included two cohorts—one with intermittent IV dosing and one with continuous oral dosing. The study included 23 women with advanced breast cancer; the best response was stable disease at 44% ($n = 8$) on the IV dosing, and there were no responses in the five patients on the oral dosing [106]. Rucaparib has been evaluated in the phase I setting in combination with various chemotherapy regimens [107].

There are currently no trials evaluating rucaparib in a phase III setting in breast cancer.

6.3.3.4 Niraparib

Niraparib (MK-4827) is an orally available PARP inhibitor. A phase I study evaluating niraparib in solid organ tumors included 12 patients with advanced breast cancer. Common side effects included hematological toxicity, fatigue, headache, abdominal pain, nausea and vomiting, and anorexia. Two of the four patients with a *BRCA* mutation who had breast cancer had a partial response to treatment [108]. Phase III study results of the BRAVO trial comparing niraparib to physician's choice of chemotherapy in *BRCA*-positive advanced breast cancer are awaited.

6.3.3.5 Talazoparib

Talazoparib is considered one of the most potent PARP inhibitors. A phase I study demonstrated a 50% response rate among *BRCA* mutation carriers with advanced breast cancer [109]. Common side effects included hematological toxicity, nausea, fatigue, and diarrhea. Results from the phase II ABRAZO study presented by Turner et al. were presented at the 2017 annual meeting of the American Society of Clinical Oncology.

The trial evaluated two cohorts—platinum naive and platinum exposed. Talazoparib demonstrated impressive response rates in both cohorts, among both *BRCA1* and *BRCA2* carriers and among both triple-negative and endocrine-responsive subtypes. There are ongoing studies evaluating talazoparib in the neo-adjuvant setting, in combination with chemotherapy in metastatic TN breast cancer and in combination with avelumab in solid organ tumors. Results from the phase III EMBRACA study comparing talazoparib and chemotherapy are awaited.

6.3.4 Future Directions

Resistance to PARP inhibitors is an area of ongoing research and is already being addressed in combination therapy clinical trial design. Some of the described resistance mechanisms include up-regulation of multi-drug resistance efflux pumps and somatic mutations of *TP53BP1* which can result in partial restoration of HR and reversion of *BRCA* mutation and restoration of BRCA function [110–112]. The specific mechanisms characteristic in *BRCA*-associated breast cancer are yet to be elucidated and characterized.

6.3.4.1 Immunotherapy

As the presence of a *BRCA* mutation leads to genetic instability leading to increased number of mutations, it has been hypothesized that this would translate into translating into more neo-antigens and that this could translate into greater susceptibility to immunotherapy regimens. Additionally, *BRCA1/2*-associated tumors are often characterized by lymphocytic infiltration, and there is emerging data correlating response rate to immunotherapy with level of tumor-infiltrating lymphocytes. There are several ongoing studies evaluating the combination of PARP inhibitors with immunotherapeutic agents.

6.3.4.2 Novel Agents

Trabectedin is a novel marine-derived agent thought to have anti-neoplastic activity in cells with deficient DNA damage repair pathways and has been shown to have promising activity

in phase II studies in *BRCA*-deficient metastatic breast cancer [113, 114] with an overall response rate of 17% in heavily pre-treated patients and 33% among the *BRCA2* carriers.

Lurbinectedin is a novel agent that, among other anti-neoplastic activities, induces double-strand DNA breaks and had been observed to have activity against homologous recombination-deficient cell lines. Encouraging phase II results were presented at the ESMO annual meeting in 2016 in *BRCA1/2*-deficient advanced breast cancer with an overall response rate of 44% in heavily pre-treated patients [115].

Sacituzumab govitecan (IMMU-132) is an anti-Trop-2-SN-38 antibody-drug conjugate that has topoisomerase I (Topo I) inhibitory activity. Pre-clinical activity in combination with PARP inhibitors in TNBC (including both *BRCA*-associated and non-*BRCA* breast cancers) suggests the combination successfully exploits synthetic lethality [116].

AZD6738 is an ATR inhibitor being evaluated in combination with a PARP inhibitor that is thought to help overcome PARP inhibitor resistance mechanisms.

There is data to suggest that c-met inhibitors in combination with PARP inhibitors may help overcome PARP inhibitor resistance [117].

In pre-clinical models G-quadruplex-interacting compounds have been found to be toxic to *BRCA1*- and *BRCA2*-deficient cells, and olaparib-resistant *BRCA*-deficient cells were found to be sensitive to these compounds and as such they are of interest for clinical studies [118].

6.4 Systemic Considerations for Other Hereditary Syndrome-Associated Breast Cancers

6.4.1 Introduction

The prevalence of a germline mutation (other than BRCA1/2) associated with increased risk of breast cancer was found to be 4.4% in women ≤45 in one study on a sequential group of patients referred for genetic testing [119] and similar prevalence seen in another series[120]. The other moderate- to high-risk penetrance genes with an established associated risk for breast cancer are *p53, PTEN, CDH1, STK11, PALB2, CHEK2, ATM, NBN*, and *NF-1* [8]. As next-generation multi-gene panels become more available and affordable, more patients are likely to undergo testing for genes other than BRCA1/2; however, the clinical implications for screening, prevention, and treatment for breast cancer resulting from these other moderate- to high-risk penetrance mutations are not well established, are still evolving, and are the subject of ongoing research.

6.4.2 Systemic Therapy Considerations

6.4.2.1 *p53* Mutation (Li-Fraumeni Syndrome)

p53 is a critical tumor suppressor gene and a germline mutation in p53 is associated with a high risk of malignancy. One study estimated that the prevalence of a germline p53 mutation among women with early-onset breast cancer and no family history was 5–8% [121]. Studies have suggested that patients with germline mutations in p53 are less susceptible to DNA-damaging cytotoxic agents [122, 123].

Novel therapeutic approaches may include MK-8776, a novel chk-1 kinase inhibitor found to radio-sensitize *p53*-deficient cancer cells [124], and MK-1775, a Wee1-kinase inhibitor found to sensitize *p53*-deficient cells to DNA-damaging agents [125].

6.4.2.2 *PTEN* Mutation (Cowden Syndrome)

PTEN is a tumor suppressor gene involved in the PI3K/AKT/mTOR pathway—targeting upstream components of the pathway including PI3K/AKT/mTOR may provide a therapeutic opportunity in these patients. A phase I/II study evaluating a PI3K inhibitor, BGT226, in patients with advanced malignancy including advanced breast cancer aimed to enrich the population for patients with Cowden syndrome; however, no reference

was made to patients with Cowden syndrome in the subsequent publication [126].

6.4.2.3 *PALB2* Mutation

PALB2 encodes a protein that is an important partner and localizer for *BRCA2* [127]. The presence of a germline *PALB2* mutation may be a consideration for trying therapies targeting synthetic lethality, and in fact it is thought the cells with LOH for *PALB2* may also have increased sensitivity to PARP inhibition. There are several trials currently recruiting evaluating PARP inhibitors in patients with solid organ tumors and a *PALB2* mutation.

6.4.2.4 *CHEK2, ATM,* and *NBN* Mutations

The cumulative lifetime risk of breast cancer before age 40 in the presence of a *CHEK2* mutation is less than 2% [128] and less than 1% in the presence of a germline mutation in *ATM/NBN. CHEK2, ATM,* and *NBN* are all involved in DNA repair pathways. Subsequently, treatment of advanced solid organ tumors in the presence of these mutations with PARP inhibitors is currently underway.

6.4.2.5 *CDH1* Mutation

In cell lines with a *CDH1* germline mutation or E-cadherin impairment, there is preclinical data suggesting resistance to taxanes, aberrant Notch-1 activation, Bcl-2 over-expression, and abnormal activation of the EFGR-signaling pathway [129–131]. Each of these could potentially have therapeutic impact; however, at present there is no robust clinical data to indicate how these biological characteristics may impact clinical management.

6.4.2.6 STK11 Mutation (Peutz-Jeghers Syndrome)

Peutz-Jeghers syndrome (PJS) is an autosomal dominant syndrome in which patients have a germline mutation in *STK11*. These patients have a high risk for developing a malignancy, particularly gastric cancer and breast cancer, with an 8% risk of developing breast cancer by age 40[132]. The mutation in *STK11* (or *LKB1*) results in aberrant mTOR pathway signaling. Studies aiming to target the mTOR pathway and evaluating everolimus in patients with PJS with advanced malignancies or polyposis were withdrawn and closed due to low enrollment.

6.5   Conclusions

Germline mutations in cancer predisposition genes are more common among young women with breast cancer; specifically, the presence of a germline *BRCA1/2* mutation is the most common germline mutation in women under the age of 40 and has therapeutic implications on the choice of systemic therapies, particularly in advanced breast cancer. Consequently, genetic testing should be encouraged soon after diagnosis in young women with breast cancer. Moderate-penetrance cancer susceptibility genes contribute to a very small percentage of early-onset breast cancers, while higher-penetrance cancer susceptibility genes are exceedingly rare. The therapeutic impact of a germline mutation in other cancer predisposition genes is still being researched.

References

1. Ford D, Easton DF, Stratton M, et al. Genetic heterogeneity and penetrance analysis of the BRCA1 and BRCA2 genes in breast cancer families. The Breast Cancer Linkage Consortium. Am J Hum Genet. 1998;62:676–89.
2. Roa BB, Boyd AA, Volcik K, Richards CS. Ashkenazi Jewish population frequencies for common mutations in BRCA1 and BRCA2. Nat Genet. 1996;14:185–7.
3. Paul A, Paul S. The breast cancer susceptibility genes (BRCA) in breast and ovarian cancers. Front Biosci (Landmark Ed). 2014;19:605–18.
4. King MC, Marks JH, Mandell JB, New York Breast Cancer Study Group. Breast and ovarian cancer risks due to inherited mutations in BRCA1 and BRCA2. Science. 2003;302:643–6.
5. Walsh T, Casadei S, Lee MK, et al. Mutations in 12 genes for inherited ovarian, fallopian tube, and peritoneal carcinoma identified by massively parallel sequencing. Proc Natl Acad Sci U S A. 2011;108:18032–7.
6. Kuchenbaecker KB, Hopper JL, Barnes DR, et al. Risks of breast, ovarian, and contralateral breast cancer for BRCA1 and BRCA2 mutation carriers. JAMA. 2017;317:2402–16.
7. Mersch J, Jackson MA, Park M, et al. Cancers associated with BRCA1 and BRCA2 mutations other than breast and ovarian. Cancer. 2015;121:269–75.
8. Easton DF, Pharoah PD, Antoniou AC, et al. Gene-panel sequencing and the prediction of breast-cancer risk. N Engl J Med. 2015;372:2243–57.
9. Rosenberg SM, Ruddy KJ, Tamimi RM, et al. BRCA1 and BRCA2 mutation testing in young women with breast cancer. JAMA Oncol. 2016;2:730–6.
10. Xu X, Weaver Z, Linke SP, et al. Centrosome amplification and a defective G2-M cell cycle checkpoint induce genetic instability in BRCA1 exon 11 isoform-deficient cells. Mol Cell. 1999;3:389–95.
11. Yu VP, Koehler M, Steinlein C, et al. Gross chromosomal rearrangements and genetic exchange between nonhomologous chromosomes following BRCA2 inactivation. Genes Dev. 2000;14:1400–6.
12. Foulkes WD, Shuen AY. In brief: BRCA1 and BRCA2. J Pathol. 2013;230:347–9.
13. Pardo B, Gomez-Gonzalez B, Aguilera A. DNA repair in mammalian cells: DNA double-strand break repair: how to fix a broken relationship. Cell Mol Life Sci. 2009;66:1039–56.
14. Venkitaraman AR. Linking the cellular functions of BRCA genes to cancer pathogenesis and treatment. Annu Rev Pathol. 2009;4:461–87.
15. Roy R, Chun J, Powell SN. BRCA1 and BRCA2: different roles in a common pathway of genome protection. Nat Rev Cancer. 2012;12:68–78.
16. Yang H, Jeffrey PD, Miller J, et al. BRCA2 function in DNA binding and recombination from a BRCA2-DSS1-ssDNA structure. Science. 2002;297:1837–48.
17. Jensen RB, Carreira A, Kowalczykowski SC. Purified human BRCA2 stimulates RAD51-mediated recombination. Nature. 2010;467:678–83.
18. Wang B, Matsuoka S, Ballif BA, et al. Abraxas and RAP80 form a BRCA1 protein complex required for the DNA damage response. Science. 2007;316:1194–8.
19. Chen L, Nievera CJ, Lee AY, Wu X. Cell cycle-dependent complex formation of BRCA1.CtIP. MRN is important for DNA double-strand break repair. J Biol Chem. 2008;283:7713–20. https://doi.org/10.1074/jbc.M710245200. Epub 2008 Jan 2
20. Zhang F, Ma J, Wu J, et al. PALB2 links BRCA1 and BRCA2 in the DNA-damage response. Curr Biol. 2009;19:524–9.
21. Tutt A, Bertwistle D, Valentine J, et al. Mutation in Brca2 stimulates error-prone homology-directed repair of DNA double-strand breaks occurring between repeated sequences. EMBO J. 2001;20:4704–16.
22. Turner N, Tutt A, Ashworth A. Hallmarks of 'BRCAness' in sporadic cancers. Nat Rev Cancer. 2004;4:814–9.

23. Caestecker KW, Van de Walle GR. The role of BRCA1 in DNA double-strand repair: past and present. Exp Cell Res. 2013;319:575–87.

24. Osorio A, de la Hoya M, Rodriguez-Lopez R, et al. Loss of heterozygosity analysis at the BRCA loci in tumor samples from patients with familial breast cancer. Int J Cancer. 2002;99:305–9.

25. Cavalli LR, Singh B, Isaacs C, et al. Loss of heterozygosity in normal breast epithelial tissue and benign breast lesions in BRCA1/2 carriers with breast cancer. Cancer Genet Cytogenet. 2004;149:38–43.

26. Konishi H, Mohseni M, Tamaki A, et al. Mutation of a single allele of the cancer susceptibility gene BRCA1 leads to genomic instability in human breast epithelial cells. Proc Natl Acad Sci U S A. 2011;108:17773–8.

27. Ludwig T, Chapman DL, Papaioannou VE, Efstratiadis A. Targeted mutations of breast cancer susceptibility gene homologs in mice: lethal phenotypes of Brca1, Brca2, Brca1/Brca2, Brca1/p53, and Brca2/p53 nullizygous embryos. Genes Dev. 1997;11:1226–41.

28. Evers B, Jonkers J. Mouse models of BRCA1 and BRCA2 deficiency: past lessons, current understanding and future prospects. Oncogene. 2006;25:5885–97.

29. Leegte B, van der Hout AH, Deffenbaugh AM, et al. Phenotypic expression of double heterozygosity for BRCA1 and BRCA2 germline mutations. J Med Genet. 2005;42:e20.

30. Spannuth WA, Thaker PH, Sood AK. Concomitant BRCA1 and BRCA2 gene mutations in an Ashkenazi Jewish woman with primary breast and ovarian cancer. Am J Obstet Gynecol. 2007;196:e6–9.

31. Greenblatt MS, Chappuis PO, Bond JP, et al. TP53 mutations in breast cancer associated with BRCA1 or BRCA2 germ-line mutations: distinctive spectrum and structural distribution. Cancer Res. 2001;61:4092–7.

32. Holstege H, Joosse SA, van Oostrom CT, et al. High incidence of protein-truncating TP53 mutations in BRCA1-related breast cancer. Cancer Res. 2009;69:3625–33.

33. Sedic M, Kuperwasser C. BRCA1-hapoinsufficiency: unraveling the molecular and cellular basis for tissue-specific cancer. Cell Cycle. 2017;15:621–7.

34. Monteiro AN. BRCA1: the enigma of tissue-specific tumor development. Trends Genet. 2003;19:312–5.

35. Elledge SJ, Amon A. The BRCA1 suppressor hypothesis: an explanation for the tissue-specific tumor development in BRCA1 patients. Cancer Cell. 2002;1:129–32.

36. Sedic M, Skibinski A, Brown N, et al. Haploinsufficiency for BRCA1 leads to cell-type-specific genomic instability and premature senescence. Nat Commun. 2015;6:7505.

37. Palacios J, Robles-Frias MJ, Castilla MA, et al. The molecular pathology of hereditary breast cancer. Pathobiology. 2008;75:85–94.

38. Mavaddat N, Barrowdale D, Andrulis IL, et al. Pathology of breast and ovarian cancers among BRCA1 and BRCA2 mutation carriers: results from the Consortium of Investigators of Modifiers of BRCA1/2 (CIMBA). Cancer Epidemiol Biomark Prev. 2012;21:134–47.

39. Lakhani SR, Van De Vijver MJ, Jacquemier J, et al. The pathology of familial breast cancer: predictive value of immunohistochemical markers estrogen receptor, progesterone receptor, HER-2, and p53 in patients with mutations in BRCA1 and BRCA2. J Clin Oncol. 2002;20:2310–8.

40. Honrado E, Benitez J, Palacios J. Histopathology of BRCA1- and BRCA2-associated breast cancer. Crit Rev Oncol Hematol. 2006;59:27–39.

41. Atchley DP, Albarracin CT, Lopez A, et al. Clinical and pathologic characteristics of patients with BRCA-positive and BRCA-negative breast cancer. J Clin Oncol. 2008;26:4282–8.

42. Molyneux G, Smalley MJ. The cell of origin of BRCA1 mutation-associated breast cancer: a cautionary tale of gene expression profiling. J Mammary Gland Biol Neoplasia. 2011;16:51–5.

43. Molyneux G, Geyer FC, Magnay FA, et al. BRCA1 basal-like breast cancers originate from luminal epithelial progenitors and not from basal stem cells. Cell Stem Cell. 2010;7:403–17.

44. Lim E, Vaillant F, Wu D, et al. Aberrant luminal progenitors as the candidate target population for basal tumor development in BRCA1 mutation carriers. Nat Med. 2009;15:907–13.

45. Saal LH, Gruvberger-Saal SK, Persson C, et al. Recurrent gross mutations of the PTEN tumor suppressor gene in breast cancers with deficient DSB repair. Nat Genet. 2008;40:102–7.

46. Eerola H, Heikkila P, Tamminen A, et al. Histopathological features of breast tumours in BRCA1, BRCA2 and mutation-negative breast cancer families. Breast Cancer Res. 2005;7:R93–100.

47. Lewin R, Sulkes A, Shochat T, et al. Oncotype-DX recurrence score distribution in breast cancer patients with BRCA1/2 mutations. Breast Cancer Res Treat. 2016;157:511–6.

48. Halpern N, Sonnenblick A, Uziely B, et al. Oncotype Dx recurrence score among BRCA1/2 germline mutation carriers with hormone receptors positive breast cancer. Int J Cancer. 2017;140:2145–9.

49. Goodwin PJ, Phillips KA, West DW, et al. Breast cancer prognosis in BRCA1 and BRCA2 mutation carriers: an International Prospective Breast Cancer Family Registry population-based cohort study. J Clin Oncol. 2012;30:19–26.

50. Rennert G, Bisland-Naggan S, Barnett-Griness O, et al. Clinical outcomes of breast cancer in carriers of BRCA1 and BRCA2 mutations. N Engl J Med. 2007;357:115–23.

51. Huzarski T, Byrski T, Gronwald J, et al. Ten-year survival in patients with BRCA1-negative and BRCA1-positive breast cancer. J Clin Oncol. 2013;31:3191–6.

52. El-Tamer M, Russo D, Troxel A, et al. Survival and recurrence after breast cancer in BRCA1/2 mutation carriers. Ann Surg Oncol. 2004;11:157–64.

53. Veronesi A, de Giacomi C, Magri MD, et al. Familial breast cancer: characteristics and outcome of BRCA 1-2 positive and negative cases. BMC Cancer. 2005;5:70.

54. Brekelmans CT, Seynaeve C, Menke-Pluymers M, et al. Survival and prognostic factors in BRCA1-associated breast cancer. Ann Oncol. 2006;17:391–400.

55. Arun B, Bayraktar S, Liu DD, et al. Response to neo-adjuvant systemic therapy for breast cancer in BRCA mutation carriers and noncarriers: a single-institution experience. J Clin Oncol. 2011;29:3739–46.

56. Bonadona V, Dussart-Moser S, Voirin N, et al. Prognosis of early-onset breast cancer based on BRCA1/2 mutation status in a French population-based cohort and review. Breast Cancer Res Treat. 2007;101:233–45.

57. Foulkes WD, Chappuis PO, Wong N, et al. Primary node negative breast cancer in BRCA1 mutation carriers has a poor outcome. Ann Oncol. 2000;11:307–13.

58. Moller P, Borg A, Evans DG, et al. Survival in prospectively ascertained familial breast cancer: analysis of a series stratified by tumour characteristics, BRCA mutations and oophorectomy. Int J Cancer. 2002;101:555–9.

59. Robson ME, Chappuis PO, Satagopan J, et al. A combined analysis of outcome following breast cancer: differences in survival based on BRCA1/BRCA2 mutation status and administration of adjuvant treatment. Breast Cancer Res. 2004;6:R8–R17.

60. Chalasani P, Livingston R. Differential chemotherapeutic sensitivity for breast tumors with "BRCAness": a review. Oncologist. 2013;18:909–16.

61. Bayraktar S, Gluck S. Systemic therapy options in BRCA mutation-associated breast cancer. Breast Cancer Res Treat. 2013;135:355–66.

62. Zhong Q, Peng HL, Zhao X, et al. Effects of BRCA1- and BRCA2-related mutations on ovarian and breast cancer survival: a meta-analysis. Clin Cancer Res. 2015;21:211–20.

63. van den Broek AJ, Schmidt MK, van't Veer LJ, et al. Worse breast cancer prognosis of BRCA1/BRCA2 mutation carriers: what's the evidence? A systematic review with meta-analysis. PLoS One. 2015;10:2015.

64. Lee EH, Park SK, Park B, et al. Effect of BRCA1/2 mutation on short-term and long-term breast cancer survival: a systematic review and meta-analysis. Breast Cancer Res Treat. 2010;122:11–25.

65. Baretta Z, Mocellin S, Goldin E, et al. Effect of BRCA germline mutations on breast cancer prognosis: a systematic review and meta-analysis. Medicine. 2016;95:e4975.

66. Tassone P, Tagliaferri P, Perricelli A, et al. BRCA1 expression modulates chemosensitivity of BRCA1-defective HCC1937 human breast cancer cells. Br J Cancer. 2003;88:1285–91.

67. Quinn JE, Kennedy RD, Mullan PB, et al. BRCA1 functions as a differential modulator of chemotherapy-induced apoptosis. Cancer Res. 2003;63:6221–8.

68. Kennedy RD, Quinn JE, Mullan PB, et al. The role of BRCA1 in the cellular response to chemotherapy. J Natl Cancer Inst. 2004;96:1659–68.

69. Foulkes WD. BRCA1 and BRCA2: chemosensitivity, treatment outcomes and prognosis. Familial Cancer. 2006;5:135–42.

70. Kriege M, Seynaeve C, Meijers-Heijboer H, et al. Sensitivity to first-line chemotherapy for metastatic breast cancer in BRCA1 and BRCA2 mutation carriers. J Clin Oncol. 2009;27:3764–71.

71. Byrski T, Gronwald J, Huzarski T, et al. Pathologic complete response rates in young women with BRCA1-positive breast cancers after neoadjuvant chemotherapy. J Clin Oncol. 2010;28:375–9.

72. Byrski T, Dent R, Blecharz P, et al. Results of a phase II open-label, non-randomized trial of cis-platin chemotherapy in patients with BRCA1-positive metastatic breast cancer. Breast Cancer Res. 2014;14:R110.

73. Wysocki PJ, Korski K, Lamperska K, et al. Primary resistance to docetaxel-based chemotherapy in meta-static breast cancer patients correlates with a high frequency of BRCA1 mutations. Med Sci Monit. 2008;14:SC7–10.

74. Byrski T, Gronwald J, Huzarski T, et al. Response to neo-adjuvant chemotherapy in women with BRCA1-positive breast cancers. Breast Cancer Res Treat. 2008;108:289–96.

75. Kriege M, Jager A, Hooning MJ, et al. The efficacy of taxane chemotherapy for metastatic breast cancer in BRCA1 and BRCA2 mutation carriers. Cancer. 2012;118:899–907.

76. Raphael J, Mazouni C, Caron O, et al. Should BRCA2 mutation carriers avoid neoadjuvant chemotherapy? Med Oncol. 2014;31:850.

77. Paluch-Shimon S, Friedman E, Berger R, et al. Neoadjuvant doxorubicin and cyclophosphamide followed by paclitaxel in triple-negative breast cancer among BRCA1 mutation carriers and non-carriers. Breast Cancer Res Treat. 2016;157:157–65.

78. Esteller M, Silva JM, Dominguez G, et al. Promoter hypermethylation and BRCA1 inactivation in sporadic breast and ovarian tumors. J Natl Cancer Inst. 2000;92:564–9.

79. Turner NC, Reis-Filho JS, Russell AM, et al. BRCA1 dysfunction in sporadic basal-like breast cancer. Oncogene. 2007;26:2126–32.

80. Carey L, Winer E, Viale G, et al. Triple-negative breast cancer: disease entity or title of convenience? Nat Rev Clin Oncol. 2010;7:683–92.

81. Curigliano G, Goldhirsch A. The triple-negative sub-type: new ideas for the poorest prognosis breast cancer. J Natl Cancer Inst Monogr. 2011;2011:108–10.

82. Telli ML, Jensen KC, Vinayak S, et al. Phase II study of gemcitabine, carboplatin, and iniparib as neoadjuvant therapy for triple-negative and BRCA1/2 mutation-associated breast cancer with assessment of a tumor-based measure of genomic instability: PrECOG 0105. J Clin Oncol. 2015;33:1895–901.

83. Telli ML, Timms KM, Reid J, et al. Homologous recombination deficiency (HRD) score predicts response to platinum-containing neoadjuvant chemotherapy in patients with triple-negative breast cancer. Clin Cancer Res. 2016;22:3764–73.

84. Telli M, McMillan A, Ford JM, et al. Homologous recombination deficiency (HRD) as a predictive biomarker of response to neoadjuvant platinum-based therapy in patients with triple negative breast cancer (TNBC): a pooled analysis. Cancer Res. 2016;76(4 Suppl):Abstract nr P3-07-12.

85. Isakoff SJ, Mayer EL, He L, et al. TBCRC009: a multicenter phase II clinical trial of platinum monotherapy with biomarker assessment in metastatic triple-negative breast cancer. J Clin Oncol. 2015;33:1902–9.

86. Silver DP, Richardson AL, Eklund AC, et al. Efficacy of neoadjuvant Cisplatin in triple-negative breast cancer. J Clin Oncol. 2010;28:1145–53.

87. von Minckwitz G, Schneeweiss A, Loibl S, et al. Neoadjuvant carboplatin in patients with triple-negative and HER2-positive early breast cancer (GeparSixto; GBG 66): a randomised phase 2 trial. Lancet Oncol. 2014;15:747–56.

88. Hahnen E, Lederer B, Hauke J, et al. Germline mutation status, pathological complete response, and disease-free survival in triple-negative breast cancer: secondary analysis of the GeparSixto Randomized Clinical Trial. JAMA Oncol. 2017;3:1378–85.

89. Carey LA. Targeted chemotherapy? Platinum in BRCA1-dysfunctional breast cancer. J Clin Oncol. 2010;28:361–3.

90. Boudin L, Goncalves A, Sabatier R, et al. Highly favorable outcome in BRCA-mutated metastatic breast cancer patients receiving high-dose chemotherapy and autologous hematopoietic stem cell transplantation. Bone Marrow Transplant. 2016;51:1082–6.

91. Pristauz G, Petru E, Stacher E, et al. Androgen receptor expression in breast cancer patients tested for BRCA1 and BRCA2 mutations. Histopathology. 2010;57:877–84.

92. Farmer H, McCabe N, Lord CJ, et al. Targeting the DNA repair defect in BRCA mutant cells as a therapeutic strategy. Nature. 2005;434:917–21.

93. Fong PC, Boss DS, Yap TA, et al. Inhibition of poly(ADP-ribose) polymerase in tumors from BRCA mutation carriers. N Engl J Med. 2009;361:123–34.

94. Tutt A, Robson M, Garber JE, et al. Oral poly(ADP-ribose) polymerase inhibitor olaparib in patients with BRCA1 or BRCA2 mutations and advanced breast cancer: a proof-of-concept trial. Lancet. 2010;376:235–44.

95. Gelmon KA, Tischkowitz M, Mackay H, et al. Olaparib in patients with recurrent high-grade serous or poorly differentiated ovarian carcinoma or triple-negative breast cancer: a phase 2, multicentre, open-label, non-randomised study. Lancet Oncol. 2011;12:852–61.

96. Kaufman B, Shapira-Frommer R, Schmutzler RK, et al. Olaparib monotherapy in patients with advanced cancer and a germline BRCA1/2 mutation. J Clin Oncol. 2015;33:244–50.

97. Dent RA, Lindeman GJ, Clemons M, et al. Phase I trial of the oral PARP inhibitor olaparib in combination with paclitaxel for first- or second-line treatment of patients with metastatic triple-negative breast cancer. Breast Cancer Res. 2013;15:R88.

98. Balmana J, Tung NM, Isakoff SJ, et al. Phase I trial of olaparib in combination with cisplatin for the treatment of patients with advanced breast, ovarian and other solid tumors. Ann Oncol. 2014;25:1656–63.

99. Lee JM, Hays JL, Annunziata CM, et al. Phase I/Ib study of olaparib and carboplatin in BRCA1 or BRCA2 mutation-associated breast or ovarian cancer with biomarker analyses. J Natl Cancer Inst. 2014;106:dju089.

100. Matulonis UA, Wulf GM, Barry WT, et al. Phase I dose escalation study of the PI3kinase pathway inhibitor BKM120 and the oral poly (ADP ribose) polymerase (PARP) inhibitor olaparib for the treatment of high-grade serous ovarian and breast cancer. Ann Oncol. 2017;28:512–8.

101. Tan AR, Toppmeyer D, Stein MN, et al. Phase I trial of veliparib, (ABT-888), a poly(ADP-ribose) polymerase (PARP) inhibitor, in combination with doxorubicin and cyclophosphamide in breast cancer and other solid tumors. J Clin Oncol. 2011;29:3041. ASCO Meeting Abstracts

102. Somlo G, Sparano JA, Cigler T, et al. ABT-888 (veliparib) in combination with carboplatin in patients with stage IV BRCA-associated breast cancer. A California Cancer Consortium Trial. J Clin Oncol. 2012;30:1010. ASCO Meeting Abstracts

103. Isakoff SJ, Overmoyer B, Tung NM, et al. A phase II trial of the PARP inhibitor veliparib (ABT888) and temozolomide for metastatic breast cancer. J Clin Oncol. 2010;28:1019. ASCO Meeting Abstracts

104. Wolf DM, Yau C, Sanil A, et al. DNA repair deficiency biomarkers and the 70-gene ultra-high risk signature as predictors of veliparib/carboplatin response in the I-SPY 2 breast cancer trial. NPJ Breast Cancer. 2017;3:31.

105. Severson TM, Wolf DM, Yau C, et al. The BRCA1ness signature is associated significantly with response to PARP inhibitor treatment versus control in the I-SPY 2 randomized neoadjuvant setting. Breast Cancer Res. 2017;19:99.

106. Drew Y, Ledermann J, Hall G, et al. Phase 2 multicentre trial investigating intermittent and continuous dosing schedules of the poly(ADP-ribose) polymerase inhibitor rucaparib in germline BRCA

mutation carriers with advanced ovarian and breast cancer. Br J Cancer. 2016;114:e21.

107. Wilson RH, Evans TJ, Middleton MR, et al. A phase I study of intravenous and oral rucaparib in combination with chemotherapy in patients with advanced solid tumours. Br J Cancer. 2017;116:884–92.

108. Sandhu SK, Schelman WR, Wilding G, et al. The poly(ADP-ribose) polymerase inhibitor niraparib (MK4827) in BRCA mutation carriers and patients with sporadic cancer: a phase 1 dose-escalation trial. Lancet Oncol. 2013;14:882–92.

109. de Bono J, Ramanathan RK, Mina L, et al. Phase I, dose-escalation, two-part trial of the PARP inhibitor talazoparib in patients with advanced germline BRCA1/2 mutations and selected sporadic cancers. Cancer Discov. 2017;7:620–9.

110. Edwards SL, Brough R, Lord CJ, et al. Resistance to therapy caused by intragenic deletion in BRCA2. Nature. 2008;451:1111–5.

111. Swisher EM, Sakai W, Karlan BY, et al. Secondary BRCA1 mutations in BRCA1-mutated ovarian carcinomas with platinum resistance. Cancer Res. 2008;68:2581–6.

112. Bouwman P, Jonkers J. Molecular pathways: how can BRCA-mutated tumors become resistant to PARP inhibitors? Clin Cancer Res. 2014;20:540–7.

113. Delaloge S, Wolp-Diniz R, Byrski T, et al. Activity of trabectedin in germline BRCA1/2-mutated metastatic breast cancer: results of an international first-in-class phase II study. Ann Oncol. 2014;25:1152–8.

114. Ghouadni A, Delaloge S, Lardelli P, et al. Higher antitumor activity of trabectedin in germline BRCA2 carriers with advanced breast cancer as compared to BRCA1 carriers: a subset analysis of a dedicated phase II trial. Breast. 2017;34:18–23.

115. BalmanaJ, Cruz, C., Arun, B. Anti-tumor activity of PM01183(lurbinectedin) in BRCA1/2 associated metastatic breast cancer patients; results of a single-agent phase II trial. In ESMO. Annals of Oncology2016; 68–99.

116. Cardillo TM, Sharkey RM, Rossi DL, et al. Synthetic lethality exploitation by an Anti-Trop-2-SN-38 antibody-drug conjugate, IMMU-132, plus PARP inhibitors in BRCA1/2-wild-type triple-negative breast cancer. Clin Cancer Res. 2017;23:3405–15.

117. Du Y, Yamaguchi H, Wei Y, et al. Blocking c-Met-mediated PARP1 phosphorylation enhances anti-tumor effects of PARP inhibitors. Nat Med. 2016;22:194–201.

118. Zimmer J, Tacconi EMC, Folio C, et al. Targeting BRCA1 and BRCA2 deficiencies with G-quadruplex-interacting compounds. Mol Cell. 2016;61:449–60.

119. Tung N, Lin NU, Kidd J, et al. Frequency of germline mutations in 25 cancer susceptibility genes in a sequential series of patients with breast cancer. J Clin Oncol. 2016;34:1460–8.

120. Tung N, Battelli C, Allen B, et al. Frequency of mutations in individuals with breast cancer referred for BRCA1 and BRCA2 testing using next-generation sequencing with a 25-gene panel. Cancer. 2015;121:25–33.

121. McCuaig JM, Armel SR, Novokmet A, et al. Routine TP53 testing for breast cancer under age 30: ready for prime time? Familial Cancer. 2012;11:607–13.

122. Weller M. Predicting response to cancer chemotherapy: the role of p53. Cell Tissue Res. 1998;292:435–45.

123. Kappel S, Janschek E, Wolf B, et al. TP53 germline mutation may affect response to anticancer treatments: analysis of an intensively treated Li-Fraumeni family. Breast Cancer Res Treat. 2015;151:671–8.

124. Bridges KA, Chen X, Liu H, et al. MK-8776, a novel chk1 kinase inhibitor, radiosensitizes p53-defective human tumor cells. Oncotarget. 2016;7:71660–72.

125. Hirai H, Iwasawa Y, Okada M, et al. Small-molecule inhibition of Wee1 kinase by MK-1775 selectively sensitizes p53-deficient tumor cells to DNA-damaging agents. Mol Cancer Ther. 2009;8:2992–3000.

126. Markman B, Tabernero J, Krop I, et al. Phase I safety, pharmacokinetic, and pharmacodynamic study of the oral phosphatidylinositol-3-kinase and mTOR inhibitor BGT226 in patients with advanced solid tumors. Ann Oncol. 2012;23:2399–408.

127. Tischkowitz M, Xia B. PALB2/FANCN: recombining cancer and Fanconi anemia. Cancer Res. 2010;70:7353–9.

128. Tung N, Domchek SM, Stadler Z, et al. Counselling framework for moderate-penetrance cancer-susceptibility mutations. Nat Rev Clin Oncol. 2016;13:581–8.

129. Ferreira AC, Suriano G, Mendes N, et al. E-cadherin impairment increases cell survival through Notch-dependent upregulation of Bcl-2. Hum Mol Genet. 2012;21:334–43.

130. Mateus AR, Seruca R, Machado JC, et al. EGFR regulates RhoA-GTP dependent cell motility in E-cadherin mutant cells. Hum Mol Genet. 2007;16:1639–47.

131. Mateus AR, Simoes-Correia J, Figueiredo J, et al. E-cadherin mutations and cell motility: a genotype-phenotype correlation. Exp Cell Res. 2009;315:1393–402.

132. Hearle N, Schumacher V, Menko FH, et al. Frequency and spectrum of cancers in the Peutz-Jeghers syndrome. Clin Cancer Res. 2006;12:3209–15.

Surgical Management of Breast Cancer in Young Women

Rosa Di Micco and Oreste Gentilini

7.1 Overview

7.1.1 Background

Historically, breast cancer in young women had poorer prognosis, higher risk of locoregional recurrence (LRR) and greater likelihood of underlying genetic mutations than breast cancer in the older counterpart. The more aggressive tumour biology has often paralleled a more aggressive surgical treatment even though this does not necessarily equate better oncologic outcomes.

The randomized controlled Milano I trial comparing quadrantectomy versus radical mastectomy found almost four times the rate of local recurrence (LR) in women younger than 45 years compared with older women in the breast conservation group, but this did not translate into a difference in breast cancer-specific survival (26.1% vs. 24.3%, $p = 0.8$) or overall survival (OS) (41.7% vs. 41.2%, $p = 1$) between the two groups after 20-year follow-up [1]. The pooled analysis of data from two large randomized trials, European Organization for Research and Treatment of Cancer (EORTC) and the Danish Breast Cancer Cooperative Group (DBCG) trials, found that women younger than 35 years who underwent breast-conserving surgery had 9.24 times the risk of LR compared with women older than 60 years with a 10-year actuarial LR rate of 35% versus 7% in mastectomy patients, but no difference in LRR free survival or OS was found [2]. These findings have been confirmed by a more recent meta-analysis of over 22,000 women aged 40 or less evaluating five population-based cohorts [3–7] and the same pooled analysis from the EORTC/DBCG [2] and concluding that mastectomy was not associated to an improved OS and distant-disease free-survival compared to breast-conserving surgery plus radiotherapy (BCT) [8].

To date, literature provides strong evidence that the surgical type does not affect survival and distant-disease occurrence in young breast cancer patients as well as in older ones. This is consistent with previous RCTs [1, 9–13] comparing mastectomy with BCT in the breast cancer population as a whole, indicating that the surgical choice for younger women should use accepted criteria without impacting outcome [14, 15].

However, the effect of the type of surgery on LRR in young breast cancer patients is still highly debated. Most of the studies reviewed by Vila et al. [8] found that BCT was associated

R. Di Micco (✉)
Breast Unit, San Raffaele University and Research Hospital, Milan, Italy

Department of Clinical Medicine and Surgery, University of Naples Federico II, Naples, Italy
e-mail: dimicco.rosa@hsr.it

O. Gentilini
Breast Unit, San Raffaele University and Research Hospital, Milan, Italy
e-mail: gentilini.oreste@hsr.it

© Springer Nature Switzerland AG 2020
O. Gentilini et al. (eds.), *Breast Cancer in Young Women*,
https://doi.org/10.1007/978-3-030-24762-1_7

with a higher rate of LR and LRR when compared with mastectomy [9, 16, 17], but in a subset analysis of 101 patients <35 years with stage I breast cancer, no significant difference was observed in the 10-year LRR rate (18% BCT vs. 19.8% mastectomy), distant metastasis and OS [18]. In particular, the study by van der Sangen et al. [5], also included in the meta-analysis, evaluated a large cohort of 1451 patients aged ≤40 years from the Eindhoven-Cancer Registry who underwent breast cancer surgery from 1988 to 2005 reporting a worse local control after BCT with a linearly increasing cumulative risk of developing a local relapse even after more than 15 years of follow-up, whereas after mastectomy a plateau was reached after 6 years. In 2016 the results from the English Prospective study of Outcomes in Sporadic versus Hereditary breast cancer (POSH) [19] on 3024 women younger than 40 years diagnosed with breast cancer between 2000 and 2008 demonstrated similar LRR in the first 18 months from mastectomy and BCT, but larger disparity at 5-year (2.6% vs. 5.3%, $p < 0.001$) and 10-year (4.9% vs. 11.7%, $p < 0.001$) follow-up with significantly higher LRR in the BCT patients.

At the same time, in the last decade, other studies on surgical management in young patients have shown a different trend. In 2017 Quan et al. [20] reporting on 1381 young (<35-year-old) patients from Ontario Cancer Registry found no statistically significant effect of surgery type on recurrence (HR = 0.9) and survival (HR = 0.98). Furthermore, they showed that distant metastatic disease represented the most common site of first failure for all women in the study regardless of the surgical approach. This high rate of distant metastases may reflect an inherent biologic difference in young women with breast cancer compared to their older counterparts, which should be maybe addressed by systemic rather than local treatment. Even in the POSH study, the frequency of LR was much lower than that of distant relapse indicating that the main hazard experienced by young patients is of distant rather than of local recurrence (752 vs. 139 events) [19]. Similarly, the retrospective analysis of 201 patients aged <35 years who underwent BCT at the European

Institute of Oncology of Milan between 1997 and 2004 showed a cumulative incidence of ipsilateral breast tumour recurrence of 12.3% at 10-year follow-up which does not justify, according to the authors, mastectomy indication based on patient's age only [21]. In addition to this, Aalders et al. [22] reached the same conclusion by evaluating data of the Netherlands Cancer Registry on contemporary rates of LR and LRR in 1000 young (<35-year-old) patients with breast cancer operated between 2003 and 2008. They found no influence of the type of surgery on the risk of LR (3.5%) and highlighted a decreasing trend in the risk of LRR (3.7%) concluding that young age itself does not imply an increased 5-year rate of LRR.

As a result the decision between BCT and mastectomy in young women with breast cancer should be based on reliable and contemporary risk estimation, as their life expectation is longer and a LR could affect their quality of life. In order to evaluate this risk, Botteri et al. [23] have recently concluded a single-centre cohort study including <40-year-old women diagnosed with early breast cancer and treated with BCT at the European Institute of Oncology in Milan from 1997 to 2010. The main objective of this study was to assess whether the safety of breast-conserving surgery has improved over time and if other components of breast cancer therapy could be identified as clinically responsible of improved outcomes. The study population included 1331 consecutive patients who underwent breast-conserving surgery followed by whole breast radiotherapy and showed a dramatic improvement in prognosis after 2005, when the use of trastuzumab was implemented in routine clinical practice. Considering that the prognosis did not improve in Her-2-positive patients only, the authors argued that the increasing use of the classification in molecular subtypes which allows more tailored therapy, general improvements in diagnostic ability and the introduction of new systemic treatments has generated a global improvement in outcomes. According to their data, the incidence of ipsilateral breast tumour recurrence decreased by 7% each year, going from 1.42 per 100 person-years in those treated up to 2002 to 0.48 per 100 person-years in those treated after 2005. Hence, the 10-year local relapse rate is 4.8%, which is much better than percentages previously reported in young women, i.e. 10.2% at 5-year follow-up and 12% at 15-year [24, 25].

To summarize, surgeons in favour of mastectomy still find that young patients are poorly represented in those historical trials, so generalization of results could be not reliable, the definition of "young" is not homogeneous, and the increased risk of LRR showed in less recent studies could already be good reasons to be more aggressive. But this is now an old misconception, and currently the reported improving outcome of BCT is achieved through a synergic pre-operative work-up working along with surgery plus radiotherapy and systemic therapy guided by tumour biology. In addition to this, breast cancer in young patients is de facto a relative uncommon condition (around 5–7% of breast cancers arises in women younger than 40), and it is acceptable that they represent a minority of those studied, but now we have sufficient data to support international guidelines specifically dedicated to young breast cancer patients.

7.1.2 Current Guidelines

Breast-conserving surgery followed by radiotherapy is currently the standard of care for early breast cancer with no difference in overall survival compared to mastectomy. As a matter of fact, the European Society of Breast Cancer Specialists (EUSOMA) working group confirmed that conservative surgery is the first option, whenever suitable, for young breast cancer patients too in the most recent international consensus guidelines for breast cancer in young women (BCY3) [26]. Nevertheless, the choice of the surgical treatment in young breast cancer patient still represents a challenge due to both the rare condition and the fact that young age is an independent risk factor for increased local recurrence [1, 12, 13, 27, 28]. In particular, some of the histopathological characteristics such as larger size, higher grade, presence of peripheral

extensive intraductal component, vascular embolies and lymphoid stroma have been related to a higher risk of LR [29].

In this scenario, there is a high risk of taking emotionally driven decisions and opting for the more aggressive, and maybe unnecessary, surgical procedure [21]. However, the worse prognosis of many young patients cannot be mitigated by a more aggressive local treatment, as more extensive surgery does not result in improved survival.

The care of young women with breast cancer should always be tailored on the single patient and her specific issues related to fertility preservation, sexuality, activities of daily living, social life, pregnancy and lactation which could affect in a way surgical decision and timing. For this reason, young breast cancer patients deserve a "special" attention and a multidisciplinary approach in order to choose the best surgical treatment.

7.2 Breast-Conserving Surgery Versus Mastectomy and the Increasing Role of Primary Systemic Therapy

In early breast cancer, breast-conserving surgery followed by radiotherapy provides the same long-term survival benefit as modified radical mastectomy in women with stage I–II breast cancer. The importance of surgical quality is supported by data showing that the completeness of excision is more important than the extent of surgery [19]. Aesthetic outcome, body image changes and the impact on sexuality may be more relevant in young women. Literature on quality of life after BCT shows good results regardless of age, and BCT is always associated to higher scores if compared to mastectomy [30, 31].

In advanced breast cancer, age alone is not a reason to prescribe more aggressive therapy, and the management should be the same as in the older breast cancer population. Likewise, young patients with inflammatory breast cancer, which is slightly more frequent in young women of African origin, follow common guidelines regardless of age.

7.2.1 Breast-Conserving Surgery

The goal of breast-conserving surgery is to provide clear radial tumour margins. There is no upper limit for tumour size, but a large tumour in a small breast is a relative contraindication since an appropriate resection would result in a poor aesthetic outcome. In these cases, as well as in the older counterpart, considering tumour biology and imaging, the primary systemic therapy (PST) could help downsize the tumour and allow less invasive surgery. When breast-conserving surgery is indicated in young patients, the tumour excision can be performed through a wide local excision removing the tumour en bloc from the subcutaneous tissue to the pectoralis fascia with macroscopically free radial margin as well as it happens for patients of any age. The involvement of radial margin is associated with significantly worse OS and disease-free survival also in studies on young patients, so attention to margins, with re-excision where appropriate, is strongly recommended [19].

Whenever poor aesthetic outcomes are expected, oncoplastic repair techniques should be offered in order to maximize cosmetic results. The use of oncoplastic techniques is very common in younger patients who seem to be more motivated to preserve their body image, despite bilateral or more complex surgery. Although modern breast surgery aims to remove the tumour while removing the smallest volume of tissue, on one hand the wish for a better symmetry can lead to more extensive surgery, i.e. bilateral oncoplastic surgery, on the other hand the wish to avoid mastectomy can lead to extend the indications for breast-conserving surgery even when mastectomy would be indicated, i.e. "extreme" oncoplasty can be performed as the last chance to have the breast saved [32, 33].

However, the worse biologic features of breast cancer in young patients suggest that many women might be treated with PST in order to reduce the mastectomy rates and, in general, to improve cosmetic and functional outcomes after smaller surgical resections in cases where major response is achieved. Another advantage of using PST might be to have more time to perform genetic testing and allow both the patient and the physician to discuss between either a therapeutic procedure alone, which might be limited and conservative, or a risk-reducing surgery (see Chap. 7). The re-assessment after PST should always evaluate the eventual inflammatory presentation at diagnosis, the response to therapy and the residual tumour burden in order to choose the best surgical indication.

7.2.2 Mastectomy

When mastectomy is indicated, skin and nipple-sparing techniques with immediate breast reconstruction are the gold standard for all breast cancer women and, even more, for young patients, except for inflammatory breast cancer for whom delayed reconstruction is generally recommended [34]. Data from UK national audit show that age is the only factor to be associated with patient responses on quality of life, showing that younger patients have higher expectations and are more prone to choose immediate reconstruction [35].

7.2.3 Axillary Surgery

Indications for sentinel node biopsy or axillary dissection and the surgical management of involved nodes in young breast cancer patients should be the same as in older patients both in upfront surgery as well as in neoadjuvant setting. There is no evidence of any differences in sentinel node biopsy outcomes related to the patient age. The optimal treatment of the axilla after primary chemotherapy remains controversial and should be tailored on the single patient regardless of age [35] (Figs. 7.1 and 7.2).

7.3 Special Situations in Young Patients

Breast cancer in young ladies could arise in special settings that are more frequently associated to the young age. In these cases, the surgical management could be slightly different.

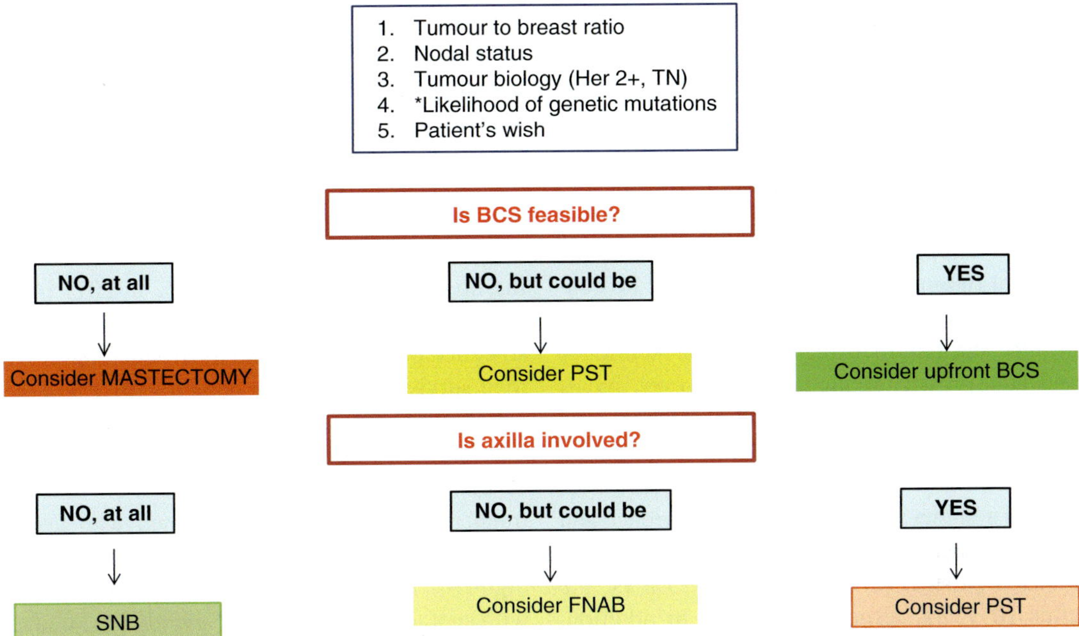

*If the information deriving from the genetic testing could change surgical indication, always take into account to wait for it, listen to the patient's wishes and consider timing for upfront surgery versus PST according to the availability of an «urgent» genetic test.
If the test is positive ALWAYS explain the alternative of bilateral risk reducing surgery

Fig. 7.1 Surgical evaluation at diagnosis

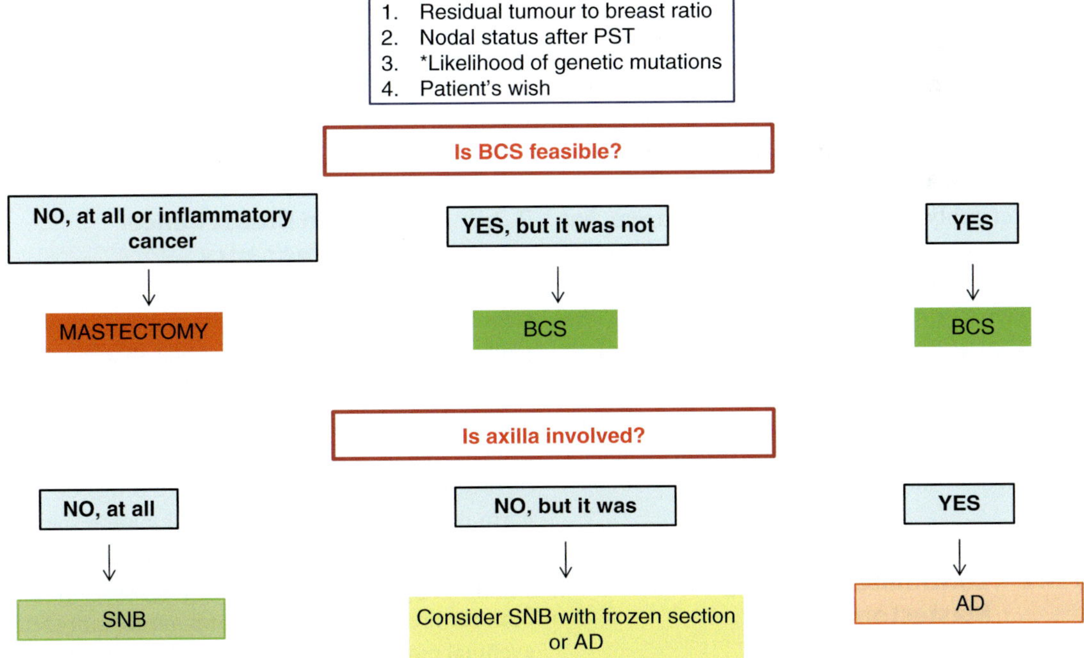

Fig. 7.2 Surgical evaluation after PST

7.3.1 High Genetic Risk

The management of young patients with breast cancer and harbouring germline BRCA mutation is very complex and has been specifically addressed in a separate and dedicated chapter (see Chap. 6).

Briefly, in patients with BRCA1/2 mutation or other strongly predisposition mutations, the bilateral risk-reducing mastectomy may be considered as part of the initial work-up, trying to balance the risk of ipsilateral breast recurrence and new primary malignancy. However, breast conservation remains a suitable option, and patients should be carefully informed that no survival benefit has been de facto demonstrated, despite a higher risk of ipsilateral recurrence and contralateral breast cancer if compared with non-mutated patients (27% vs. 4% and 25% vs. 1% after 10 years, respectively) [36]. In addition, prophylactic salpingo-oophorectomy should be discussed from the age of 35 provided that the woman has completed the family planning and should preferably be done before the age of 40 especially in BRCA1 mutation carriers, always taking into account the patient's wishes and family history [37, 38]. In high-risk women who opted for breast conservation, prophylactic salpingo-oophorectomy can reduce both the risk of in-breast tumour recurrence (HR:1.37, $p = 0.19$) and, as well as tamoxifen, contralateral breast cancer occurrence [39]. Every young woman with breast cancer should be offered genetic counselling preferably before starting any treatment, but if she is not ready to consider genetic issues at diagnosis, it is advisable to treat the cancer first and then to offer counselling again during the follow-up. For all surgical decisions, and particularly for risk-reducing mastectomy, patients must be properly counselled and given adequate time to decide. Once an informed decision is made by the patient, it should be respected [34].

7.3.2 Contralateral Prophylactic Mastectomy

Despite no survival advantage, more and more young women with unilateral breast cancer are choosing to undergo contralateral prophylactic mastectomy (CPM), even without a known hereditary predisposition to the disease. Young age at diagnosis has been identified as a predictor of likelihood to undergo CPM [40–44]. A recent analysis of California Cancer Registry data documented an increase in bilateral mastectomy rates above all in women under 40 climbing up from 3.6% in 1998 to 33% in 2011 [45]. A recent SEER analysis showed that anxiety, the so-called piece of mind and the desire to improve their survival are the most common drivers in the patient's choice for CPM, although this means that lots of young women overestimate their risk of contralateral cancer [46]. The risk of contralateral disease in young women who tested negative for BRCA1/2 mutations, even with a high-risk family history, is similar to patients with sporadic breast cancer. Nevertheless, if after receiving proper and thorough information based on current available data on prognosis, surgical complications and psychological consequences, the young patient shows a strong motivation to undergo prophylactic surgery, this preference should be respected [47]. These data suggest that young women need to be very carefully informed about the risks and benefits of surgery, highlighting that the risk of systemic recurrence, which is not affected by the surgical choice, exceeds the risk of developing a contralateral cancer [48].

7.3.3 Surgery in Breast Cancer During Pregnancy

If breast cancer occurs during pregnancy, the young patient should be well informed that abortion does not improve prognosis and that the cancer as well as its treatment will not affect the foetus' health. Surgery can be safely performed during any stage of pregnancy, and most anaesthetic drugs do not harm the foetus [49]. The surgical choice should not be affected by the pregnancy but must follow the same guidelines as for non-pregnant women both for breast conservation and mastectomy and eventual reconstruction [50, 51]. However, in case of breast conservation, radiotherapy should be delayed to post-delivery time [52]. Mastectomy is not recommended solely on the basis of pregnancy and delay in time to radiotherapy. Furthermore, immediate reconstruction with tissue expander, even if prolonging surgery duration is not associated with adverse obstetrical or foetal outcomes, it can be safely used as a bridge to leave open all reconstructive options. Even sentinel node biopsy is feasible during pregnancy, as the estimated absorbed doses are widely below the 0.1–0.2 Gy foetal threshold absorbed dose [53]. It is recommended to inject colloid in the morning (1-day protocol) to minimize radiation exposure, while blue dye is not recommended due to the potential risk of anaphylactic maternal reaction [54].

7.3.4 Surgery in Locoregional Relapse

The recommendations for young women do not differ from those for the general population. An isolated LR after BCT should be treated by mastectomy, but, whenever possible, a second breast-conserving surgery could be offered to the patient after an informed decision-making process. To date, results from the CALOR study [55] suggest to consider also chemotherapy in women with HR-negative tumours and isolated LR, although the second isolated LR portends poor prognosis [56]. In case of LR, based on expert opinion level of evidence, endocrine therapy and trastuzumab could also be recommended in ER+ and Her2+ disease, respectively [34].

References

1. Veronesi U, Cascinelli N, Mariani L, Greco M, Saccozzi R, Luini A, et al. Twenty-year follow-up of a randomized study comparing breast-conserving surgery with radical mastectomy for early breast cancer. N Engl J Med. 2002;347(16):1227–32.
2. Voogd AC, Nielsen M, Peterse JL, Blichert-Toft M, Bartelink H, Overgaard M, et al. Differences in risk factors for local and distant recurrence after breast-conserving therapy or mastectomy for stage I and II breast cancer: pooled results of two large European randomized trials. J Clin Oncol. 2001;19(6):1688–97.
3. Kroman N, Holtveg H, Wohlfahrt J, Jensen MB, Mouridsen HT, Blichert-Toft M, et al. Effect of breast-conserving therapy versus radical mastectomy on prognosis for young women with breast carcinoma. Cancer. 2004;100(4):688–93.
4. Bantema-Joppe EJ, de Munck L, Visser O, Willemse PH, Langendijk JA, Siesling S, et al. Early-stage young breast cancer patients: impact of local treatment on survival. Int J Radiat Oncol Biol Phys. 2011;81(4):e553–9.
5. van der Sangen MJ, van de Wiel FM, Poortmans PM, Tjan-Heijnen VC, Nieuwenhuijzen GA, Roumen RM, et al. Are breast conservation and mastectomy equally effective in the treatment of young women with early breast cancer? Long-term results of a population-based cohort of 1,451 patients aged ≤ 40 years. Breast Cancer Res Treat. 2011;127(1):207–15.
6. Mahmood U, Morris C, Neuner G, Koshy M, Kesmodel S, Buras R, et al. Similar survival with breast conservation therapy or mastectomy in the management of young women with early-stage breast cancer. Int J Radiat Oncol Biol Phys. 2012;83(5):1387–93.
7. Jeon YW, Choi JE, Park HK, Kim KS, Lee JY, Suh YJ. Impact of local surgical treatment on survival in young women with T1 breast cancer: long-term results of a population-based cohort. Breast Cancer Res Treat. 2013;138(2):475–84.
8. Vila J, Gandini S, Gentilini O. Overall survival according to type of surgery in young (≤40 years) early breast cancer patients: a systematic meta-analysis comparing breast-conserving surgery versus mastectomy. Breast. 2015;24(3):175–81.
9. Arriagada R, Lê MG, Guinebretière JM, Dunant A, Rochard F, Tursz T. Late local recurrences in a randomised trial comparing conservative treatment with total mastectomy in early breast cancer patients. Ann Oncol. 2003;14(11):1617–22.
10. Blichert-Toft M, Nielsen M, Düring M, Møller S, Rank F, Overgaard M, et al. Long-term results of breast conserving surgery vs. mastectomy for early stage invasive breast cancer: 20-year follow-up of the Danish randomized DBCG-82TM protocol. Acta Oncol. 2008;47(4):672–81.
11. Fisher B, Anderson S, Bryant J, Margolese RG, Deutsch M, Fisher ER, et al. Twenty-year follow-up of a randomized trial comparing total mastectomy, lumpectomy, and lumpectomy plus irradiation for the treatment of invasive breast cancer. N Engl J Med. 2002;347(16):1233–41.
12. Poggi MM, Danforth DN, Sciuto LC, Smith SL, Steinberg SM, Liewehr DJ, et al. Eighteen-year results in the treatment of early breast carcinoma with mastectomy versus breast conservation therapy: the National Cancer Institute Randomized Trial. Cancer. 2003;98(4):697–702.
13. van Dongen JA, Voogd AC, Fentiman IS, Legrand C, Sylvester RJ, Tong D, et al. Long-term results of a randomized trial comparing breast-conserving therapy with mastectomy: European Organization for Research and Treatment of Cancer 10801 trial. J Natl Cancer Inst. 2000;92(14):1143–50.

14. Cao JQ, Olson RA, Tyldesley SK. Comparison of recurrence and survival rates after breast-conserving therapy and mastectomy in young women with breast cancer. Curr Oncol. 2013;20(6):e593–601.

15. Ye JC, Yan W, Christos PJ, Nori D, Ravi A. Equivalent survival with mastectomy or breast-conserving surgery plus radiation in young women aged <40 years with early-stage breast cancer: a National Registry-based Stage-by-Stage Comparison. Clin Breast Cancer. 2015;15(5):390–7.

16. Fodor J, Mózsa E, Zaka Z, Polgár C, Major T. Local relapse in young (< or = 40 years) women with breast cancer after mastectomy or breast conserving surgery: 15-year results. Magy Onkol. 2005;49(3):203, 205–8

17. Bantema-Joppe EJ, van den Heuvel ER, de Munck L, de Bock GH, Smit WG, Timmer PR, et al. Impact of primary local treatment on the development of distant metastases or death through locoregional recurrence in young breast cancer patients. Breast Cancer Res Treat. 2013;140(3):577–85.

18. Beadle BM, Woodward WA, Tucker SL, Outlaw ED, Allen PK, Oh JL, et al. Ten-year recurrence rates in young women with breast cancer by locoregional treatment approach. Int J Radiat Oncol Biol Phys. 2009;73(3):734–44.

19. Maishman T, Cutress RI, Hernandez A, Gerty S, Copson ER, Durcan L, et al. Local recurrence and breast oncological surgery in young women with breast cancer: the POSH Observational Cohort Study. Ann Surg. 2017;266:165–72.

20. Quan ML, Paszat LF, Fernandes KA, Sutradhar R, McCready DR, Rakovitch E, et al. The effect of surgery type on survival and recurrence in very young women with breast cancer. J Surg Oncol. 2017;115(2):122–30.

21. Gentilini O, Botteri E, Rotmensz N, Toesca A, De Oliveira H, Sangalli C, et al. Breast-conserving surgery in 201 very young patients (<35 years). Breast. 2010;19(1):55–8.

22. Aalders KC, Postma EL, Strobbe LJ, van der Heiden-van der Loo M, Sonke GS, Boersma LJ, et al. Contemporary locoregional recurrence rates in young patients with early-stage breast cancer. J Clin Oncol. 2016;34(18):2107–14.

23. Botteri E, Veronesi P, Vila J, Rotmensz N, Galimberti V, Thomazini MV, et al. Improved prognosis of young patients with breast cancer undergoing breast-conserving surgery. Br J Surg. 2017;104:1802–10.

24. Bartelink H, Horiot JC, Poortmans P, Struikmans H, Van den Bogaert W, Barillot I, et al. Recurrence rates after treatment of breast cancer with standard radiotherapy with or without additional radiation. N Engl J Med. 2001;345(19):1378–87.

25. Fisher ER, Anderson S, Tan-Chiu E, Fisher B, Eaton L, Wolmark N. Fifteen-year prognostic discriminants for invasive breast carcinoma: National Surgical Adjuvant Breast and Bowel Project Protocol-06. Cancer. 2001;91(8 Suppl):1679–87.

26. Paluch-Shimon S, Pagani O, Partridge AH, Bar-Meir E, Fallowfield L, Fenlon D, et al. Second international consensus guidelines for breast cancer in young women (BCY2). Breast. 2016;26:87–99.

27. Fisher B, Jeong JH, Anderson S, Bryant J, Fisher ER, Wolmark N. Twenty-five-year follow-up of a randomized trial comparing radical mastectomy, total mastectomy, and total mastectomy followed by irradiation. N Engl J Med. 2002;347(8):567–75.

28. Miles RC, Gullerud RE, Lohse CM, Jakub JW, Degnim AC, Boughey JC. Local recurrence after breast-conserving surgery: multivariable analysis of risk factors and the impact of young age. Ann Surg Oncol. 2012;19(4):1153–9.

29. Partridge AH, Pagani O, Abulkhair O, Aebi S, Amant F, Azim HA, et al. First international consensus guidelines for breast cancer in young women (BCY1). Breast. 2014;23(3):209–20.

30. O'Connell RL, DiMicco R, Khabra K, O'Flynn EA, deSouza N, Roche N, et al. Initial experience of the BREAST-Q breast-conserving therapy module. Breast Cancer Res Treat. 2016;160:79–89.

31. King TA. Selecting local therapy in the young breast cancer patient. J Surg Oncol. 2011;103(4):330–6.

32. Silverstein MJ, Savalia N, Khan S, Ryan J. Extreme oncoplasty: breast conservation for patients who need mastectomy. Breast J. 2015;21(1):52–9.

33. Silverstein MJ. Radical mastectomy to radical conservation (extreme oncoplasty): a revolutionary change. J Am Coll Surg. 2016;222(1):1–9.

34. Paluch-Shimon S, Pagani O, Partridge AH, Abulkhair O, Cardoso MJ, Dent RA, et al. ESO-ESMO 3rd international consensus guidelines for breast cancer in young women (BCY3). Breast. 2017;35:203–17.

35. National Mastectomy and Breast Reconstruction Audit. 2011. http://www.hscic.gov.uk/catalogue/PUB02731/clin-audi-supp-prog-mast-brea-reco-2011-rep1.pdf2011.

36. Garcia-Etienne CA, Barile M, Gentilini OD, Botteri E, Rotmensz N, Sagona A, et al. Breast-conserving surgery in BRCA1/2 mutation carriers: are we approaching an answer? Ann Surg Oncol. 2009;16(12):3380–7.

37. Domchek SM, Friebel TM, Singer CF, Evans DG, Lynch HT, Isaacs C, et al. Association of risk-reducing surgery in BRCA1 or BRCA2 mutation carriers with cancer risk and mortality. JAMA. 2010;304(9):967–75.

38. Bernstein JL, Thomas DC, Shore RE, Robson M, Boice JD, Stovall M, et al. Contralateral breast cancer after radiotherapy among BRCA1 and BRCA2 mutation carriers: a WECARE study report. Eur J Cancer. 2013;49(14):2979–85.

39. Pierce LJ, Levin AM, Rebbeck TR, Ben-David MA, Friedman E, Solin LJ, et al. Ten-year multi-institutional results of breast-conserving surgery and radiotherapy in BRCA1/2-associated stage I/II breast cancer. J Clin Oncol. 2006;24(16):2437–43.

40. Tuttle TM, Barrio AV, Klimberg VS, Giuliano AE, Chavez-MacGregor M, Buum HA, et al. Guidelines

for guidelines: an assessment of the American Society of breast surgeons contralateral prophylactic mastectomy consensus statement. Ann Surg Oncol. 2017;24(1):1–2.

41. Yao K, Stewart AK, Winchester DJ, Winchester DP. Trends in contralateral prophylactic mastectomy for unilateral cancer: a report from the National Cancer Data Base, 1998–2007. Ann Surg Oncol. 2010;17(10):2554–62.

42. Arrington AK, Jarosek SL, Virnig BA, Habermann EB, Tuttle TM. Patient and surgeon characteristics associated with increased use of contralateral prophylactic mastectomy in patients with breast cancer. Ann Surg Oncol. 2009;16(10):2697–704.

43. King TA, Sakr R, Patil S, Gurevich I, Stempel M, Sampson M, et al. Clinical management factors contribute to the decision for contralateral prophylactic mastectomy. J Clin Oncol. 2011;29(16):2158–64.

44. Jones NB, Wilson J, Kotur L, Stephens J, Farrar WB, Agnese DM. Contralateral prophylactic mastectomy for unilateral breast cancer: an increasing trend at a single institution. Ann Surg Oncol. 2009;16(10):2691–6.

45. Kurian AW, Lichtensztajn DY, Keegan TH, Nelson DO, Clarke CA, Gomez SL. Use of and mortality after bilateral mastectomy compared with other surgical treatments for breast cancer in California, 1998–2011. JAMA. 2014;312(9):902–14.

46. Rosenberg SM, Tracy MS, Meyer ME, Sepucha K, Gelber S, Hirshfield-Bartek J, et al. Perceptions, knowledge, and satisfaction with contralateral prophylactic mastectomy among young women with breast cancer: a cross-sectional survey. Ann Intern Med. 2013;159(6):373–81.

47. Cardoso F, Loibl S, Pagani O, Graziottin A, Panizza P, Martincich L, et al. The European Society of breast cancer specialists recommendations for the management of young women with breast cancer. Eur J Cancer. 2012;48(18):3355–77.

48. Rosenberg SM, Partridge AH. Management of breast cancer in very young women. Breast. 2015;24(Suppl 2):S154–8.

49. Moran BJ, Yano H, Al Zahir N, Farquharson M. Conflicting priorities in surgical intervention for cancer in pregnancy. Lancet Oncol. 2007;8(6):536–44.

50. Amant F, Deckers S, Van Calsteren K, Loibl S, Halaska M, Brepoels L, et al. Breast cancer in pregnancy: recommendations of an international consensus meeting. Eur J Cancer. 2010;46(18):3158–68.

51. Lohsiriwat V, Peccatori FA, Martella S, Azim HA, Sarno MA, Galimberti V, et al. Immediate breast reconstruction with expander in pregnant breast cancer patients. Breast. 2013;22(5):657–60.

52. Toesca A, Gentilini O, Peccatori F, Azim HA, Amant F. Locoregional treatment of breast cancer during pregnancy. Gynecol Surg. 2014;11(4):279–84.

53. Gentilini O, Cremonesi M, Toesca A, Colombo N, Peccatori F, Sironi R, et al. Sentinel lymph node biopsy in pregnant patients with breast cancer. Eur J Nucl Med Mol Imaging. 2010;37(1):78–83.

54. Loibl S, Schmidt A, Gentilini O, Kaufman B, Kuhl C, Denkert C, et al. Breast cancer diagnosed during pregnancy: adapting recent advances in breast cancer care for pregnant patients. JAMA Oncol. 2015;1(8):1145–53.

55. Aebi S, Gelber S, Anderson SJ, Láng I, Robidoux A, Martín M, et al. Chemotherapy for isolated locoregional recurrence of breast cancer (CALOR): a randomised trial. Lancet Oncol. 2014;15(2):156–63.

56. Wapnir IL, Gelber S, Anderson SJ, Mamounas EP, Robidoux A, Martín M, et al. Poor prognosis after second locoregional recurrences in the CALOR Trial. Ann Surg Oncol. 2017;24(2):398–406.

Elżbieta Senkus

8.1 Outcomes of Locoregional Therapies in Young Breast Cancer Patients

Breast cancer in young women is associated with higher risk of locoregional recurrence, even if corrected for stage and tumor characteristics. This phenomenon is observed in case of both breast-conserving therapy (BCT) and mastectomy [1–3]. In a series comprising 3602 women enrolled in three European Organisation for Research and Treatment of Cancer (EORTC) trials who had undergone breast conservation (55%) or mastectomy (45%) for early-stage breast cancer, age and breast conservation were independent risk factors for isolated locoregional recurrence [2].

Large retrospective series of patients treated with BCT in the last 20 years consistently report significantly higher incidence of local failures among younger patients [4, 5], as well as age-related differences in outcomes of patients treated between 1970 and 1990 [6]. In a series of 758 patients ≤40 years from southern Netherlands, treated between 1988 and 2002, 5- and 10-year local recurrence rates were as high as 9% and 17.9% [7]. These numbers have, however, improved significantly in later cohorts of patients, mostly due to improved effective-

ness of adjuvant systemic therapies: in another study from the same setting, 5-year local recurrence rates in patients ≤40 years decreased from 9.8% for women treated between 1988 and 1998 to 3.3% for those treated between 2006 and 2010 [8].

Age was also the only independent prognostic factor for local control ($P = 0.0001$) in the EORTC "boost versus no boost" trial (Fig. 8.1), and the largest absolute improvement from the use of additional radiation dose (boost) to the tumor bed occurred in patients aged 40 years or less. In this large (5569 patients) randomized study, however, improvements in local control related to the use of higher radiation dose did not translate into survival benefit [9, 10]. Interestingly, the effect of age on local recurrence was not observed in the triple-negative breast cancer (TNBC) subtype in a series of 1930 patients from the Memorial Sloan Kettering Cancer Center (MSKCC) [11].

In mastectomized patients the negative impact of age on locoregional recurrence was demonstrated in 4 of 11 studies included in the systematic review by Kent et al. [12]. Among patients enrolled in 13 International Breast Cancer Study Group (IBCSG) randomized trials, age <40 years (together with involvement of ≥4 lymph nodes and inadequate axillary surgery) was the main determinant of >15% risk of locoregional recurrence [13].

Importantly, no difference in long-term outcomes is observed in mastectomized patients,

E. Senkus (✉)
Department of Oncology & Radiotherapy, Medical University of Gdańsk, Gdańsk, Poland
e-mail: elsenkus@gumed.edu.pl

© Springer Nature Switzerland AG 2020
O. Gentilini et al. (eds.), *Breast Cancer in Young Women*,
https://doi.org/10.1007/978-3-030-24762-1_8

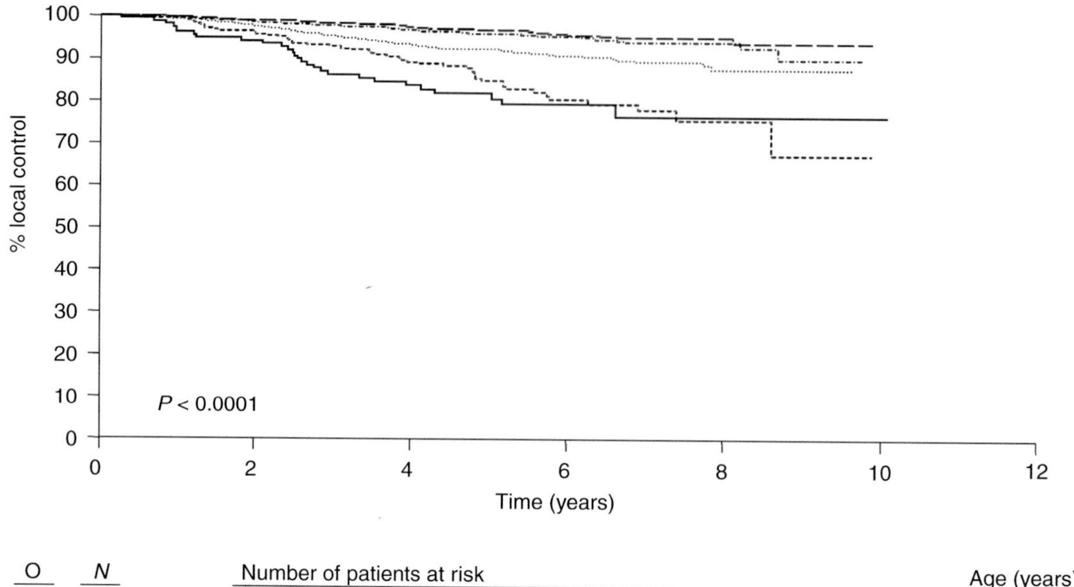

O	N	Number of patients at risk					Age (years)
28	156	137	95	46	9	1	——— ≤ 35
48	314	285	200	90	17	0	------- 36 – 40
109	1407	1316	912	407	75	0	·········· 41 – 50
75	1885	1768	1220	525	102	0	--·--·-- 51 – 60
58	1807	1694	1237	518	85	0	——— > 60

Fig. 8.1 Local recurrence rate according to age in the EORTC "boost vs no boost" trial [10]

compared to those undergoing BCT. Indeed, young BCT patients generally demonstrate higher locoregional recurrence rates, compared to those treated with mastectomy [2, 14, 15]. In spite of that, in a systematic meta-analysis (22,598 patients 40 years old or younger from five population-based studies) and one pooled analysis of two clinical trials (10,898 BCT patients and 11,700 mastectomy patients), after adjustments for tumor size and nodal status, no difference in the risk of death was found between the two groups, with a nonsignificant 10% lower risk in BCT patients (HR 0.9) (Fig. 8.2) [16]. Similarly, in the Dutch series of 536 T1N0-3M0 patients ≤40 years, even though the risk of locoregional recurrence was almost threefold higher in those undergoing BCT, this did not translate into an increased risk of distant metastases or death [15]. On the contrary, significantly higher breast cancer-specific and overall survival rates were observed for stage IIB patients aged 20–34 years from the Surveillance, Epidemiology, and End Results (SEER) Program database, treated with BCT, compared to mastectomy without radio-

therapy [17]. No differences in long-term outcomes were observed for stages I and IIA and for patients aged 35–39 years [17]. Inferior survival was also observed in node-positive T1 patients aged <40 years treated with mastectomy versus those undergoing BCT (HR 1.91). In this series postmastectomy chest wall radiotherapy was used only in case of positive margins or multifocality or when locoregional radiotherapy was used for positive apical lymph nodes or extensive extra nodal growth [18]. The most plausible explanation for superior outcomes in BCT patients is the almost universal use of radiotherapy in this population. These data provide strong support for offering BCT to all suitable patients, regardless of age. Younger patients are at higher risk of locoregional failure, but more extensive surgery is not able to improve the risk of distant failure or death.

In young patients treated with conservative breast surgery, increased risk of local recurrence, compared to older patients, was observed predominantly in luminal A and HER2-positive subtypes and the highest absolute risk was present in

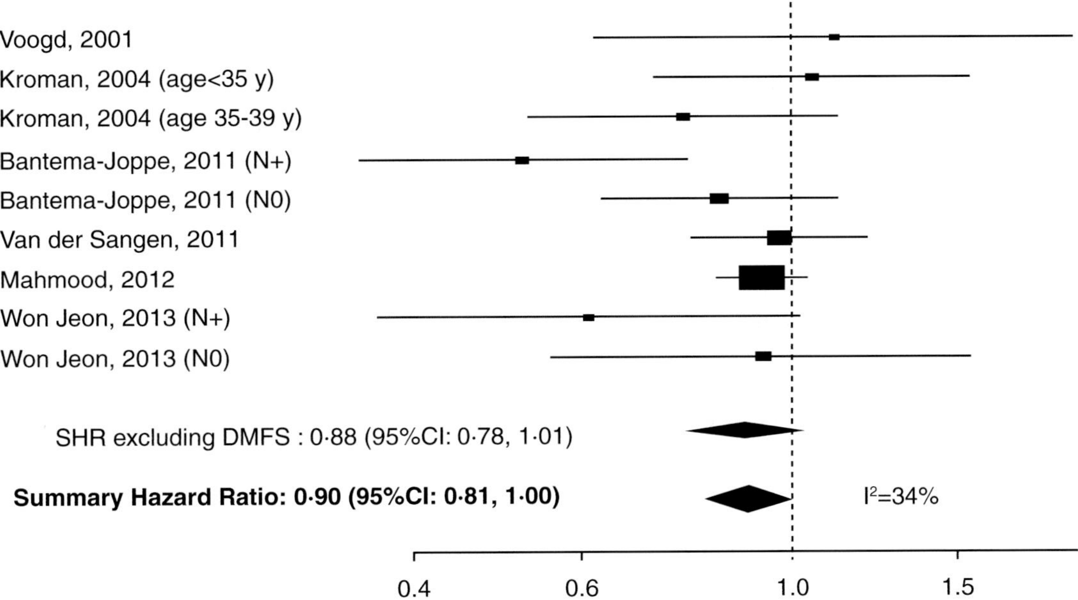

Fig. 8.2 Survival outcomes in young patients (≤40) undergoing BCS vs mastectomy [16]. *SHR* summary hazard ratio, *DMFS* Distant metastasis free survival, *CI* confidence interval

HER2-positive and triple-negative patients aged ≤40 years [19]. In another series of 524 patients treated with mastectomy or BCT, the prognostic value of age for the risk of locoregional recurrence was limited to luminal A tumors, and no difference was seen in luminal B and non-luminal subtypes [3].

Prognosis in BCT-treated patients developing ipsilateral breast tumor recurrence is better than that observed in case of local recurrence after mastectomy. In a series of 124 patients with an isolated local recurrence in the breast following breast-conserving surgery and radiotherapy for early-stage breast cancer diagnosed at the age of 40 years or younger, 10-year local control rate was 95%, distant recurrence-free survival rate 61%, and overall survival rate 73% [20]. Better prognosis is observed in patients developing local recurrence more than 5 years after BCT (HR 0.53), with lesions 2 cm or smaller (HR 0.35) and with local recurrences detected by breast imaging (versus symptomatic ones) (HR 0.27) [20]. Interestingly, although young patients develop local failures more often than the older ones, their prognosis following local recurrence and overall survival seem to be better, compared to the older population [21, 22].

The age at diagnosis matters even among "young" patients: in a series of 167 T1-2 patients aged 26–45, treated with BCT, including brachytherapy boost, age ≤35 was associated with a threefold increase in the risk of local failure, together with high tumor grade and negative hormone receptor status. Importantly, also in this series, increased local recurrence rate did not translate into increase in the risk of distant metastases and death [23].

8.2 Role and Technical Aspects of Radiotherapy in Young Breast Cancer Patients

Increased risk of local recurrence after BCT in younger women provides a rationale for the use of more "aggressive" radiotherapy. Indeed, the

EORTC "boost versus no boost" trial demonstrated the largest absolute benefit from additional radiation dose to the tumor bed in patients aged <40, although the relative risk reduction was similar among all age groups [9]. As a result, use of tumor bed boost in women <50 is uniformly recommended by most guidelines [24, 25]. As the local recurrence risk is higher in young patients, even with use of standard dose boost, there are attempts to improve these results by further escalation of the radiation dose. The optimal tumor bed dose in patients ≤50 has been tested in the "young boost" trial, comparing standard boost of 16 Gy to 26 Gy, and the results are awaited [26].

Fractionation regimen in young breast cancer patients should not differ from those used in older patients. The 2018 American Society for Radiation Oncology (ASTRO) guidelines for whole-breast irradiation clearly state that there is no evidence indicating deleterious effects of moderately hypofractionated whole-breast irradiation in younger patients; thus the decisions regarding its use should be made regardless of age [27].

Because of increased local failure rate and because young patients are not only at risk of true recurrence, but also of second primary cancers within the conserved breast, the policy of limiting the irradiation volume only to the tumor bed (partial breast irradiation—PBI) is generally not recommended in young women. According to the guidelines of the Groupe Européen de Curiethérapie-European Society for Therapeutic Radiology and Oncology (GEC-ESTRO) and ASTRO, PBI is considered appropriate and safe only in the age group >50 (without other defined risk factors) and women ≤40 are clearly defined as "unsuitable" for PBI [28, 29]. Also the American Brachytherapy Society considers PBI acceptable only in women ≥50 years old [30]. In the retrospective series of 183 patients aged 40–50 from Japan, however, no difference in the risk of in-breast recurrence was observed between those undergoing PBI using multicatheter brachytherapy and whole-breast irradiation [31].

Postmastectomy radiotherapy (PMRT) is routinely recommended in all patients with four or more involved lymph nodes; the role of PMRT in patients with one to three involved nodes remains disputable, and there is no agreement between the major guidelines, with recommendations varying from routine use in all node-positive patients [24, 32] to the use only in those with additional risk factors [25, 33, 34].

As young mastectomy patients have higher locoregional failure rates, the relative reduction in breast cancer mortality due to postmastectomy radiotherapy is more pronounced in the youngest age groups, although the relative decline in the locoregional recurrence risk is similar in all age groups [35]. In a retrospective series of 382 patients aged ≤35 from the Ontario Cancer Registry treated with mastectomy between 1994 and 2003, after a median follow-up of only 2.72 years, an isolated local recurrence occurred in 15% of patients, and regional in 17%; postmastectomy radiotherapy was able to decrease this risk by almost 50% (HR 0.54), without an effect on distant recurrences or death without recurrence [36]. Significant benefit from postmastectomy radiotherapy in terms of locoregional control and overall survival, despite more advanced disease stages, was observed among 107 stage IIA–IIIC patients <35 years treated at MD Anderson with doxorubicin-based neoadjuvant chemotherapy and mastectomy [37].

Young mastectomy patients share risk factors for locoregional failure with older age groups: primary tumor size and nodal stage, as well as lack of radiotherapy and appropriate adjuvant systemic therapy [38]. While postmastectomy radiotherapy seems substantiated in the vast majority, if not all young node-positive patients, some data also suggest benefit from irradiation in the node-negative population. In a study of 502 T1-2N0 patients treated with mastectomy, after a median follow-up of 77 months, local recurrence rates in patients >40 and ≤40 were 1.7 and 7%, respectively; prognostic factors for locoregional recurrence in patients ≤40 included tumor size and presence of lymphatic vascular invasion [39]. In a series of 1136 node-negative T1–T2 breast cancer cases treated with mastectomy without PMRT at Massachusetts General Hospital between 1980 and 2004, locoregional recurrence risk was twice higher in patients ≤50. When combined with two or more other risk factors, such as tumor size ≥ 2 cm, presence of lymphatic vascular invasion, close or positive margins, and absence of adjuvant systemic treatment, locoregional recurrence rate was as high as almost 20% [40]. Surprisingly, no beneficial effect of postmastectomy radiotherapy on cause-specific and overall survival was demonstrated among 1104 pT3N0 patients from the SEER database, although in patients younger than 40, a trend for benefit was observed [41].

Locoregional irradiation was demonstrated to improve long-term outcomes in two large randomized studies (EORTC 22922/10925 and MA.20) [42, 43]. Neither of these studies, however, demonstrated any aberrations from the generally observed trends in treatment efficacy in young patients. No effect of age was observed in the French study assessing the role of internal mammary node irradiation [44]. On the contrary, in the Danish prospective population study, in which only patients with right-sided tumors received internal mammary node irradiation, and which demonstrated an overall survival improvement from this procedure, an obvious trend for more relative benefit in younger age groups was observed, adding up to the generally higher absolute "background" risk of recurrence in these patients [45]. Interestingly, in a series of over 8000 patients enrolled in 13 randomized IBCSG trials, young age was a risk factor for chest wall and axillary, but not supraclavicular, failures [13].

Ductal carcinoma in situ (DCIS) is relatively infrequent in young women, being predominantly a screen-detected condition (most countries provide screening mammography from the age of 50), but, if observed, is associated with high local failure risk. Among 1607 women treated for DCIS in Ontario between 1994 and 2003 with breast-conserving surgery and radiotherapy, the 10-year cumulative local recurrence rate for patients younger than 45 years was 27%, significantly higher than for older age groups—for each year of increase in age, the local recurrence rate decreased by 4%. The use of tumor bed boost had no impact on tumor control. On multivariate analysis age less than 45 years was one of the strongest predictors of any local recurrence, invasive and non-

invasive [46]. In a series of 143 DCIS patients from William Beaumont Hospital in Royal Oak, Michigan, treated with BCT, at median follow-up of 19.3 years, the 20-year actuarial rate of recurrence in 31 patients ≤ 45 was 26.7%, including 20.4% of invasive recurrences. Most of recurrences (23.3%) occurred within the first 10 years after treatment [47]. A Rare Cancer Network study collected data on 373 DCIS patients ≤ 45. After median follow-up of 72 months, the local relapse-free survival was 63% for patients aged ≤ 39 years and 81% for those aged 40–45 years. Conservative surgery without adjuvant radiotherapy resulted in unacceptable 54% 10-year local recurrence rate. Adjuvant irradiation without tumor bed boost was associated with reduction in the risk of local relapse (28% 10-year local recurrence rate), and further improvement was seen it those given additional dose to the tumor bed (14% 10-year local recurrence rate)—$p < 0.0001$ (Fig. 8.3) [48].

8.3 Utilization of Radiotherapy in Young Breast Cancer Patients

In spite of generally higher risk of local failure, young patients seem to be the population most often exposed to suboptimal local treatments. In 317,596 patients from the US National Cancer Database, in the youngest age group (≤ 35 years), the adjusted odds ratio of having a mastectomy (versus patients aged 61–64) exceeded 2; higher frequency of mastectomy was also seen in other "younger" patients. Worryingly, young women treated with conservative surgery were less likely to receive radiation (OR 0.69 for women ≤ 35). On the contrary, the probability of receiving postmastectomy radiotherapy, both when indicated and when there were no indications for adjuvant irradiation, was higher among younger patients [49]. Reasons for underuse of radiation among younger women with breast cancer were explored in a cohort of 21,008 patients from the MarketScan Database. The only non-socioeconomic factor contributing to lower probability of receiving radiotherapy as part of BCT was having at least one child aged less than 7 years [50].

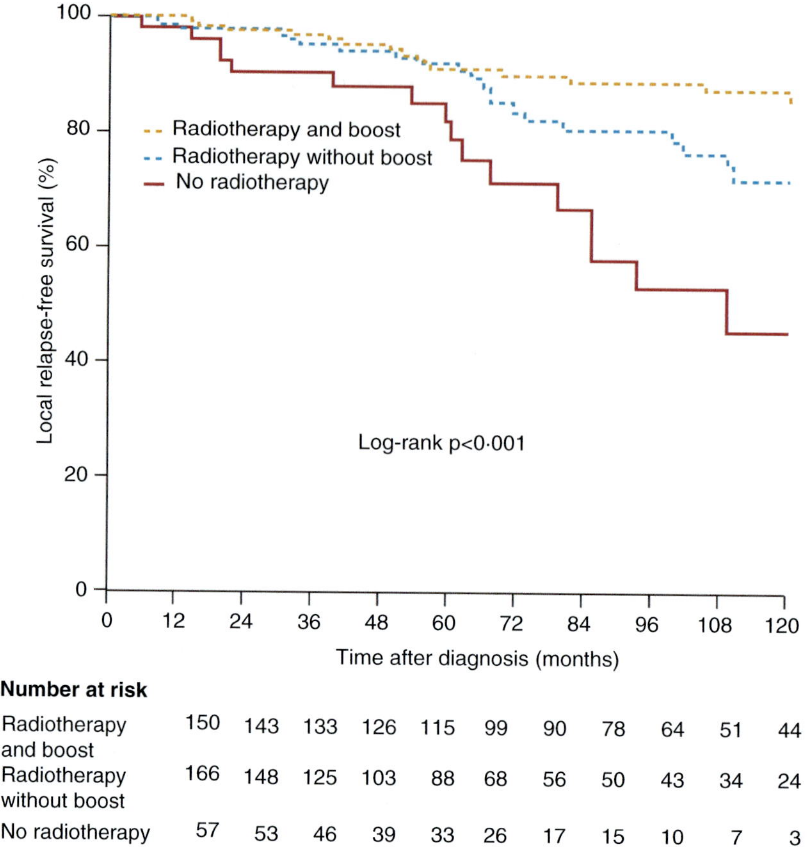

Fig. 8.3 Local relapse-free survival in young DCIS patients undergoing breast conservation by treatment group [48]

Number at risk

Radiotherapy and boost	150	143	133	126	115	99	90	78	64	51	44
Radiotherapy without boost	166	148	125	103	88	68	56	50	43	34	24
No radiotherapy	57	53	46	39	33	26	17	15	10	7	3

8.4 Complications of Radiotherapy in Young Breast Cancer Patients

Young women, due to expected long posttreatment survival, are also at larger risk of long-term treatment toxicities. Indeed, among the participants of the Women's Environmental, Cancer, and Radiation Epidemiology (WECARE) study, women <40 who received >1.0 Gy of absorbed dose to the correspondent quadrant of the contralateral breast had a 2.5-fold greater risk for contralateral breast cancer (CBC) than unexposed women; this risk increase was not observed in women >40 [51]. Similar observation was made in 7425 breast cancer survivors from two Dutch institutions. The risk of CBC was increased 1.5-fold in women <45 treated with postlumpectomy radiotherapy compared with those who had postmastectomy radiotherapy; this was explained by differences in radiation dose to the contralateral breast from direct electron field and tangential fields [52]. The relative risk of medially located CBC in this young population increased by 0.37 per each additional Gy of average radiation dose to the medial part of the contralateral breast [52].

A nonsignificant trend for increased risk of cardiovascular mortality among younger patient cohorts irradiated for cancer of the left breast was observed in the analysis of 308,861 US women from SEER cancer registries [53]. On the contrary, in the EORTC "boost" study, the only cohort which did not experience increased risk of severe fibrosis related to the administration of additional tumor bed dose was patients younger than 41 years [9].

8.5 Conclusions

Young patients are at increased risk of locoregional recurrence irrespective of type of surgery. Long-term outcomes after BCT are at least equal and possibly superior to mastectomy, which may be related to lesser use of radiotherapy in mastectomized patients. Age, as a risk factor for locoregional failure, should be taken into account when considering indications for postmastectomy or regional irradiation. However, as young patients may be at increased risk of long-term treatment toxicities of radiotherapy, meticulous care should be given to the use of optimal irradiation techniques.

References

1. Laurberg T, Alsner J, Tramm T, Jensen V, Lyngholm CD, Christiansen PM, Overgaard J. Impact of age, intrinsic subtype and local treatment on long-term local-regional recurrence and breast cancer mortality among low-risk breast cancer patients. Acta Oncol. 2017;56(1):59–67.
2. de Bock GH, van der Hage JA, Putter H, Bonnema J, Bartelink H, van de Velde CJ. Isolated locoregional recurrence of breast cancer is more common in young patients and following breast conserving therapy: long-term results of European Organisation for Research and Treatment of Cancer studies. Eur J Cancer. 2006;42(3):351–6.
3. Kim SW, Chun M, Han S, Jung YS, Choi JH, Kang SY, Yim H, Kang SH. Young age is associated with increased locoregional recurrence in node-positive breast cancer with luminal subtypes. Cancer Res Treat. 2017;49(2):484–93.
4. Braunstein LZ, Taghian AG, Niemierko A, Salama L, Capuco A, Bellon JR, Wong JS, Punglia RS, MacDonald SM, Harris JR. Breast-cancer subtype, age, and lymph node status as predictors of local recurrence following breast-conserving therapy. Breast Cancer Res Treat. 2017;161(1):173–9.
5. Arvold ND, Taghian AG, Niemierko A, Abi Raad RF, Sreedhara M, Nguyen PL, Bellon JR, Wong JS, Smith BL, Harris JR. Age, breast cancer subtype approximation, and local recurrence after breast-conserving therapy. J Clin Oncol. 2011;29(29):3885–91.
6. Harrold EV, Turner BC, Matloff ET, Pathare P, Beinfield M, McKhann C, Ward BA, Haffty BG. Local recurrence in the conservatively treated breast cancer patient: a correlation with age and family history. Cancer J Sci Am. 1998;4(5):302–7.
7. van der Leest M, Evers L, van der Sangen MJ, Poortmans PM, van de Poll-Franse LV, Vulto AJ, Nieuwenhuijzen GA, Brenninkmeijer SJ, Creemers GJ, Voogd AC. The safety of breast-conserving therapy in patients with breast cancer aged < or = 40 years. Cancer. 2007;109(10):1957–64.
8. van Laar C, van der Sangen MJ, Poortmans PM, Nieuwenhuijzen GA, Roukema JA, Roumen RM, Tjan-Heijnen VC, Voogd AC. Local recurrence following breast-conserving treatment in women aged 40 years or younger: trends in risk and the impact on prognosis in a population- based cohort of 1143 patients. Eur J Cancer. 2013;49(15):3093–101.
9. Bartelink H, Maingon P, Poortmans P, Weltens C, Fourquet A, Jager J, Schinagl D, Oei B, Rodenhuis C, Horiot JC, Struikmans H, Van Limbergen E, Kirova Y, Elkhuizen P, Bongartz R, Miralbell R, Morgan D, Dubois JB, Remouchamps V, Mirimanoff RO, Collette S, Collette L. European Organisation for Research and Treatment of Cancer Radiation Oncology and Breast Cancer Groups. Whole-breast irradiation with or without a boost for patients treated with breast-conserving surgery for early breast cancer: 20-year follow-up of a randomised phase 3 trial. Lancet Oncol. 2015;16(1):47–56.
10. Vrieling C, Collette L, Fourquet A, Hoogenraad WJ, Horiot JC, Jager JJ, Bing Oei S, Peterse HL, Pierart M, Poortmans PM, Struikmans H, Van den Bogaert W, Bartelink H, EORTC Radiotherapy, Breast Cancer Groups. Can patient-, treatment- and pathology-related characteristics explain the high local recurrence rate following breast-conserving therapy in young patients? Eur J Cancer. 2003;39(7):932–44.
11. Radosa JC, Eaton A, Stempel M, Khander A, Liedtke C, Solomayer EF, Karsten M, Pilewskie M, Morrow M, King TA. Evaluation of local and distant recurrence patterns in patients with triple-negative breast cancer according to age. Ann Surg Oncol. 2017;24(3):698–704.
12. Kent C, Horton J, Blitzblau R, Koontz BF. Whose disease will recur after mastectomy for early stage, node-negative breast cancer? A systematic review. Clin Breast Cancer. 2015;15(6):403–12.
13. Karlsson P, Cole BF, Chua BH, Price KN, Lindtner J, Collins JP, Kovács A, Thürlimann B, Crivellari D, Castiglione-Gertsch M, Forbes JF, Gelber RD, Goldhirsch A, Gruber G, International Breast Cancer Study Group. Patterns and risk factors for locoregional failures after mastectomy for breast cancer: an International Breast Cancer Study Group report. Ann Oncol. 2012;23(11):2852–8.
14. van der Sangen MJ, van de Wiel FM, Poortmans PM, Tjan-Heijnen VC, Nieuwenhuijzen GA, Roumen RM, Ernst MF, Tutein Nolthenius-Puylaert MC, Voogd AC. Are breast conservation and mastectomy equally effective in the treatment of young women with early breast cancer? Long-term results of a population-based cohort of 1,451 patients aged ≤40 years. Breast Cancer Res Treat. 2011;127(1):207–15.
15. Bantema-Joppe EJ, van den Heuvel ER, de Munck L, de Bock GH, Smit WG, Timmer PR, Dolsma WV, Jansen L, Schröder CP, Siesling S, Langendijk

JA, Maduro JH. Impact of primary local treatment on the development of distant metastases or death through locoregional recurrence in young breast cancer patients. Breast Cancer Res Treat. 2013;140(3):577–85.

16. Vila J, Gandini S, Gentilini O. Overall survival according to type of surgery in young (≤40 years) early breast cancer patients: a systematic meta-analysis comparing breast-conserving surgery versus mastectomy. Breast. 2015;24(3):175–81.

17. Ye JC, Yan W, Christos PJ, Nori D, Ravi A. Equivalent survival with mastectomy or breast-conserving surgery plus radiation in young women aged < 40 years with early-stage breast cancer: a national registry-based stage-by-stage comparison. Clin Breast Cancer. 2015;15(5):390–7.

18. Bantema-Joppe EJ, de Munck L, Visser O, Willemse PH, Langendijk JA, Siesling S, Maduro JH. Early-stage young breast cancer patients: impact of local treatment on survival. Int J Radiat Oncol Biol Phys. 2011;81(4):e553–9.

19. Kim HJ, Han W, Yi OV, Shin HC, Ahn SK, Koh BS, Moon HG, You JH, Son BH, Ahn SH, Noh DY. Young age is associated with ipsilateral breast tumor recurrence after breast conserving surgery and radiation therapy in patients with HER2-positive/ER-negative subtype. Breast Cancer Res Treat. 2011;130(2):499–505.

20. van der Sangen MJ, Poortmans PM, Scheepers SW, Lemaire BM, van Berlo CL, Tjan-Heijnen VC, Voogd AC. Prognosis following local recurrence after breast conserving treatment in young women with early breast cancer. Eur J Surg Oncol. 2013;39(8):892–8.

21. Courdi A, Doyen J, Gal J, Chamorey E. Local recurrence after breast cancer affects specific survival differently according to patient age. Oncology. 2010;79(5–6):349–54.

22. Miles RC, Gullerud RE, Lohse CM, Jakub JW, Degnim AC, Boughey JC. Local recurrence after breast-conserving surgery: multivariable analysis of risk factors and the impact of young age. Ann Surg Oncol. 2012;19(4):1153–9.

23. Guinot JL, Baixauli-Perez C, Soler P, Tortajada MI, Moreno A, Santos MA, Mut A, Gozalbo F, Arribas L. High-dose-rate brachytherapy boost effect on local tumor control in young women with breast cancer. Int J Radiat Oncol Biol Phys. 2015;91(1):165–71.

24. Senkus E, Kyriakides S, Ohno S, Penault-Llorca F, Poortmans P, Rutgers E, Zackrisson S, Cardoso F, ESMO Guidelines Committee. Primary breast cancer: ESMO Clinical Practice Guidelines for diagnosis, treatment and follow-up. Ann Oncol. 2015;26(Suppl 5):v8–30.

25. https://www.nccn.org/professionals/physician_gls/pdf/breast.pdf. Accessed 16 Jul 2017.

26. https://clinicaltrials.gov/ct2/show/NCT00212121. Accessed 16 Jul 2017.

27. Smith BD, Bellon JR, Blitzblau R, Freedman G, Haffty B, Hahn C, Halberg F, Hoffman K, Horst K, Moran J, Patton C, Perlmutter J, Warren L, Whelan T, Wright JL, Jagsi R. Radiation therapy for the whole breast: executive summary of an American Society for Radiation Oncology (ASTRO) evidence-based guideline. Pract Radiat Oncol. 2018;8(3):145–52.

28. Polgár C, Van Limbergen E, Pötter R, Kovács G, Polo A, Lyczek J, Hildebrandt G, Niehoff P, Guinot JL, Guedea F, Johansson B, Ott OJ, Major T, Strnad V. GEC-ESTRO breast cancer working group. patient selection for accelerated partial-breast irradiation (APBI) after breast-conserving surgery: recommendations of the Groupe Européen de Curiethérapie-European Society for Therapeutic Radiology and Oncology (GEC-ESTRO) breast cancer working group based on clinical evidence (2009). Radiother Oncol. 2010;94(3):264–73.

29. Correa C, Harris EE, Leonardi MC, Smith BD, Taghian AG, Thompson AM, White J, Harris JR. Accelerated partial breast irradiation: executive summary for the update of an ASTRO evidence-based consensus statement. Pract Radiat Oncol. 2017;7(2):73–9.

30. Shah C, Vicini F, Wazer DE, Arthur D, Patel RR. The American Brachytherapy Society consensus statement for accelerated partial breast irradiation. Brachytherapy. 2013;12(4):267–77.

31. Sato K, Mizuno Y, Fuchikami H, Kato M, Shimo T, Kubota J, Takeda N, Inoue Y, Seto H, Okawa T. Impact of young age on local control after partial breast irradiation in Japanese patients with early stage breast cancer. Breast Cancer. 2017;24(1):79–85.

32. Wenz F, Sperk E, Budach W, Dunst J, Feyer P, Fietkau R, Haase W, Harms W, Piroth MD, Sautter-Bihl ML, Sedlmayer F, Souchon R, Fussl C, Sauer R, Breast Cancer Expert Panel of the German Society of Radiation Oncology (DEGRO). DEGRO practical guidelines for radiotherapy of breast cancer IV: radiotherapy following mastectomy for invasive breast cancer. Strahlenther Onkol. 2014;190(8):705–14.

33. Recht A, Comen EA, Fine RE, Fleming GF, Hardenbergh PH, Ho AY, Hudis CA, Hwang ES, Kirshner JJ, Morrow M, Salerno KE, Sledge GW Jr, Solin LJ, Spears PA, Whelan TJ, Somerfield MR, Edge SB. Postmastectomy radiotherapy: an American Society of Clinical Oncology, American Society for Radiation Oncology, and Society of Surgical Oncology Focused Guideline Update. J Clin Oncol. 2016;34(36):4431–42.

34. Curigliano G, Burstein HJ, Winer EP, Gnant M, Dubsky P, Loibl S, Colleoni M, Regan M, Piccart-Gebhart M, Senn H-J, Thürlimann B, on behalf of the Panel Members of the St Gallen International Expert Consensus on the Primary Therapy of Early Breast Cancer 2017. De-escalating and escalating treatments for early stage breast cancer: the St. Gallen International Expert Consensus Conference on the Primary Therapy of Early Breast Cancer 2017. Ann Oncol. 2017;28(8):1700–12.

35. EBCTCG (Early Breast Cancer Trialists' Collaborative Group), McGale P, Taylor C, Correa C, Cutter D, Duane F, Ewertz M, Gray R, Mannu G, Peto R, Whelan T, Wang Y, Wang Z, Darby S. Effect of radiotherapy after mastectomy and axillary surgery on 10-year recurrence and 20-year breast can-

cer mortality: meta-analysis of individual patient data for 8135 women in 22 randomised trials. Lancet. 2014;383(9935):2127–35.

36. Quan ML, Osman F, McCready D, Fernandes K, Sutradhar R, Paszat L. Postmastectomy radiation and recurrence patterns in breast cancer patients younger than age 35 years: a population-based cohort. Ann Surg Oncol. 2014;21(2):395–400.

37. Garg AK, Oh JL, Oswald MJ, Huang E, Strom EA, Perkins GH, Woodward WA, Yu TK, Tereffe W, Meric-Bernstam F, Hahn K, Buchholz TA. Effect of postmastectomy radiotherapy in patients <35 years old with stage II–III breast cancer treated with doxorubicin-based neoadjuvant chemotherapy and mastectomy. Int J Radiat Oncol Biol Phys. 2007;69(5):1478–83.

38. Lammers EJ, Huibers P, van der Sangen MJ, van de Poll-Franse LV, Poortmans PM, Ernst MF, Lemaire BM, Meijs CM, Nuytinck HK, Voogd AC. Factors contributing to improved local control after mastectomy in patients with breast cancer aged 40 years or younger. Breast. 2010;19(1):44–9.

39. Yildirim E, Berberoglu U. Can a subgroup of node-negative breast carcinoma patients with T1-2 tumor who may benefit from postmastectomy radiotherapy be identified? Int J Radiat Oncol Biol Phys. 2007;68(4):1024–9.

40. Abi-Raad R, Boutrus R, Wang R, Niemierko A, Macdonald S, Smith B, Taghian AG. Patterns and risk factors of locoregional recurrence in T1-T2 node negative breast cancer patients treated with mastectomy: implications for postmastectomy radiotherapy. Int J Radiat Oncol Biol Phys. 2011;81(3):e151–7.

41. Yan W, Christos P, Nori D, Chao KS, Ravi A. Is there a cause-specific survival benefit of postmastectomy radiation therapy in women younger than age 50 with T3N0 invasive breast cancer? A SEER database analysis: outcomes by receptor status/race/age: analysis using the NCI Surveillance, Epidemiology, and End Results (SEER) database. Am J Clin Oncol. 2013;36(6):552–7.

42. Poortmans PM, Collette S, Kirkove C, Van Limbergen E, Budach V, Struikmans H, Collette L, Fourquet A, Maingon P, Valli M, De Winter K, Marnitz S, Barillot I, Scandolaro L, Vonk E, Rodenhuis C, Marsiglia H, Weidner N, van Tienhoven G, Glanzmann C, Kuten A, Arriagada R, Bartelink H, Van den Bogaert W, EORTC Radiation Oncology and Breast Cancer Groups. Internal mammary and medial supraclavicular irradiation in breast cancer. N Engl J Med. 2015;373(4):317–27.

43. Whelan TJ, Olivotto IA, Parulekar WR, Ackerman I, Chua BH, Nabid A, Vallis KA, White JR, Rousseau P, Fortin A, Pierce LJ, Manchul L, Chafe S, Nolan MC, Craighead P, Bowen J, McCready DR, Pritchard KI, Gelmon K, Murray Y, Chapman JA, Chen BE, Levine MN, MA.20 Study Investigators. Regional nodal irradiation in early-stage breast cancer. N Engl J Med. 2015;373(4):307–16.

44. Hennequin C, Bossard N, Servagi-Vernat S, Maingon P, Dubois JB, Datchary J, Carrie C, Roullet B, Suchaud JP, Teissier E, Lucardi A, Gerard JP, Belot A, Iwaz J, Ecochard R, Romestaing P. Ten-year survival results of a randomized trial of irradiation of internal mammary nodes after mastectomy. Int J Radiat Oncol Biol Phys. 2013;86(5):860–6.

45. Thorsen LB, Offersen BV, Danø H, Berg M, Jensen I, Pedersen AN, Zimmermann SJ, Brodersen HJ, Overgaard M, Overgaard J. DBCG-IMN: a population-based cohort study on the effect of internal mammary node irradiation in early node-positive breast cancer. J Clin Oncol. 2016;34(4):314–20.

46. Kong I, Narod SA, Taylor C, Paszat L, Saskin R, Nofech-Moses S, Thiruchelvam D, Hanna W, Pignol JP, Sengupta S, Elavathil L, Jani PA, Done SJ, Metcalfe S, Rakovitch E. Age at diagnosis predicts local recurrence in women treated with breast-conserving surgery and postoperative radiation therapy for ductal carcinoma in situ: a population-based outcomes analysis. Curr Oncol. 2014;21(1):e96–e104.

47. Vicini FA, Shaitelman S, Wilkinson JB, Shah C, Ye H, Kestin LL, Goldstein NS, Chen PY, Martinez AA. Long-term impact of young age at diagnosis on treatment outcome and patterns of failure in patients with ductal carcinoma in situ treated with breast-conserving therapy. Breast J. 2013;19(4):365–73.

48. Omlin A, Amichetti M, Azria D, Cole BF, Fourneret P, Poortmans P, Naehrig D, Miller RC, Krengli M, Gutierrez Miguelez C, Morgan D, Goldberg H, Scandolaro L, Gastelblum P, Ozsahin M, Dohr D, Christie D, Oppitz U, Abacioglu U, Gruber G. Boost radiotherapy in young women with ductal carcinoma in situ: a multicentre, retrospective study of the Rare Cancer Network. Lancet Oncol. 2006;7(8):652–6.

49. Freedman RA, Virgo KS, Labadie J, He Y, Partridge AH, Keating NL. Receipt of locoregional therapy among young women with breast cancer. Breast Cancer Res Treat. 2012;135(3):893–906.

50. Pan IW, Smith BD, Shih YC. Factors contributing to underuse of radiation among younger women with breast cancer. J Natl Cancer Inst. 2014;106(1):djt340.

51. Stovall M, Smith SA, Langholz BM, Boice JD Jr, Shore RE, Andersson M, Buchholz TA, Capanu M, Bernstein L, Lynch CF, Malone KE, Anton-Culver H, Haile RW, Rosenstein BS, Reiner AS, Thomas DC, Bernstein JL, Women's Environmental, Cancer, and Radiation Epidemiology Study Collaborative Group. Dose to the contralateral breast from radiotherapy and risk of second primary breast cancer in the WECARE study. Int J Radiat Oncol Biol Phys. 2008;72(4):1021–30.

52. Hooning MJ, Aleman BM, Hauptmann M, Baaijens MH, Klijn JG, Noyon R, Stovall M, van Leeuwen FE. Roles of radiotherapy and chemotherapy in the development of contralateral breast cancer. J Clin Oncol. 2008;26(34):5561–8.

53. Darby SC, McGale P, Taylor CW, Peto R. Long-term mortality from heart disease and lung cancer after radiotherapy for early breast cancer: prospective cohort study of about 300,000 women in US SEER cancer registries. Lancet Oncol. 2005;6(8):557–65.

Timing and Type of Breast Reconstruction in Young Breast Cancer Patients

Rosa Di Micco and Oreste Gentilini

9.1 Background

The time a young breast cancer patient spends from the diagnosis to the end of treatment usually covers a limited period of her lifetime compared to the remaining part of her life when the healthy woman has to deal with the fear of recurrence and the aesthetic outcome of breast cancer surgery.

Breast reconstruction is an important component in the final recovery of many breast cancer patients and is a main contributor to the quality of life of the post-breast cancer patient. An unreconstructed mastectomy defect as well as a poorly executed reconstruction may serve as a constant reminder of the previous cancer. Therefore, the more aesthetic and natural a reconstructed breast appears and feels, the more completely a breast cancer patient will recover. Blondeel et al. [1] have masterfully explained how to surgically create an attractive breast through a reproducible three-step principle based on three important anatomical entities of the breast:

- The footprint, or the interface of the posterior surface of the breast with the thoracic wall;
- the conus of the breast, or the principal shape and volume made up by the mammary gland in normal breasts;
- the envelope of the breast consisting of the skin and subcutaneous fat.

The systematic approach for recreating the female breast after mastectomy consists of creating the breast footprint on the chest wall, placing a proper conus on the footprint and re-draping the appropriate skin envelope over the conus [2].

The appropriate timing and type of breast reconstruction are considerations in young as well as in older breast cancer patients. However young women have different physiologic and psychological characteristics than older ones, requiring a specific therapeutic approach both in the therapeutic and reconstructive phases. Young breast cancer patients have a more youthful breast structure and are generally in good health; thus the full spectrum of reconstructive options should be offered. Nevertheless, various factors can influence a young woman's decision about reconstructive techniques such as finding a life partner, planning a family, beginning a career or having a highly active lifestyle. Furthermore, young patients are often well informed about prognosis, risk factors and surgical alternatives, as well as more willing to ask for mastectomy in lieu of breast-conserving therapy believing it to

R. Di Micco
Breast Unit, San Raffaele University and Research Hospital, Milan, Italy

Department of Clinical Medicine and Surgery, University of Naples Federico II, Naples, Italy
e-mail: dimicco.rosa@hsr.it

O. Gentilini (✉)
Breast Unit, San Raffaele University and Research Hospital, Milan, Italy
e-mail: gentilini.oreste@hsr.it

© Springer Nature Switzerland AG 2020
O. Gentilini et al. (eds.), *Breast Cancer in Young Women*,
https://doi.org/10.1007/978-3-030-24762-1_9

be a more definitive risk reduction strategy [3]. The role of the surgical oncologist is to recommend the surgical procedure which best suits the individual patient's situation from the oncological perspective; if mastectomy is required, he/she will explain whether mastectomy will be radical or modified radical and whether skin and eventually the nipple-areola complex can be spared. In this preoperative phase, a first discussion about timing could be started; the surgeon could illustrate the possibility of an immediate or a delayed breast reconstruction according to the breast cancer staging, the eventual need for adjuvant radiotherapy and chemotherapy.

Subsequently, all the options of the reconstructive repertoire will be discussed with the patient choosing the technique which best suits her according to her comorbidities, body characteristics, personal habits and activities, as well as smoking and drug abuse, along with specific complications and disadvantages.

The choice of the most appropriate breast reconstruction is based on oncological needs, surgeon's advice and patient's desire and should always be discussed in a multidisciplinary setting.

9.2 Timing of Breast Reconstruction

Breast reconstruction can be performed as an immediate procedure, at the time of mastectomy, or as a delayed procedure, after adjuvant chemotherapy and/or radiotherapy. As an alternative, the immediate-delayed procedure provides an immediate reconstruction with a temporary implant, and after an average 6-month period from the end of adjuvant treatment (chemotherapy and/or radiotherapy), a definitive implant or an autologous flap can replace the expander.

Several factors impact the choice and timing of breast reconstruction. Immediate breast reconstruction should be reserved for patients with stage I or II disease who are at low risk of requiring post-mastectomy radiotherapy (PMRT). The aesthetic outcomes of immediate reconstruction are superior to those of delayed reconstruction due to the retention of the natural skin enve-

lope and, eventually, of the nipple-areola complex. However, when PMRT is planned, delayed reconstruction with total autologous reconstruction remains the gold standard whenever possible; otherwise immediate-delayed reconstruction with temporary implant placed at the time of mastectomy usually results in less complication than radiating a definitive implant, although this issue remains controversial [4, 5].

9.2.1 Immediate Reconstruction

The majority of women undergoing mastectomy for breast cancer are eligible for immediate breast reconstruction (IBR), but reconstruction rates remain low, less than 15% in all but the most specialized cancer centres around the world due to patient-related and adjuvant therapy-related factors as well as clinician beliefs [6]. Young breast cancer patients are more motivated than their older counterparts to receive IBR, willing to preserve their body image at the expense of a higher complication rate and a more complex surgery [3]. IBR can be based both on implant placement and autologous reconstruction; the surgeon and the patient will decide together which type of reconstruction suits better the single case. PMRT is traditionally regarded as a contraindication to IBR with implants due to a three-time higher rate of implant-related complications (i.e. capsular contracture, infection, fibrosis), resulting in poor aesthetic outcome [7]. However, recent studies demonstrate that immediate implant-based reconstruction in the setting of PMRT, despite imperfect results, shows acceptable aesthetic outcomes and complication rates, with a high level of patient satisfaction and low decisional regret [8]. Similarly, autologous reconstruction can suffer from a higher rate of complications (i.e. fat necrosis, flap contracture, skin fibrosis) but still lower than implant-based breast reconstruction followed by PMRT [9]. At the time of mastectomy, both definitive and temporary implants can be placed; according to the local conditions and the surgeon's evaluation, in cases when a temporary implant is placed, a second procedure is mandatory to complete the breast reconstruction (see Sect. 2.3).

9.2.2 Delayed Reconstruction

Delayed breast reconstruction is performed in a separate stage after mastectomy, requiring complete wound healing at the end of the adjuvant treatment (not including hormonal therapy). It can be offered as an alternative to immediate reconstruction, particularly when PMRT is planned, in order to reduce the complication rate after RT, whilst it is still mandatory in cases of inflammatory breast cancer [10, 11]. However, more recent data on immediate reconstruction in cases of inflammatory breast cancer suggest that this opportunity could be offered in selected cases, despite a higher complication rate, with no difference in survival [12, 13]. The routine practice is to wait at least 30–40 days from the end of chemotherapy and 6 months from radiotherapy. Autologous tissue reconstruction allows for replacement of irradiated skin and a more natural-appearing, ptotic breast [13]. Tissue expander-based reconstruction is avoided after radiation therapy because of the high risk of wound healing problems and capsular contracture, with its associated pain and physical deformity [14]. However if implant-based reconstruction is preferred, even after PMRT, nourishing the mastectomy site with several sessions of lipofilling before placing the implant, or transferring normal, nonirradiated tissue to the breast, even if to cover an implant, reduces the complication rate and the rate of reconstruction failure [14].

9.2.3 Delayed-Immediate Reconstruction

Delayed-immediate reconstruction is always feasible and represents a two-step procedure to reconstruct the breast immediately with a temporary implant (i.e. a tissue expander) and then, after a period of inflation, to complete the reconstructive phase with a definitive implant or autologous tissue. The tissue expander for the breast was developed in the setting of total mastectomy where no skin was available at the end of the oncological procedure to cover the definitive implant. Today, the indications for the expander placement are extended: to all cases when the skin available is not enough to reconstruct a large-sized breast; when skin flap viability, pectoralis muscle coverage or generally local conditions at the end of the mastectomy are not safe enough to support the placement of a definitive implant; in most centres, when PMRT is planned; and when choice between implant-based and autologous reconstruction is not clear yet. The placement of a tissue expander can give more time to the patient and/or the surgeon to decide while preserving the skin spared during the primary surgery [8, 15, 16].

9.3 Type of Breast Reconstruction

The choice of the most suitable type of breast reconstruction is mainly based on optimal patient selection. The young breast cancer patient usually has a wider choice compared to the older counterpart, but each technique should match her clinical history, physical characteristics and personal desire. In general, there are two types of breast reconstruction:

- Autologous reconstruction requiring that tissue coming from the same patient is utilized to reconstruct the breast;
- Implant-based reconstruction implying that a prosthesis is used to rebuild the breast volume.

In any kind of breast reconstruction, each patient should be informed that the final result cannot be achieved after one single operation; it represents indeed, a pathway towards the restoration of the body image and could require secondary corrections. The goal of the first operation, regardless of which technique is used, is to obtain a basic shape, and later, the reconstructed breast can be ameliorated, with nipple reconstruction, scar revision, volume adjustments or shape corrections, and the contralateral breast is made symmetric, if not done before [2].

9.3.1 Implant-Based Breast Reconstruction

In the USA approximately 80% of reconstructions are performed using prosthetic devices, with the vast majority performed immediately at the time of mastectomy [17, 18]. The vast majority of patients, including young breast cancer patients, have successful implant-based reconstructions and an overall quicker recovery compared with autologous reconstruction. However, infections occur at a higher rate than with most elective surgery procedures. An ongoing debate concerns the best approach to implant-based reconstruction, i.e. whether it should be a one-stage (direct to implant) or a two-stage (tissue expander and then implant) procedure. Advocates for the one-stage technique emphasize a low revision rate, fewer operations, reduced overall cost and excellent patient satisfaction [19–21]. On the other side, advocates for the two-stage technique highlight the improved patient satisfaction based on recontouring and selecting an ideal prosthesis for the second procedure, reduced capsular contracture in the setting of PMRT, a lower unplanned revision rate and excellent patient outcomes [22, 23]. Success with either technique is ultimately based on proper patient selection, surgical technique and surgeon's experience. Therefore, it is mandatory to be clear with patients that smoking, diabetes, obesity or vascular diseases can increase the complication rates [19, 22].

A *definitive implant* can be placed when there are enough skin and good muscle coverage; this means that in IBR a conservative mastectomy should be performed; thus the skin as well as total or partial muscle coverage should be available. These conditions are common in small-breasted patients. As the breast volume or ptosis increases, when a conservative mastectomy is performed, the only possibility to have an immediate implant-based reconstruction is to use an acellular dermal matrix (ADM) or mesh in order to complete the muscular pocket inferiorly and grant good implant coverage of the lower pole ptosis or, alternatively, place the implant pre-pectorally by using specific porcine dermal matrices [19, 24–26]. As a second choice,

a delayed-immediate breast reconstruction can be realized by placing a *tissue expander* at the time of mastectomy (or later in cases when a delayed implant-based reconstruction is desired) and then replacing the temporary implant with a definitive one at least 6 months after the end of radiotherapy or chemotherapy or 1 month after the completion of expansion when no adjuvant treatment is planned. The second stage usually allows for: precise positioning of the inframammary fold; capsulotomy to release soft tissue, thus increasing breast projection and ptosis; and re-evaluation of the breast height and width to achieve maximal symmetry with the contralateral breast [22]. In some selected cases, a definitive expander can be placed at the time of primary surgery and then filled with saline or air, and once the ideal volume has been reached, the injection port is removed under local anaesthesia [27].

Describing in depth the surgical techniques by which implant-based breast reconstruction can be performed is beyond the scope of this chapter; however some data on last-generation devices available could interest the reader in order to offer the young breast cancer patient the widest choice possible. US data on implant-based reconstruction show that in the vast majority of cases, ADMs are used. Current innovations in the ever-changing landscape of implant-based breast reconstruction can be summarized into two types of devices: *biologic and synthetic mesh*. Biologic meshes include human-derived ADM (i.e. AlloDerm, Megaderm, hMatrix, DermaMatrix, DermACELL, etc.) and nonhuman sources called xenografts, derived from porcine dermis, foetal bovine dermis or bovine pericardium (i.e. Braxon, Permacol, Protexa, Strattice, SurgiMend, Tutomesh, Veritas, etc.) [28]. Despite the large plethora of processing differences, outcome parity is frequently encountered in both comparative and single-cohort study [29, 30]. The only randomized controlled trial on ADMs, the BREASTrial, showed no significant difference in complication rates between two different ADMs. Synthetic meshes include permanent meshes (i.e. TiLOOP Bra, a titanium-coated polypropylene mesh) or absorbable meshes (i.e. Vicryl Mesh, SERI scaffold,

TIGR Matrix). The only randomized controlled trial comparing synthetic and biologic mesh in the IBR setting found a similar complication rate, with higher rates of severe complications and failure in the ADM cohort [31]. A recent systematic review by Cabalag et al. [32] suggests the use of ADM to expand the submuscular pocket both in a single-stage setting, where direct-to-implant breast reconstruction is facilitated with an improved cosmesis and a better definition of the inframammary fold, and in the two-stage setting to shorten the expansion time. However, in the ADM-assisted single-stage procedure, the overall complication rate is lower than in the traditional two-stage submuscular approach, despite an increased rate of mastectomy flap necrosis [19, 33, 34]. Conversely, in ADM-assisted two-stage expander-to-implant reconstruction, the outcomes are inferior due to a higher rate of seroma, infection and mastectomy flap necrosis when compared to non-ADM two-stage reconstruction [35–37]. To date, differences in sourcing and processing of matrices seem less important than technique and experience of the surgeon using them. There is some evidence suggesting that ADM may ameliorate capsular contracture; the reported protective effects of ADMs in irradiated tissue are inconsistent [28, 32].

9.3.2 Autologous Breast Reconstruction

Tissue for autologous breast reconstruction can be harvested from different sites with different degrees of complexity according to the individual patient's body habitus and fat deposits. The breast volume can be restored through fat grafting, using pedicled flaps or free flaps according to local and systemic conditions as well as patient expectations. Compared to implant-based reconstruction, autologous reconstruction provides a soft, warm, pliable breast which follows natural changes of the body (i.e. weight gain/loss, ptosis, etc.). Despite requiring more complex or multiple surgeries, longer time and higher risks to achieve final results, autologous breast reconstruction

reliably maintains its original characteristics over time and ensures long-lasting outcomes which could be more appealing for young breast cancer patients. In the UK report from 2007 to 2014, the use of free flap procedures increased from 17 to 21%, while pedicled flap use decreased from 50 to 22% of all IBR [16].

Once a patient's preference for autologous reconstruction is assessed, the donor site tissue suitability is fundamental in the decision-making process. The available donor site tissues must be tested on the abdomen, buttock or inner thigh through the "pinch test" [38] in order to guide operative planning and select the patient according to her wishes, risk factors and specific complications, the setting in which the surgeon works, resources available and the surgeon's technical expertise.

9.3.2.1 Fat Grafting

Fat grafting is a available tool in breast surgery, having an important role both in breast-conserving surgery to treat cosmetic sequelae, and in breast reconstruction as a complement to refine the aesthetic result, as well as in pure aesthetic surgery [39, 40]. The total breast reconstruction with fat grafts appears as the ideal reconstructive technique, being easy to perform, with low impact on the patient's body integrity besides being reproducible, fully autologous and with minimal scars and a low complication rate along with the additional benefit of liposuction. However, it is a multiple-stage surgery and usually requires balancing of the contralateral breast. It can be offered alone when the breast envelope has been preserved or after skin expansion with tissue expander, BRAVA system, or with abdominal advancement flap [41–45]. The ideal candidate is a patient with small- to moderate-sized breasts and enough donor sites, motivated to undergo four to five lipomodelling sessions, even more for previously irradiated breasts. Good results are derived from appropriate patient selection and greater surgical experience with fat grafting. Over time, enthusiasm for this technique has decreased, and it appears suitable only for very selected patients who accept multiple surgeries and are not willing or suitable for other surgery.

9.3.2.2 Pedicled Flaps

- Latissimus Dorsi (LD) Flap: is the historical myocutaneous flap used for autologous breast reconstruction since the 1970s, because it is simple to harvest and safe, both in partial and total breast reconstruction, similarly in primary and secondary surgery [46, 47]. Currently, the standard LD is not the first choice in breast reconstruction and is less and less used as a single procedure as it represents the lifeboat to fallback procedure when other types of reconstruction have failed. An ideal candidate for LD flap is a lady with small breast volume and excess tissue laterally and upwards across the midback. LD flap volume can be increased by harvesting an "extended" LD flap, lipofilling the flap before insetting or adding an implant or tissue expander [48–50]. However, the quality of the aesthetic result can at times be less than desired and complications at the donor site can be troublesome [51]. In particular, young patients should be informed of the extra scarring on the back and functional impairment on the shoulder and arm that LD flap limits in some activities such as mountain climbing, skiing and swimming [52].

- More recent muscle-sparing LD flaps [53–55] and pedicled perforator flaps deriving from the same area, i.e. thoracodorsal artery perforator (TAP) [56, 57], lateral thoracic artery perforator (LTAP) [58] and lateral intercostal artery perforator (LICAP) [59], being muscle and nerve sparing could lead to less morbidity. Nevertheless, sparing the muscle means also decreasing the flap volume, so they are mainly utilized in partial rather than in total breast reconstruction, where additional autologous or prosthetic volume is required.

- Transverse Rectus Abdominis Myocutaneous (TRAM) Flap is another historical myocutaneous flap to be used after radical mastectomy in order to restore breast volume at the expense of weakening the abdominal wall [60]. This flap, despite being safe and easy to harvest, yields a high rate of donor site complication (i.e. abdominal hernia or bulge, fat necrosis, flap loss) [61]. For these reasons, TRAM flap should not be recommended as the first choice in young breast cancer patients, and it is losing ground in favour of muscle-sparing and free TRAM flaps. However, it still remains a good option of autologous reconstruction, particularalry if delayed, in centres where microsurgical expertise is not common yet and the ideal candidates remain obese, active smokers, previously irradiated patients who are also good candidates to abdominoplasty [62].

9.3.2.3 Free Flaps

- Deep Inferior Epigastric Artery Perforator (DIEAP) currently represents the gold standard of autologous breast reconstruction in breast centres where microsurgery is performed [63]. This flap offers the patient the same advantages as the TRAM flap and discards the most important disadvantages of the myocutaneous flap by preserving the continuity of the rectus muscle and so granting a higher abdominal physical well-being according to patient-reported outcomes [64]. The donor site morbidity is reduced, a sensate reinnervation is possible, postoperative pain is less, recovery is quicker and hospital stay is reduced. The more complex nature of this type of surgery, leading to increased operating time, is balanced by the more permanent and gratifying results achieved [65, 66]. Nevertheless the advantages and cost-effectiveness of this surgery are evident only when patients are carefully selected based on perforator anatomy and surgery is performed by experienced surgeons [67]. Most women who have had or will have mastectomy are possible candidates for a DIEAP flap, provided that a good donor site is available, and also larger breast volume can be rebuilt. Absolute contraindications are very rare: previous abdominoplasty or abdominal liposuction or active smoking. Relative contraindications include large abdominal incisions, and preoperative angio-CT is mandatory to assess the presence and location of perforator vessels [68, 69]. This flap can be offered both in immediate and delayed reconstruction, as first or second choice after previous failure or expander placement. If additional volume is required, a "stacked" DIEAP flap can be harvested or an implant can be added underneath [70, 71]. Of course, this flap requires longer and more complex surgery, but in high-volume centres and in expert hands, results could be excellent, with a flap failure rate less than 2% [65, 66, 72]. Significantly higher risks of complications (flap necrosis, fat necrosis, delayed wound healing, donor site morbidity) are associated with age, BMI, immediate reconstruction, bilateral procedures and radiation [64].

- Superficial Inferior Epigastric Artery (SIEA) Flap is raised from the same donor site of DIEAP but on a different vascular pedicle. However, despite minor donor site morbidity and a quicker harvesting, it is still less frequently performed due to the low reliability of its vascular pedicle being of sufficient calibre in 24–70% of patients [73]. The current use of preoperative imaging has promoted the use of the SIEA flap in selected cases when vascular anatomy is compatible with free tissue transfer [72].

When the abdomen is not viable as a donor for autologous reconstruction, the second flap of choice has to be found in buttock and thigh flaps, always according to surgeon's preference and patient's anatomy.

- Superior Gluteal Artery Perforator (SGAP) Flap is suitable for both uni- and bilateral breast reconstruction due to its consistency, volume and reliable anatomy. Ideal candidates are patients with breast weight of 200–600 g. However, the contour defect produced in the upper buttock could be significant, the scar is difficult to hide and in a thin patient there is a loss of padding [74].
- Inferior Gluteal Artery Perforator (IGAP) Flap is similarly a good flap for breast reconstruction. The ideal candidate is someone with saddlebag deformity, since body contour would be improved with the surgery. The scar is well concealed in the natural depression of the inferior gluteal crease and the round shape of the buttock is preserved. The displeasing sensation of sitting on the scar must be considered, and there is a slight increase in the risk of dehiscence and injury of the posterior femoral cutaneous and sciatic nerve [75].
- Profunda Artery Perforator (PAP) Flap provides soft and pliable tissue from a relatively plentiful donor site even in those patients with inadequate abdominal tissue. The scar is well hidden in the gluteal crease, and this flap allows the surgeon to rebuild a volume of 300–400 g with some limitation in large-breasted women. The skin paddle, due to its location, tends to be slightly darker in pigmentation when compared to breast skin, which could impact in delayed reconstruction where no breast skin is available any more and the flap needs to be inset with its own skin. Due to its versatility and effectiveness, it is currently the second choice flap in several centres where microsurgical autologous reconstruction is routinely performed [72, 76].

- Transverse Myocutaneous Gracilis (TMG) or Transverse Upper Gracilis (TUG) Flaps are two myocutaneous flaps taking the whole or the upper part of the gracilis muscle, respectively. They are a good and reliable alternative in autologous breast reconstruction, being easier to harvest even for less experienced microsurgeons. Donor site morbidity is minimal and the resulting scar is well hidden as in a thigh lift. However, perforator flaps are more and more preferred due to the absence of muscle sacrifice, lower complication rate and improving learning curve of breast microsurgeons [76, 77].
- Lumbar Artery Perforator (LAP) Flap is a promising alternative to the gluteal flaps, even in lean patients, as it takes advantage of the fatty tissue of the "love handles" overlying the iliac crest and the buttock area where fair amounts of tissue can be harvested. The scar and the donor site can be hidden and do not distort the contour, as this is essentially the same area routinely excised in a traditional buttock lift. This is one of the newest types of perforator flaps for breast reconstruction and is performed in very few centres, yet [78–81].

Other alternative flaps like septocutaneous tensor fascia latae (TFL), deep circumflex iliac artery (DCIA) and anterolateral thigh (ALT) are only occasionally used.

9.3.3 Composite Breast Reconstruction

The wording "composite breast reconstruction" has been recently reported to define a composite approach in breast reconstruction where an implant is used in combination with fat grafting. This technique can not only lower the volume and surface area of foreign material (the prosthesis) but also transform the implant-based reconstruction into a more natural looking breast with less visible and palpable implant edges. Additionally, adding fat allows changing the position of the implant to a more prepectoral position as the subcutaneous layers of the mastectomy flaps can be thickened by grafted fat. This is a variation on the two-stage implant-based breast reconstruction, as the expander is placed in the primary procedure, then inflated and step-by step deflated as long as mastectomy flaps are lipofilled. During the last lipofilling section, the expander is removed and a small implant placed to provide extra projection, volume and shape [82]. Results are very encouraging; indeed many centres were already combining fat grafting and implant-based reconstruction, defining this reconstructive system as "hybrid breast reconstruction", being both autologous and implant-based [83].

Presently, based on the evidence reported, surgeons contemplating breast reconstruction on a young breast cancer patient should consider the following: patient's preferences, cancer prognosis and risk factors; the setting in which the surgeon works; resources available; the evidence avaiable; and, equally important, the surgeon's technical expertise.

Despite the limited good-quality data regarding the impact of radiation therapy on complication rates between the different types of autologous reconstruction, radiation therapy is known to affect the complication rates in the setting of any type of reconstruction, but, if feasible, autologous breast reconstruction gives better outcomes. A multidisciplinary approach is the key in planning breast reconstruction after mastectomy; preoperative multidisciplinary meeting and optimal patient's selection are of paramount importance to discuss all the alternatives and choose the best options to offer the individual patient.

References

1. Blondeel PN, et al. Shaping the breast in aesthetic and reconstructive breast surgery: an easy three-step principle. Plast Reconstr Surg. 2009;123(2):455–62.
2. Blondeel PN, et al. Shaping the breast in aesthetic and reconstructive breast surgery: an easy three-step principle. Part II--breast reconstruction after total mastectomy. Plast Reconstr Surg. 2009;123(3):794–805.
3. Ellsworth WA, et al. Breast reconstruction in women under 30: a 10-year experience. Breast J. 2011;17(1):18–23.
4. Cordeiro PG, et al. Irradiation after immediate tissue expander/implant breast reconstruction: outcomes, complications, aesthetic results, and satisfaction among 156 patients. Plast Reconstr Surg. 2004;113(3):877–81.
5. Cowen D, et al. Immediate post-mastectomy breast reconstruction followed by radiotherapy: risk factors for complications. Breast Cancer Res Treat. 2010;121(3):627–34.
6. Brennan ME, Spillane AJ. Uptake and predictors of post-mastectomy reconstruction in women with breast malignancy--systematic review. Eur J Surg Oncol. 2013;39(6):527–41.
7. Barry M, Kell MR. Radiotherapy and breast reconstruction: a meta-analysis. Breast Cancer Res Treat. 2011;127(1):15–22.
8. Brennan ME, et al. Immediate expander/implant breast reconstruction followed by post-mastectomy radiotherapy for breast cancer: aesthetic, surgical, satisfaction and quality of life outcomes in women with high-risk breast cancer. Breast. 2016;30:59–65.
9. Clarke-Pearson EM, et al. Comparison of irradiated versus nonirradiated DIEP flaps in patients undergoing immediate bilateral DIEP reconstruction with unilateral postmastectomy radiation therapy (PMRT). Ann Plast Surg. 2013;71(3):250–4.
10. Costa SD, et al. Neoadjuvant chemotherapy shows similar response in patients with inflammatory or locally advanced breast cancer when compared with operable breast cancer: a secondary analysis of the GeparTrio trial data. J Clin Oncol. 2010;28(1):83–91.
11. Dawood S, et al. International expert panel on inflammatory breast cancer: consensus statement for standardized diagnosis and treatment. Ann Oncol. 2011;22(3):515–23.
12. Patel SA, et al. Immediate breast reconstruction for women having inflammatory breast cancer in the United States. Cancer Med. 2018;7:2887.
13. Simpson AB, et al. Immediate reconstruction in inflammatory breast cancer: challenging current care. Ann Surg Oncol. 2016;23(Suppl 5):642–8.
14. Chang DW, Barnea Y, Robb GL. Effects of an autologous flap combined with an implant for breast reconstruction: an evaluation of 1000 consecutive reconstructions of previously irradiated breasts. Plast Reconstr Surg. 2008;122(2):356–62.

15. Kronowitz SJ. Delayed-immediate breast reconstruction: technical and timing considerations. Plast Reconstr Surg. 2010;125(2):463–74.
16. Mennie JC, et al. National trends in immediate and delayed post-mastectomy reconstruction procedures in England: a seven-year population-based cohort study. Eur J Surg Oncol. 2017;43(1):52–61.
17. Albornoz CR, et al. A paradigm shift in U.S. breast reconstruction: increasing implant rates. Plast Reconstr Surg. 2013;131(1):15–23.
18. Cemal Y, et al. A paradigm shift in U.S. breast reconstruction: part 2. The influence of changing mastectomy patterns on reconstructive rate and method. Plast Reconstr Surg. 2013;131(3):320e–6e.
19. Salzberg CA, et al. An 8-year experience of direct-to-implant immediate breast reconstruction using human acellular dermal matrix (AlloDerm). Plast Reconstr Surg. 2011;127(2):514–24.
20. Colwell AS. Direct-to-implant breast reconstruction. Gland Surg. 2012;1(3):139–41.
21. Colwell AS, et al. Breast reconstruction following nipple-sparing mastectomy: predictors of complications, reconstruction outcomes, and 5-year trends. Plast Reconstr Surg. 2014;133(3):496–506.
22. Pusic AL, Cordeiro PG. Breast reconstruction with tissue expanders and implants: a practical guide to immediate and delayed reconstruction. Semin Plast Surg. 2004;18(2):71–7.
23. Spear SL, et al. Two-stage prosthetic breast reconstruction using AlloDerm including outcomes of different timings of radiotherapy. Plast Reconstr Surg. 2012;130(1):1–9.
24. Reitsamer R, Peintinger F. Prepectoral implant placement and complete coverage with porcine acellular dermal matrix: a new technique for direct-to-implant breast reconstruction after nipple-sparing mastectomy. J Plast Reconstr Aesthet Surg. 2015;68(2):162–7.
25. Antony AK, et al. Acellular human dermis implantation in 153 immediate two-stage tissue expander breast reconstructions: determining the incidence and significant predictors of complications. Plast Reconstr Surg. 2010;125(6):1606–14.
26. Winters ZE, Colwell AS. Role of acellular dermal matrix-assisted implants in breast reconstruction. Br J Surg. 2014;101(5):444–5.
27. Becker H, Zhadan O. Filling the Spectrum expander with air-a new alternative. Plast Reconstr Surg Glob Open. 2017;5(10):e1541.
28. Kim JYS, Mlodinow AS. What's new in acellular dermal matrix and soft-tissue support for prosthetic breast reconstruction. Plast Reconstr Surg. 2017;140(5S Advances in Breast Reconstruction):30S–43S.
29. Cheng A, Saint-Cyr M. Comparison of different ADM materials in breast surgery. Clin Plast Surg. 2012;39(2):167–75.
30. Hinchcliff KM, et al. Comparison of two cadaveric acellular dermal matrices for immediate breast reconstruction: a prospective randomized trial. J Plast Reconstr Aesthet Surg. 2017;70(5):568–76.
31. Gschwantler-Kaulich D, et al. Mesh versus acellular dermal matrix in immediate implant-based breast reconstruction – a prospective randomized trial. Eur J Surg Oncol. 2016;42(5):665–71.
32. Cabalag MS, et al. Alloplastic adjuncts in breast reconstruction. Gland Surg. 2016;5(2):158–73.
33. Macadam SA, Lennox PA. Acellular dermal matrices: use in reconstructive and aesthetic breast surgery. Can J Plast Surg. 2012;20(2):75–89.
34. Jansen LA, Macadam SA. The use of AlloDerm in postmastectomy alloplastic breast reconstruction: part I. A systematic review. Plast Reconstr Surg. 2011;127(6):2232–44.
35. Kim JY, et al. A meta-analysis of human acellular dermis and submuscular tissue expander breast reconstruction. Plast Reconstr Surg. 2012;129(1):28–41.
36. Hoppe IC, et al. Complications following expander/implant breast reconstruction utilizing acellular dermal matrix: a systematic review and meta-analysis. Eplasty. 2011;11:e40.
37. Sbitany H, Serletti JM. Acellular dermis-assisted prosthetic breast reconstruction: a systematic and critical review of efficacy and associated morbidity. Plast Reconstr Surg. 2011;128(6):1162–9.
38. Alamouti R, Hachach Haram N, Farhadi J. A novel grading system to assess donor site suitability in autologous breast reconstruction. J Plast Reconstr Aesthet Surg. 2015;68(6):e129–30.
39. Delay E, Guerid S. The role of fat grafting in breast reconstruction. Clin Plast Surg. 2015;42(3):315–23. vii
40. Hitier M, et al. Tolerance and efficacy of lipomodelling as an element of breast symmetry in breast reconstruction. Ann Chir Plast Esthet. 2014;59(5):311–9.
41. Delay E, Delaporte T, Sinna R. Breast implant alternatives. Ann Chir Plast Esthet. 2005;50(5):652–72.
42. Delay E, Meruta AC, Guerid S. Indications and controversies in total breast reconstruction with lipomodeling. Clin Plast Surg. 2018;45(1):111–7.
43. Khouri RK, et al. Aesthetic applications of Brava-assisted megavolume fat grafting to the breasts: a 9-year, 476-patient, multicenter experience. Plast Reconstr Surg. 2014;133(4):796–807. discussion 808–9
44. Kosowski TR, Rigotti G, Khouri RK. Tissue-engineered autologous breast regeneration with Brava®-assisted fat grafting. Clin Plast Surg. 2015;42(3):325–37. viii
45. Rigotti G, et al. Autologous fat grafting in breast cancer patients. Breast. 2012;21(5):690.
46. Schneider WJ, Hill HL, Brown RG. Latissimus dorsi myocutaneous flap for breast reconstruction. Br J Plast Surg. 1977;30(4):277–81.
47. Clough KB, Kroll SS, Audretsch W. An approach to the repair of partial mastectomy defects. Plast Reconstr Surg. 1999;104(2):409–20.
48. Johns N, et al. Autologous breast reconstruction using the immediately lipofilled extended latissimus dorsi flap. J Plast Reconstr Aesthet Surg. 2018;71(2):201–8.
49. Mushin OP, Myers PL, Langstein HN. Indications and controversies for complete and implant-enhanced latissimus dorsi breast reconstructions. Clin Plast Surg. 2018;45(1):75–81.

50. Branford OA, et al. Subfascial harvest of the extended latissimus dorsi myocutaneous flap in breast reconstruction: a comparative analysis of two techniques. Plast Reconstr Surg. 2013;132(4):737–48.

51. Hammond DC. Latissimus dorsi flap breast reconstruction. Plast Reconstr Surg. 2009;124(4):1055–63.

52. Losken A, et al. Outcomes evaluation following bilateral breast reconstruction using latissimus dorsi myocutaneous flaps. Ann Plast Surg. 2010;65(1):17–22.

53. Colohan S, et al. The free descending branch muscle-sparing latissimus dorsi flap: vascular anatomy and clinical applications. Plast Reconstr Surg. 2012;130(6):776e–87e.

54. Bailey SH, et al. The low transverse extended latissimus dorsi flap based on fat compartments of the back for breast reconstruction: anatomical study and clinical results. Plast Reconstr Surg. 2011;128(5):382e–94e.

55. Rusby JE, et al. Immediate latissimus dorsi miniflap volume replacement for partial mastectomy: use of intra-operative frozen sections to confirm negative margins. Am J Surg. 2008;196(4):512–8.

56. Thomsen JB, Gunnarsson GL. The evolving breast reconstruction: from latissimus dorsi musculocutaneous flap to a propeller thoracodorsal fasciocutaneous flap. Gland Surg. 2014;3(3):151–4.

57. Santanelli F, et al. Total breast reconstruction using the thoracodorsal artery perforator flap without implant. Plast Reconstr Surg. 2014;133(2):251–4.

58. McCulley SJ, et al. Lateral thoracic artery perforator (LTAP) flap in partial breast reconstruction. J Plast Reconstr Aesthet Surg. 2015;68(5):686–91.

59. Hamdi M, et al. The lateral intercostal artery perforators: anatomical study and clinical application in breast surgery. Plast Reconstr Surg. 2008;121(2):389–96.

60. Millard DR. Breast reconstruction after a radical mastectomy. Plast Reconstr Surg. 1976;58(3):283–91.

61. Knox AD, et al. Comparison of outcomes following autologous breast reconstruction using the DIEP and pedicled TRAM flaps: a 12-year clinical retrospective study and literature review. Plast Reconstr Surg. 2016;138(1):16–28.

62. Jones G. The Pedicled TRAM flap in breast reconstruction. In: Veronesi U, et al., editors. Breast cancer. New York: Springer; 2017. p. 465–83.

63. Reid AW, et al. An international comparison of reimbursement for DIEAP flap breast reconstruction. J Plast Reconstr Aesthet Surg. 2015;68(11):1529–35.

64. Erdmann-Sager J, et al. Complications and patient-reported outcomes after abdominal-based breast reconstruction: results of the mastectomy reconstruction outcomes consortium (MROC) study. Plast Reconstr Surg. 2018;141(2):271–81.

65. Blondeel N, et al. The donor site morbidity of free DIEP flaps and free TRAM flaps for breast reconstruction. Br J Plast Surg. 1997;50(5):322–30.

66. Blondeel PN. One hundred free DIEP flap breast reconstructions: a personal experience. Br J Plast Surg. 1999;52(2):104–11.

67. Krishnan NM, et al. The cost effectiveness of the DIEP flap relative to the muscle-sparing TRAM flap in postmastectomy breast reconstruction. Plast Reconstr Surg. 2015;135(4):948–58.

68. Granzow JW, et al. Breast reconstruction with the deep inferior epigastric perforator flap: history and an update on current technique. J Plast Reconstr Aesthet Surg. 2006;59(6):571–9.

69. Roostaeian J, et al. The effect of prior abdominal surgery on abdominally based free flaps in breast reconstruction. Plast Reconstr Surg. 2014;133(3):247e–55e.

70. Pennington DG. The stacked DIEP flap. Plast Reconstr Surg. 2011;128(4):377e–8e. author reply 378e

71. DellaCroce FJ, Sullivan SK, Trahan C. Stacked deep inferior epigastric perforator flap breast reconstruction: a review of 110 flaps in 55 cases over 3 years. Plast Reconstr Surg. 2011;127(3):1093–9.

72. Healy C, Allen RJ. The evolution of perforator flap breast reconstruction: twenty years after the first DIEP flap. J Reconstr Microsurg. 2014;30(2):121–5.

73. Rozen WM, et al. The SIEA angiosome: interindividual variability predicted preoperatively. Plast Reconstr Surg. 2009;124(1):327–8. author reply 328–30

74. LoTempio MM, Allen RJ. Breast reconstruction with SGAP and IGAP flaps. Plast Reconstr Surg. 2010;126(2):393–401.

75. Allen RJ, Levine JL, Granzow JW. The in-the-crease inferior gluteal artery perforator flap for breast reconstruction. Plast Reconstr Surg. 2006;118(2):333–9.

76. Hunter JE, et al. Evolution from the TUG to PAP flap for breast reconstruction: comparison and refinements of technique. J Plast Reconstr Aesthet Surg. 2015;68(7):960–5.

77. Bodin F, et al. The transverse musculo-cutaneous gracilis flap for breast reconstruction: how to avoid complications. Microsurgery. 2016;36(1):42–8.

78. de Weerd L, et al. Autologous breast reconstruction with a free lumbar artery perforator flap. Br J Plast Surg. 2003;56(2):180–3.

79. Hamdi M, et al. Lumbar artery perforator flap: an anatomical study using multidetector computed tomographic scan and surgical pearls for breast reconstruction. Plast Reconstr Surg. 2016;138(2):343–52.

80. Honart JF, et al. Lumbar artery perforator flap for breast reconstruction. Ann Chir Plast Esthet. 2018;63(1):25–30.

81. Peters KT, et al. Early experience with the free lumbar artery perforator flap for breast reconstruction. J Plast Reconstr Aesthet Surg. 2015;68(8):1112–9.

82. Sommeling CE, et al. Composite breast reconstruction: implant-based breast reconstruction with adjunctive lipofilling. J Plast Reconstr Aesthet Surg. 2017;70(8):1051–8.

83. Nava MB, Catanuto G, Rocco N. Hybrid breast reconstruction. Minerva Chir. 2018;73(3):329–33.

Tailoring Chemotherapy and Biological Treatment in Young Patients with EBC

Dario Trapani and Giuseppe Curigliano

Young breast cancer (YBC) patients seem to display unique features, possibly defining a distinct subtype with specific phenotypical, molecular, and prognostic characteristics. Moreover, a breast cancer diagnosis in a woman under 40 implies specific issues of care like fertility preservation, genetic risk definition, and psychological, sociological, relational topics with a clear impact on educational, personal, and career trajectories.

In a series of women with newly diagnosed stage I to III breast cancer from National Comprehensive Cancer Network, younger women were more likely to be nonwhite, more educated, and employed or in school. In addition, YBCs had more advanced stages at diagnosis and higher grade, with prevalent luminal B, triple-negative, and HER2 (human epidermal growth factor receptor 2) subtypes. Accordingly, younger women were more likely to receive chemotherapy compared with the older group [2]. In stratified analyses, age ≤40 years was associated with statistically significant increases in risk of breast cancer death among women with luminal A (hazard ratio (HR) 2.1) and luminal B (HR 1.4) disease. However, in a subset of patients with HER2-overexpressing breast cancer receiving adjuvant chemotherapy with or without trastuzumab, young age was neither prognostic nor predictive of short-term outcomes [3]. Similarly, in a fully adjusted model of YBCs, there was no difference in survival among women younger than 40 years (HR 1, 3), aged 41 to 50 (HR 0.9), 61 to 70 (HR 0.8), or >70 years (HR 1.0) compared with women aged 51 to 60 years [2].

Some explanations may be provided to justify this difference of prognosis. First, chemotherapy-induced amenorrhea (CIA) is less likely to occur in younger patients. This may have an impact on survival of hormone-sensitive breast cancer since estrogen deprivation is associated with an improved outcome in endocrine-responding tumors. Despite differences between studies and the retrospective nature of some reports, a correlation between survival and CIA has been demonstrated repeatedly. In a series of 1103 women receiving an anthracycline-based regimen, patients who achieved amenorrhea had a significantly better outcome compared with those who did not (+15% of disease-free survival, DFS; +21% of overall survival, OS). As expected, the incidence of amenorrhea did not show an influence on survival in the hormone receptor-negative subgroup [4].

Further, young age seems to predict a decreased adherence to adjuvant endocrine therapy [5]. On average, youngest, oldest, nonwhite, and mastectomy-treated patients have sig-

D. Trapani · G. Curigliano (✉)
IEO, European Institute of Oncology IRCCS, Milano, Italy

Department of Oncology and Hemato-Oncology, University of Milano, Milan, Italy
e-mail: dario.trapani@ieo.it;
giuseppe.curigliano@ieo.it

nificantly lower rates of adherence to adjuvant tamoxifen prescription; indeed, overall adherence was shown to be decreased up to 50% by year 4 of therapy. Adjuvant hormone therapy non-adherence, including discontinuation, is associated with an increased mortality with an estimated decrease of 7% in 10-year survival rate for less adherent women.

Importantly, in women with luminal disease, younger age may have a prognostic significance that reflects lower adherence to endocrine therapy; a unique biology of tumors arising in younger patients may have a role, as well. Accordingly, age should not be the single decisional parameter to prescribe or recommend an aggressive adjuvant chemotherapy, and several prognostic features must be taken into account in the treatment planning. Indeed, when advising an adjuvant cytotoxic chemotherapy, long-term side effect impact on health must be balanced against the benefit in terms of breast cancer survival gain.

Currently, clinical, pathological, and molecular factors are invoked in adjuvant chemotherapy choice for early YBC: lymph node involvement (N), tumor size (T), age, histological grade (G), human epidermal growth factor receptor 2 (HER2), Ki-67 (surrogate of proliferative index), estrogen (ER) and progesterone receptor (PgR) status, and genomic prognostic signatures of recurrence.

10.1 Clinicopathological Features of Prognostic Significance

10.1.1 Tumor Size

Tumor size is a recognized independent prognostic factor for breast cancer. In a dataset consisting of 9938 early breast cancer patients with a median follow-up of 11 years by the European Organisation for Research and Treatment of Cancer (EORTC), a subgroup analysis for YBC has been performed. At univariate analysis, pathological tumor size ($T > 2$ cm), histological grade, estrogen receptor status, and molecular subtype were significantly associated with OS

and distant recurrence-free survival. However, at multivariate analysis, molecular subtype was more strongly associated with OS and distant recurrence-free survival. However, tumor size and nodal status remained independent prognostic factors for disease outcome in young breast cancer patients [6]. Moreover, in the same series, no clear benefit of adjuvant treatment was confirmed for small, node-negative YBC ($T < 1$ cm) from adjuvant chemotherapy.

10.1.2 Nodal Status

Lymph node involvement is one of the major independent determinants of prognosis.

Breast cancer spreading to regional lymph nodes affects cancer-specific OS up to 15% at 5 years. However, pN1mi metastases (i.e., micrometastases greater than 0.2 mm and/or more than 200 cells, but none greater than 2.0 mm) seem not to provide a prognostic change in survival [7], and the presence of nodal micrometastases does not provide an adjunctive information in adjuvant treatment decision.

10.1.3 Grading

Tumor grading defines the growth patterns and degree of differentiation of cancer cells, reflecting how closely they resemble normal breast epithelial cells. The grading system mostly recognized and recommended by scientific society is the Nottingham Elston-Ellis classification [8].

Tumor grading has been introduced with the aim of predicting tumor behavior, as an adjunctive and reproducible feature in prognostic considerations and treatment decisions. In the Nottingham series [9], histological grade was shown to be an independent predictor of survival, particularly for the hormone-sensitive breast cancers not overexpressing HER-2. Thus, tumor grading may provide decisional prognostic information for a subgroup of patients in which the decision of an adjuvant chemotherapy may be controversial such as lymph node-negative, very young, hormone receptor- positive

YBC. However, histological tumor grading significance is not universally recognized as a crucial parameter for adjuvant therapy decisions; moreover, its evaluation is recommended by AJCC, but it does not impact on in breast cancer staging according to TNM system [10].

10.2 Multiparametric Tools for Prognostic Definition

10.2.1 Adjuvant! Online

A first attempt to evaluate objectively multiple prognostic tumor features in order to provide a more personalized approach to early breast cancer treatment has been provided by Adjuvant! Online. Adjuvant! was designed as a Web-based tool to estimate the absolute benefit of adjuvant treatment for an individual patient. The factors considered for the estimation are age, concomitant comorbidities, ER status, tumor grade and size, and lymph node status (Fig. 10.1). The referee source arises from a SEER databank. However, when applied to EBC in patients younger than 40 years, Adjuvant! overestimated OS by 4.2% ($p = 0.04$) and breast-specific OS by 4.7% ($p = 0.01$) [11].

10.2.2 Intrinsic Subtypes and Clinicopathological Definitions

Breast cancer gene profiling and clustering have identified primarily four subtypes, luminal A, luminal B, HER2-enriched, and TNBC [12]. However, intrinsic molecular subtypes of breast cancer are evaluated in clinical practice through a surrogate definition of immunohistochemically defined subtypes, according to St. Gallen 2013 (Fig. 10.2).

Luminal A-like tumors are defined as ER- and PgR-positive and HER2-negative staining with a low proliferation index (Ki-67); luminal B-like are ER-positive/HER2-negative or HER2-positive with high proliferation index and/or low PgR staining. HER2-enriched subtype surrogate presents a HER2 overexpression but is negative for ER and PgR. Lastly, triple-negative tumors lack the expression of ER, PgR, and HER2. A practical proposed threshold for "high and low" Ki-67 is 20%, according to the 14th St. Gallen expert consensus. However, as discussed for tumor grade, the predictive significance of Ki-67 is often questioned and the role in the adjuvant therapy decision not universally accepted; moreover, its evaluation is not routinely recommended by AJCC and it is not considered in breast cancer staging according to TNM system [10, 13].

Each intrinsic tumor subtype is associated with particular clinical, pathological, demographic characteristics as well as a specific prognosis. However, the hierarchical clustering of breast cancer may have some limitations at the single patient level, and further attempts to assess the individual risk have been made (Fig. 10.3).

10.2.3 Prosigna Breast Cancer Prognostic Gene Signature Assay (PAM50)

The first tool for intrinsic subtype definition used in a clinical series is PAM50. PAM50 is a quantitative real-time 50-gene PCR (qRT-PCR) assay that can be performed using RNA extracted from formalin-fixed, paraffin-embedded (FFPE) archival samples. Interestingly, this test has introduced the concept of a prognostic signature and, then, the idea to estimate a "risk of recurrence score" (ROR-PT) to be applied in clinical series to get prognostic information with a possible predictive role, thus assisting in the decision for adjuvant chemotherapy.

In a correlative analysis of CALGB (Alliance) 9741 adjuvant breast cancer trial (2x2 factorial dose-dense and sequential anthracycline/taxane chemotherapy versus traditional and concomitant schedule), the prognostic value of PAM50 intrinsic subtype was greater than estrogen receptor/HER2 immunohistochemistry classification. Moreover, proliferation and ROR-PT considered as continuous variables were demonstrated to be strongly prognostic for tumor relapse. For proliferation score, a 0.5-unit change corresponded to an 18% increase in risk of recurrence; for

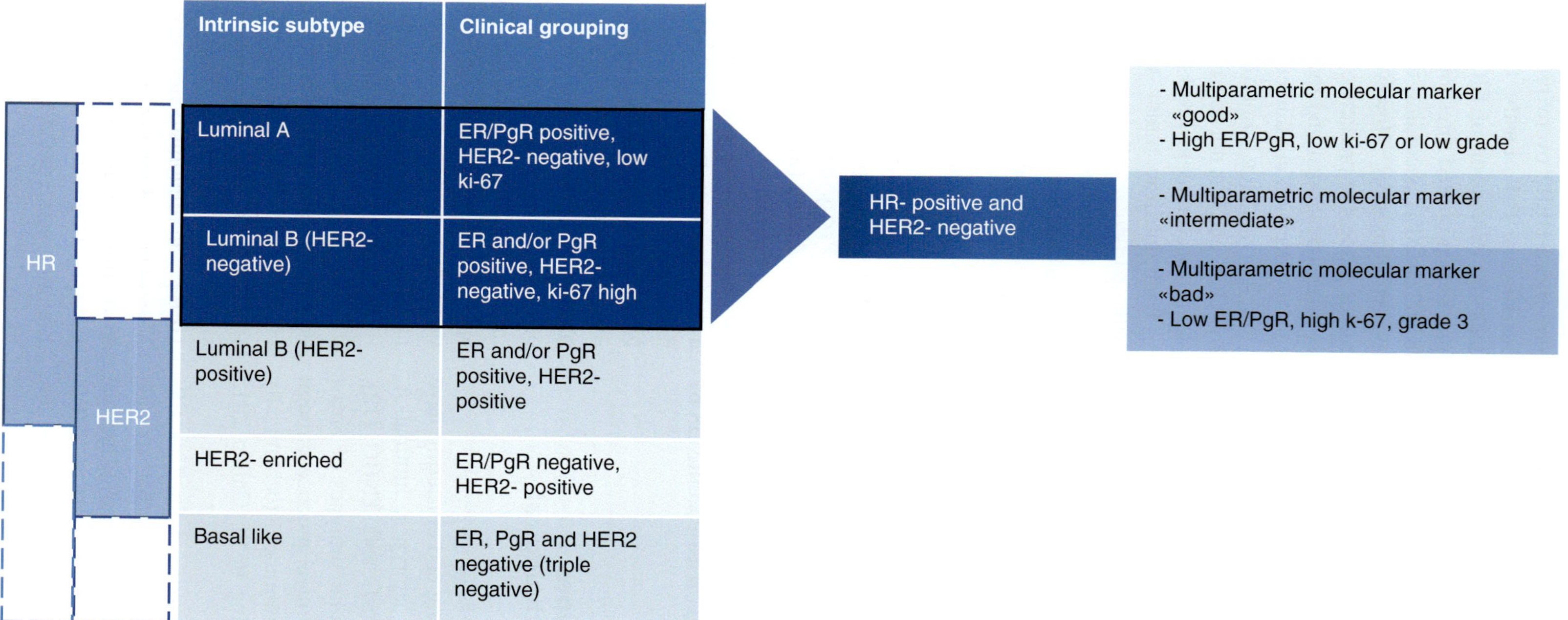

Fig. 10.1 Prospective trials exploring the prognostic and predictive role of different multiparametric tests for adjuvant treatment choice. pN and pT describe primary tumor and node involvement according to TNM 7th edition, *RS* recurrence score, *HT* hormone therapy, *CT* chemotherapy, *IDFS* invasive disease-free survival, *DDFS* distant disease-free survival, *OS* overall survival, *DFS* disease-free survival, *MFS* metastasis-free survival

	Oncotype Dx	MammaPrint	PAM50	Adjuvant!online
Method	Reverse transcription polymerase chain reaction (RT-PCR)	DNA microarray	Quantitative real-time PCR (qRT-PCR)	Web-based risk-assessment programme
Variables for prognostic risk definition	21 genes	70 genes	50 genes	Age Comorbidity ER status Tumor grade Tumor size Positive nodes
Histological sample	formalin-fixed, paraffin-embedded (FFPE)	Fresh frozen tissue	formalin-fixed, paraffin-embedded (FFPE)	Pathological report according to ASCO/CAP guidelines
Risk score	RS (low,int, high)	Prognostic signature (good, poor)	Definition of molecular Intrinsic subtypes ROR-PT (low,int, high)	Estimates 10-years DFS and OS

Fig. 10.2 Definition of breast cancer subtypes. Intrinsic subtypes can be defined by genomic assays only (i.e., PAM50). Clinical grouping table reports the clinicopathological definition according to 2011 St. Gallen Consensus. On the right, a new proposal from St. Gallen 2017 refines the HR-positive, HER2-negative disease definition according to clinicopathological and molecular risk of recurrence through multiparametric genomic tests. Some genomic tests report an intermediate risk score of recurrence (i.e., Oncotype DX), while other tests contemplate a "good" and a "poor" signature (i.e., MammaPrint). Tumor histological grade is defined according to Elston-Ellis modification of the Scarff-Bloom-Richardson grading system (Nottingham grading system). *HR* hormone receptor, *HER2* human epidermal growth factor receptor 2, *ER* estrogen receptor, *PgR* progesterone receptor. Ki-67 is intended as MIB1 labeling index

ROR-PT score, a 10-unit change corresponded to a 12% increase in risk of recurrence [14].

In the following series, ROR score has been categorized as low, intermediate, or high risk. It has been shown in TransATAC study that ROR score may provide further prognostic information for early distant recurrence and add substantial prognostic information for late distant recurrence. In particular, the inclusion of the ROR score resulted in a highly statistically significant addition of prognostic information in both node-positive and node-negative breast cancer patients [15]. However, these data have been obtained in postmenopausal breast cancer patients and may not be applicable to premenopausal YBC.

10.2.4 Oncotype DX

The 21-gene recurrence predictive tool is one of the most widely used assays for hormone-sensitive breast cancer recurrence prediction. Oncotype DX has been validated in a prospective clinical trial both in pre- and postmenopausal women, ER-positive and node-negative, thus offering a prognostic tool useful for YBC.

The 21-gene assay is based on a reverse transcription polymerase chain reaction (RT-PCR) on RNA isolated from paraffin-embedded breast cancer tissues.

Oncotype DX has been validated in population of patients enrolled in the NSABP B-14 trial of adjuvant tamoxifen in 668 patients with available archival tissue [16]. The 10-year distant recurrence risk for patients treated with tamoxifen was 7% for those with a low recurrence score (RS), 14% for those with an intermediate RS, and 31% for those with high RS.

The value of Oncotype DX has been proven in a prospective clinical trial, TAILORx (the Trial Assigning Individualized Options for Treatment (Rx)). In this study, more than 30% of

	TAILORx	Plan B	MINDACT
Multiparametric test	Oncotype DX		Mamma Print
Risk score definition	RS: -Low (<11) -Intermediate (11-25) -High (>25)	RS: -Low (≤11) -Intermediate(12-25) -High (>25)	Prognostic signature: -Good -Poor
Study design	-Lowrisk: HT -Intermediate risk: HT vs CT+HT -High risk: CT + HT	-Lowrisk: HT -Intermediate and High risk: CT + HT	-low clinical and genetic risk: HT -high clinical and genetic risk: CT + HT -discordant genetic and clinical risk: HT Vs CT+HT
Study population	30-36% are premenopausal 5% are under 40 years	Median age: 56 years	1,8% are under 35 years 34% are under 50 years
T-stage	1.1 to 5.0 cm in the greatest diameter (or 0.6 −1.0 if intermediate and high tumor grade)	-pT1-4 (node positive) -T>2cm (high risk, node negative)	T1-T3
N-stage	Node negative	Node positive and high-risk node negative tumors	Node negative and 1-3 N+ (pN1)
Outcome	RS<11 group: (5-year) -IDFS: 93,8% -DDFS:99,3% -OS: 98%	RS ≤ 11 group: (3 year) -DFS:98% RS 12-25: -DFS:98% RS>25: -DFS:92%	Discordant group (high clinical risk and low genomic risk): -CT+HT → MFS (5 years): 95,9% -HT → MFS: 94,4%

Fig. 10.3 Clinicopathological and molecular tools of clinical utility for the definition of recurrence risk in ER-positive/HER2-negative breast cancer. *RS* recurrence score, *ROR-PT* risk of recurrence score, *ER* estrogen receptor, *DFS* disease-free survival, *OS* overall survival

the patients were premenopausal and 5% under 40 years. The trial enrolled pre- and postmenopausal, ER-positive and HER2-negative breast cancer patients with tumors of 1.1–5.0 cm in the greatest diameter (or 0.6–1.0 cm if intermediate and high tumor grade) who met established guidelines for the consideration of adjuvant chemotherapy on the basis of clinicopathological features. Patients were assigned to receive endocrine therapy without chemotherapy if they had a recurrence score of 0–10 (low RS), indicating a very low risk of recurrence [17]. In the low RS cohort, the rate of invasive disease-free survival at 5 years was 93.8%; the rate of freedom from recurrence of breast cancer at a distant site at 5 years was 99.3%, the rate of freedom from recurrence at 5 years was 98.7%, and the rate of overall survival at 5 years was 98.0%. Thus, a low RS is able to detect an excellent prognostic group of ER-positive and node-negative breast cancer patients who can be treated with surgical resection (and radiation therapy, if indicated) and adjuvant endocrine therapy alone, omitting systemic chemotherapy. Interestingly, this prognostic tool may spare excessive cytotoxic adjuvant chemotherapy that would offer a minimal or no survival benefit and a certain toxicity. In the population of low RS, breast cancer had a median tumor diameter of 1.5 cm, an intermediate grade, and ER-positive staining; in clinical decision-making, without considering Oncotype DX score, these patients may represent a major challenge in advising for adjuvant chemotherapy, particularly for premenopausal and very young patients. For patients with midrange recurrence score of 11–25 (intermediate RT), hormonal adjuvant therapy was non-inferior to chemotherapy combined with endocrine therapy, with regard to the invasive disease-free survival and OS, around 84% and nearly 94% at 9 years, respectively [18]. However, the subgroup analysis of the patients younger than 50 years with a RS in the range 16–25 revealed a possible clinical relevant benefit from chemotherapy, generating a hypothesis to refine the prognostic and predictive characterization across the continuous RS. Eventually, recurrence score offers an objective tool for treatment decisions and de-escalation choice in low RS and certain intermediate RS YBC patients. In a phase 3 clinical trial by West German Study Group (PlanB), female patients with node-positive or high-risk (T2, grades 2 and 3, or age < 35 years old) node-negative HER2-negative early breast cancer, after adequate surgical treatment, with no evidence of distant metastases, were enrolled to receive an adjuvant chemotherapy. After an ad hoc amendment, chemotherapy was omitted on the basis of RS ≤ 11, corresponding to 15.3% of pN0 breast cancers. For node-negative and 1 to 3 N+ patients with low RS, PlanB results confirm the TAILORx conclusions, in a node-negative patient cohort: only 2% of the patients had a recurrence within 3 years in the low RS (≤11) group and no chemotherapy, despite being high risk by traditional parameters and possibly candidate to an adjuvant systemic cytotoxic candidates for chemotherapy. These results, indeed, provided the first prospective data in patients with both node-negative and node-positive breast cancer where RS results had been used in decision-making. Also, a high 3-year DFS (98%) in chemotherapy-treated patients with intermediate RS (12 to 25) and poorer 3-year DFS (92%) in chemotherapy-treated patients with RS >25 were reported [19]. In an attempt to complete the picture, an ongoing clinical trial is addressing the same question for node-positive (1–3 positive nodes) breast cancer with a RS ≤25 (RxPONDER Trial, Rx for Positive Node, Endocrine-Responsive Breast Cancer, NCT01272037).

10.2.5 MammaPrint

The MammaPrint (70-gene signature) assay uses microarray technology to identify high- and low-risk signatures of tumor recurrence in two groups, "good" and "poor" prognoses. MammaPrint has been preliminarily validated by an independent consortium (TRANSBIG), in a network of 40 partners and 21 countries [20]. In the multivariate analysis, MammaPrint provided the most valuable prognostic information for N0 early-stage breast cancer patients compared with traditional clinicopathological criteria.

MINDACT (Microarray In Node-negative and 1–3 positive lymph node Disease may Avoid ChemoTherapy) evaluated MammaPrint in a prospective trial to define the prognostic and predictive role of this genomic signature. The trial enrolled patients with T1–T3 (operable) ER-positive, HER2-negative breast cancer with up to three positive axillary lymph nodes (pN0, pN1), to receive adjuvant chemotherapy and endocrine therapy (high clinical and genomic score) or endocrine therapy alone (low clinical and genomic score). Clinical risk of recurrence was evaluated according to Adjuvant! Online tool, considering tumor size, grading, age, and lymph node involvement; 70-gene signature was used to determine the genomic risk or recurrence. Patients with discordant results for clinical and genomic score were randomized to receive chemotherapy followed by hormone therapy or no chemotherapy. Around 2% of the patients were less than 35 years old and almost one third of the population was under 50 year.

In the discordant group of patient with high clinical risk (candidate for adjuvant chemotherapy) and low genomic risk, chemotherapy administration provided an adjunct 1.5% in 5-year metastasis-free survival (95.9% versus 94.4%, HR 0.78; $p = 0.27$). However, MINDACT demonstrated that the use of a genomic risk strategy might reduce the use of adjuvant chemotherapy up to 46% of cases, with an overall survival rate of 94.7% at 5 years in patients not receiving adjuvant chemotherapy. On this point, the low genomic risk group consisting of 48% of node-positive patients, 93% of grade 2 and 3 tumors in patients younger than 50 years in one third of the cases, thus refining the patients' selection for adjuvant treatment decisions in some apparently clinical high-risk tumors [21].

The clinical implementation of genomic tools for risk prediction in breast cancer patients represents now a challenging area for clinicians, in the selection of the most appropriate tool according to the clinical presentation. Some of these tools have been validated only in postmenopausal patients, and the extrapolation for premenopausal indications should not be automatic and is truly discouraged. However, though results are emerging from different approaches for the prediction of the risk, like EndoPredict/EPclin, Breast Cancer Index, Mammostrat, MammaTyper, BreastPRS, or BreastOncPx, few have been specifically validated in premenopausal patients [22]. EPclin, for instance, was built as a composite tool that includes the prognostic information retrieved from the EndoPredict 8-gene mRNA-based assay and selected clinicopathological features, namely, tumor dimension and lymph node involvement, in an attempt to integrate classical and novel prognostic information. The threshold to discern high and low risk of recurrence is for EPclin Risk Score 3.3 [23]. The validation of the tool relies on the GEICAM 9906 cohort, where more than half of the sensitive population was premenopausal. Patients diagnosed with tumors scored lower than 3.3 showed an absolute reduced risk of distant metastasis of 28%. Moreover, the use of Breast Cancer Index, an 11-gene-expression-based assay, was developed to provide information on both early and late recurrence, potentially informing on decisions regarding extended adjuvant hormone treatment in the higher-risk breast cancer population [24].

10.3 HER2-Overexpressing Breast Cancer

Adjuvant treatment for HER2-overexpressing YBC follows the general recommendations for breast cancer treatment. HER2-targeting agents in the adjuvant setting have not provided different benefits in premenopausal and postmenopausal women, keeping a survival benefit in young patients, as well [3].

10.3.1 ExteNet

ExteNet is a randomized, multicenter, placebo-controlled phase 3 trial of anti-HER2 treatment extension with neratinib for 1 year, after 1 year of trastuzumab as adjuvant therapy in HER2-overexpressing early breast cancer. The study population consist of about 40% of patients under 50 years of age of which 4% were very young women (<35 years); indeed, nearly 50% of the population was premenopausal. After 2 years from the randomization, neratinib appeared to provide an improvement in invasive disease-free survival (HR = 0.67; $p = 0.0091$). An absolute gain of 2.3% in 2-year DFS was shown. According to a pre-specified subgroup analysis, neratinib added a clear advantage in DFS in ER-positive breast cancer (HR 0.51; $p = 0.0013$) but not in ER-negative disease (HR 0.93; $p = 0.74$). However, neratinib treatment was characterized by diarrhea as the most common treatment adverse event: up to 40% of the population exposed to the experimental compound had a grade 3 diarrhea event and 33% a grade 2 event. This inconvenient safety profile might have affected therapy adherence, thus reducing neratinib median dose intensity to 82% versus 98% in the placebo group [25]. On this topic, an interesting supportive care experience to increase the compliance to the treatment with neratinib has been conducted in a phase 2 trial [26]. Prophylactic treatment with loperamide and budesonide has been shown to reduce the rate of grade 3 diarrhea by 25% with a decrease of all-grade diarrhea of 30%.

10.3.2 APHINITY

The APHINITY trial intended to demonstrate an advantage in survival by incorporating pertuzumab to standard adjuvant treatment with chemotherapy and 1-year trastuzumab in early HER2-overexpressing breast cancer. Nearly 14% of the patients enrolled were under 40 years old; 4805 patients were randomized in a 1:1 design to standard or double blockade containing adjuvant regimen. After 3 years from randomization, 94.1% of pertuzumab-treated patients were disease-free, with an absolute advantage of 0.9% over trastuzumab-only treatment group (HR 0.81; $P = 0.045$). The improvement was more pronounced in patients with node-positive and hormone receptor-negative disease, with an absolute difference of 1.8% and 2.3%, respectively. However, OS data were not mature at the first interim analysis [27].

10.3.3 De-intensified Regimens

The only positive published trial of treatment de-intensification for HER2-overexpressing early breast cancer was provided by Tolaney et al., in the APT trial [28]. Treatment consisted of an anthracycline-free regimen of weekly paclitaxel and trastuzumab for 12 weeks followed by trastuzumab for 12 months of total anti-HER2 exposure. Patients enrolled in this single-arm trial were pT1c in 42% of cases with the majority of tumors smaller than 2 cm (more than 90%) and node-negative disease. Although stage I HER2-positive early breast cancers are considered as good prognosis, a minimal risk of recurrence remains and adjuvant *trastuzumab*-containing regimen is advised. The 3-year primary analysis showed a disease-free survival rate of 98.7%. A subsequent analysis demonstrated a 7-year DFS of 93.3% [29]. A better prognosis for ER-positive disease has been described with an adjunct 3.9% in survival over ER-negative disease. More recently, the long-awaited results of the PERSEPHONE trial have been presented, revealing the non-inferiority of 6 months' versus standard 12 months' exposure to trastuzumab in breast cancer patients, as adjuvant treatment [30]. Subgroup analysis suggested a possible role of shorter trastuzumab treatment in lower-risk HER2 positive patients. However, a half of the patients enrolled received a regimen containing anthracycline plus taxane and only 10% were spared anthracyclines. Accordingly, data on 6-month trastuzumab associated with shorter adjuvant cytotoxic chemotherapy without anthracyclines (i.e. weekly paclitaxel for 12 administration) cannot be recommended, and patients eligible to shorter trastuzumab should receive a standard 6-month chemotherapy.

10.4 Triple-Negative Breast Cancer

In the absence of clinically validated pharmacological targets, cytotoxic chemotherapy is the only adjuvant therapy option including anthracyclines, taxanes, alkylators, anti-metabolites, and platinum compounds. Though young patients presenting with triple-negative breast cancer are more likely to be carriers of a germline mutation of the BRCA genes, the use of targeted agents blocking the poly (ADP-ribose) polymerase in the early setting is not yet supported by clinical trials, failing to show an increase in tumor response in the neoadjuvant setting, when combined with poly-chemotherapy [31]. Indeed, in an attempt to optimize the delivery of cytotoxic chemotherapy and improve patient outcomes, dose-dense regimens have been increasingly implemented, relying on the concept that a narrower chemotherapy-free interval reduces the cancer re-growth and population of resistant clones, as modeled in the study of Gompertzian kinetics [32]. In accordance, a recent individual patient data meta-analysis from the Early Breast Cancer Trialists' Collaborative Group (EBCTCG) showed a significant reduction of breast cancer recurrence, including triple-negative subtype, with the use of a 2-week instead of the standard 3-week schedule, reporting an absolute reduction in breast cancer mortality of +2, 3% at 10 years [33]. These data support the consideration of a dose-dense regimen in selected YBC patients.

10.4.1 CREATE-X

The CREATE-X trial was designed to test the role of extending post-surgical chemotherapy with capecitabine in patients who had received neoadjuvant chemotherapy for HER2-negative early breast cancer and did not achieve a pathological complete response. Nine hundred ten patients were enrolled of which nearly 60% were premenopausal. The trial was terminated early for benefit. The final analysis showed an absolute gain in DFS of 6.5% by extending adjuvant treatment with capecitabine after 5 years of observation (HR 0.70; $P = 0.01$). Similarly, an increase in OS was evident with 89.2% of capecitabine group patients alive at 5 years versus 83.6% in the control group (HR 0.59; $p = 0.01$). In the subtype analysis, triple-negative breast cancer patients appeared to get the greatest benefit from capecitabine treatment with an absolute gain in DFS of 13.7% (HR 0.58) and of 8.5% in OS. In the subgroup analysis, the magnitude of the benefit was preserved in premenopausal women as well as in patients under 50 years of age [34].

10.4.2 Very Early TNBC

Stage I breast cancer comprises a heterogeneous group of patients with small (<1 cm) node-negative tumors with a recognized excellent prognosis. However, subtype considerations must be done among pT1a and pT1b tumors. In a large cohort of patients, Vaz-Luis et al. examined prospectively a cohort of breast cancer patients within the National Comprehensive Cancer Network Database, including 4113 women with T1a and T1b pN0 breast cancer. TNBC pT1a patients showed a 5-year DFS of 93% after locoregional treatment, without a systemic cytotoxic chemotherapy [35]. According to these and similar data, the 16th St. Gallen panelists almost unanimously recommended against routine pre-scription of adjuvant chemotherapy in pT1a pN0 TNBC, regardless of proliferation index (Ki-67), grading, and age. By pT1b breast tumors, adjuvant treatment must be discussed taking into account adverse pathological and demographic features. Therefore, one must consider the risk of death during breast cancer adjuvant chemotherapy (less than 1%) and a non-negligible risk of hospitalization for adverse events management related to systemic chemotherapy against the absolute benefit in terms of survival gain. In this age group, long-term side effects of adjuvant chemotherapy should also be part of the treatment decision algorithm.

10.5 Conclusions

Tailoring adjuvant treatment for early breast cancer in young patients is a major issue (Fig. 10.4). Young age must not be considered alone as the single feature to decide for an aggressive systemic treatment in breast cancer women. A multiparametric evaluation of the disease, taking into account demographic, pathological, and molecular characteristics, must be considered. A strategy of intensification and de-intensification has to be tailored for the individual patient, never forgetting that often an escalation strategy may be complicated by side effects, both mild and severe.

Currently, molecular-based tools can offer an additional decisional parameter in some challenging clinical settings, thus providing a crucial refinement for a personalized approach.

Settings of possible intensification and de-intensification of adjuvant systemic therapies vary across different breast cancer subtypes, as depicted above. Further results are awaited from ongoing clinical trial of (neo)adjuvant treatment in early YBC, both in the escalation and de-escalation direction in terms of extension (more time), intensification (more drugs, higher dose), and de-intensification (less treatment or omission). Therefore, further studies are warranted in terms of epidemiological evidences, special settings management, prospective results from targeted approaches, and innovative clinical trial designs with stronger academic translational

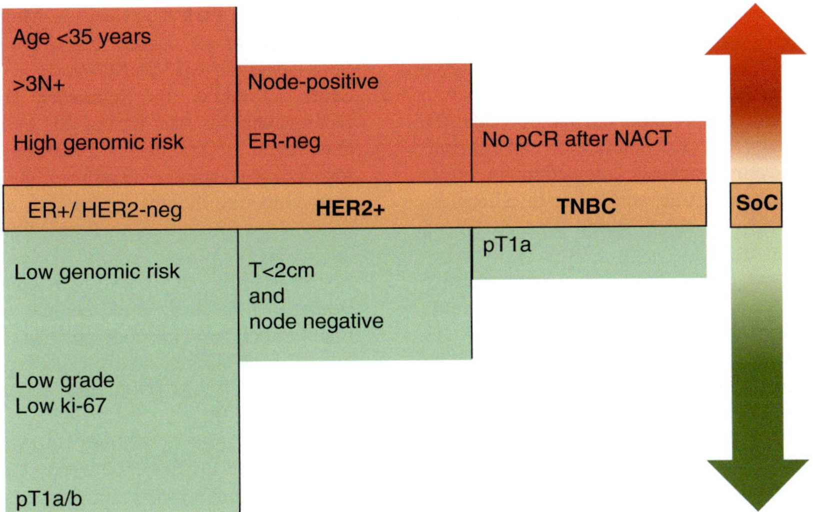

Fig. 10.4 Tailoring adjuvant treatment for early breast cancer in young patients. Settings of possible intensification and de-intensification of adjuvant systemic therapies across different breast cancer subtypes. Very young women (<35 years) may be considered for an adjuvant treatment with an aromatase inhibitor with OS when the disease is at high risk; however, age cannot be considered alone for intensification of the treatment. Hormone therapy intensification may be provided by a deeper estrogen suppression with aromatase inhibitor, ovarian suppression, or an extended regimen up to 10 years of tamoxifen. A chemo-intensification may be proposed in TNBC with the capecitabine extension regimen in high-risk, post-neoadjuvant setting. A biological escalation is proposable as double-blockade treatment with pertuzumab and trastuzumab or neratinib anti-HER2 extension. De-intensification chemotherapy may contemplate the omission of systemic cytotoxic treatment (i.e., low-risk HR+ tumors and pT1a TNBC) or a de-intensified regimen (i.e., anthracycline-free/3-month regimen for HER2-positive small tumors). See the text for major details. N+, lymph nodes involved. *ER* estrogen receptor, *HER2* human epidermal growth factor receptor 2, *TNBC* triple-negative breast cancer. T and N categories are reported according to TNM 7th edition. *pCR* pathological complete response, *NACT* neoadjuvant chemotherapy, *SoC* standard of care, for SoC it is intended a standard approach of treatment of breast cancer in the early setting i.e. surgery with 6-mo (neo)adjuvant chemotherapy and complementary radiation therapy, in case of conservative breast cancer. The image intends to emphasize that, in general, some patients may require risk- adapted escalated or de- escalated therapies, according to key prognostic factors

background in order to spare futile or noxious treatments.

References

1. Women and Health. Today's evidence, tomorrow's agenda. Geneva: World Health Organization; 2008.
2. Partridge AH, Hughes ME, Warner ET, Ottesen RA, Wong YN, Edge SB, et al. Subtype-dependent relationship between young age at diagnosis and breast cancer survival. J Clin Oncol. 2016;34(27):3308–14.
3. Partridge AH, Gelber S, Piccart-Gebhart MJ, Focant F, Scullion M, Holmes E, et al. Effect of age on breast cancer outcomes in women with human epidermal growth factor receptor 2-positive breast cancer: results from a herceptin adjuvant trial. J Clin Oncol. 2013;31:2692–8.
4. Walshe JM, Denduluri N, Swain SM. Amenorrhea in premenopausal women after adjuvant chemotherapy for breast cancer. J Clin Oncol. 2006;24:5769–79.
5. Partridge AH, Wang PS, Winer EP, Avorn J. Nonadherence to adjuvant tamoxifen therapy in women with primary breast cancer. J Clin Oncol. 2003;21:602–6.
6. Van der Hage JA, Mieog JS, van de Velde CJ, Putter H, Bartelink H, van de Vijver MJ. Impact of established prognostic factors and molecular subtype in very young breast cancer patients: pooled analysis of four EORTC randomized controlled trials. Breast Cancer Res. 2011;13(3):R68.
7. Andersson Y, Frisell J, Sylvan M, de Boniface J, Bergkvist L. Breast cancer survival in relation to the metastatic tumor burden in axillary lymph nodes. J Clin Oncol. 2010;28(17):2868–73.
8. Elston CW, Ellis IO. Pathological prognostic factors in breast cancer I. The value of histological grade in breast cancer: experience from a large study with long-term follow-up. Histopathology. 1991;19:403–10.
9. Rakha EA, El-Sayed ME, Lee AH, Elston CW, Grainge MJ, Hodi Z, et al. Prognostic significance of Nottingham histologic grade in invasive breast carcinoma. J Clin Oncol. 2008;26:3153–8.

10. Edge SB, Compton CC. The American Joint Committee on Cancer: the 7th edition of the AJCC cancer staging manual and the future of TNM. Ann Surg Oncol. 2010;17(6):1471–4.

11. Mook S, Schmidt MK, Rutgers EJ, van de Velde AO, Visser O, Rutgers SM, et al. Calibration and discriminatory accuracy of prognosis calculation for breast cancer with the online Adjuvant! Program: a hospital-based retrospective cohort study. Lancet Oncol. 2009;10(11):1070–6.

12. Cancer Genome Atlas Network. Comprehensive molecular portraits of human breast tumours. Nature. 2012;490(7418):61–70.

13. Goldhirsch A, et al. Personalizing the treatment of women with early breast cancer: highlights of the St Gallen International Expert Consensus on the Primary Therapy of Early Breast Cancer 2013. Ann Oncol. 2013;24:2206–23.

14. Liu MC, Pitcher BN, Mardis ER, Davies SR, Friedman PN, Snider JE, et al. PAM50 gene signatures and breast cancer prognosis with adjuvant anthracycline- and taxane-based chemotherapy: correlative analysis of C9741 (Alliance). NPJ Breast Cancer. 2016;2:15023.

15. Gnant M, Sestak I, Filipits M, Dowsett M, Balic M, Lopez- Knowles E, et al. Identifying clinically relevant prognostic subgroups of postmenopausal women with node-positive hormone receptor-positive early-stage breast cancer treated with endocrine therapy: a combined analysis of ABCSG-8 and ATAC using the PAM50 risk of recurrence score and intrinsic subtype. Ann Oncol. 2015;26:1685–91.

16. Paik S, Shak S, Tang G, Kim C, Baker J, Cronin M, et al. A multigene assay to predict recurrence of tamoxifen-treated, node-negative breast cancer. N Engl J Med. 2004;351(27):2817–26.

17. Sparano JA, Gray RJ, Makower DF, Pritchard KI, Albain KS, Hayes DF, et al. Prospective validation of a 21-gene expression assay in breast cancer. N Engl J Med. 2015;373(21):2005–14.

18. Sparano JA, Gray RJ, Makower DF, Pritchard KI, Albain KS, Hayes DF, et al. Adjuvant chemotherapy guided by a 21-gene expression assay in breast cancer. N Engl J Med. 2018;379:111–21.

19. Gluz O, Nitz UA, Christgen M, Kates RE, Shak S, Clemens M, et al. West German study group phase III plan B trial: first prospective outcome data for the 21-gene recurrence score assay and concordance of prognostic markers by central and local pathology assessment. J Clin Oncol. 2016;34(20):2341–9.

20. Buyse M, Loi S, van't Veer L, Viale G, Delorenzi M, Glas AM, et al. TRANSBIG Consortium. Validation and clinical utility of a 70-gene prognostic signature for women with node-negative breast cancer. J Natl Cancer Inst. 2006;98(17):1183–92.

21. Cardoso F, van't Veer LJ, Bogaerts J, Slaets L, Viale G, Delaloge S, et al. 70-Gene signature as an aid to treatment decisions in early-stage breast cancer. N Engl J Med. 2016;375(8):717–29.

22. Fayanju OM, Park KU, Lucci A. Molecular genomic testing for breast cancer: utility for surgeons. Ann Surg Oncol. 2018;25(2):512–9.

23. Sanft T, Aktas B, Schroeder B, Bossuyt V, DiGiovanna M, Abu-Khalaf M, et al. Prospective assessment of the decision-making impact of the breast cancer index in recommending extended adjuvant endocrine therapy for patients with early-stage ER-positive breast cancer. Breast Cancer Res Treat. 2015;154(3):533–41.

24. Martin M, Brase JC, Calvo L, Krappmann K, Ruiz-Borrego M, Fisch K, et al. Clinical validation of the EndoPredict test in node-positive, chemotherapy-treated ER+/HER2- breast cancer patients: results from the GEICAM 9906 trial. Breast Cancer Res. 2014;16(2):R38.

25. Chan A, Delaloge S, Holmes FA, Moy B, Iwata H, Harvey VJ, et al. ExteNET Study Group. Neratinib after trastuzumab-based adjuvant therapy in patients with HER2-positive breast cancer (ExteNET): a multicentre, randomised, double-blind, placebo-controlled, phase 3 trial. Lancet Oncol. 2016;17(3):367–77.

26. Barcenas C, Olek E, Hunt D, Tripathy D, Ibrahim E, Wilkinson M, et al. Incidence and severity of diarrhea with neratinib + intensive loperamide prophylaxis in patients (pts) with HER2+ early-stage breast cancer (EBC): Interim analysis from the multicenter, open-label, phase II control trial. CONTROL (PUMA-NER-6201). Presented at: 2016 San Antonio Breast Cancer Symposium; December 6–10, 2016, San Antonio, TX. Abstract P2-11-03.

27. Von Minckwitz G, Procter M, de Azambuja E, Zardavas D, Benyunes M, Viale G, et al. Adjuvant pertuzumab and trastuzumab in early HER2-positive breast cancer. N Engl J Med. 2017;377:122–31.

28. Tolaney SM, Barry WT, Dang CT, Yardley DA, Moy B, Marcom K, et al. Adjuvant paclitaxel and trastuzumab for node-negative, HER2-positive breast cancer. N Engl J Med. 2015;372:134–41.

29. Tolaney SM, Barry WT, Guo H, Dillon D, Dang CT, Yardley DA, et al. Seven-year (yr) follow-up of adjuvant paclitaxel (T) and trastuzumab (H) (APT trial) for node-negative, HER2-positive breast cancer (BC). J Clin Oncol. 2017. (Suppl; abstr 511;35:511.

30. Earl HM, Hiller L, Vallier AL, Loi S, Howe D, Higgins HB, et al. PERSEPHONE: 6 versus 12 months (m) of adjuvant trastuzumab in patients (pts) with HER2 positive (+) early breast cancer (EBC): randomised phase 3 non-inferiority trial with definitive 4-year (yr) disease-free survival (DFS) results. J Clin Oncol. 2018. (suppl; abstr 506;36:506.

31. Loibl S, O'Shaughnessy J, Untch M, Sikov WM, Rugo HS, McKee MD, et al. Addition of the PARP inhibitor veliparib plus carboplatin or carboplatin alone to standard neoadjuvant chemotherapy in triple-negative breast cancer (BrighTNess): a randomised, phase 3 trial. Lancet Oncol. 2018;19(4):497–509.

32. Norton L. A Gompertzian model of human breast cancer growth. Cancer Res. 1988;48(24, pt 1):7067–71.

33. Early Breast Cancer Trialists' Collaborative Group (EBCTCG). Increasing the dose intensity of chemotherapy by more frequent administration or sequential scheduling: a patient-level meta-analysis of 37,298 women with early breast cancer in 26 randomised trials. The lancet 2019.
34. Masuda N, Lee SJ, Ohtani S, Im YH, Lee ES, Yokota I, et al. Adjuvant capecitabine for breast cancer after preoperative chemotherapy. N Engl J Med. 2017;376(22):2147–59.
35. Vaz-Luis I, Ottesen RA, Hughes ME, Mamet R, Burstein HJ, Edge SB, et al. Outcomes by tumor subtype and treatment pattern in women with small, node-negative breast Cancer: a multi-institutional study. J Clin Oncol. 2014;32(20):2142–50.

Endocrine Treatment of Young Patients with EBC

Olivia Pagani

11.1 Introduction

Despite several series have shown young women are more likely to develop breast cancer subtypes associated with unfavorable prognosis [1–5], premenopausal women have hormone receptor-positive (HR+) disease in about 60% of cases [3] and early stages at diagnosis in the majority of cases [4]. A significant and growing proportion of young patients with HR+ breast cancer, treated with modern adjuvant endocrine therapy (ET), with or without chemotherapy, have excellent long-term outcomes. The oncologist is therefore challenged to precisely assess the risk of relapse according to currently available predictive and prognostic factors in order to offer the most appropriate therapeutic option to the individual patient, considering also potential side effects, quality of life (QoL), family planning, and patient's preferences. The definition of the individual risk of recurrence by clinical, immunohistochemical, and genomic parameters, when available, can identify patients more likely to benefit from the different treatment strategies. Age, nodal status, tumor size, degree of HR posi-

tivity, human epidermal growth factor receptor 2 (HER2) expression, and proliferation (defined by either Ki67 or grade) are essential components of the risk algorithm.

Premenopausal women are underrepresented in the clinical studies evaluating the prognostic information of gene expression signatures, particularly in node-positive disease [6, 7]. In the TAILORx study [8], only 4% of women in the low-risk group were <40 years: nonetheless, women belonging to the low-risk score group, who received ET alone, had an excellent outcome [99% 5-year distant recurrence-free interval (DRFI)]. In the MINDACT trial [9], only 6.2% of the study population was <40 years, 1.8% <35 years: patients who were at high clinical but low genomic risk had a 94.7% 5-year DRFI with ET alone. These small numbers prevent to clearly estimate the efficiency of gene expression signatures to discriminate young women with low-versus high-risk of recurrence [10], especially in node-positive disease: additional data are eagerly needed, but the available evidence reinforce the concept that not all young women with HR+ disease deserve adjuvant chemotherapy and their prognosis can be excellent with ET alone.

Tamoxifen for 5 years has been the standard adjuvant ET in young women for decades [11]. In the last few years, the range of adjuvant endocrine strategies in young women with EBC has broadened: in particular, the extension of tamoxifen to 10 years and the addition of ovarian function

O. Pagani (✉)
Institute of Oncology of Southern Switzerland,
Geneva University Hospitals, Swiss Group for
Clinical Cancer Research (SAKK), and International
Breast Cancer Study Group (IBCSG),
Lugano, Viganello, Switzerland
e-mail: olivia.pagani@eoc.ch

© Springer Nature Switzerland AG 2020
O. Gentilini et al. (eds.), *Breast Cancer in Young Women*,
https://doi.org/10.1007/978-3-030-24762-1_11

suppression (OFS) to tamoxifen or aromatase inhibitors (AIs) have been incorporated in the standard therapeutic armamentarium [10, 12–14]. Single-agent AIs are contraindicated in premenopausal women because of the loop stimulation of ovarian function through the increase of the hypothalamic secretion of GnRHs [15]. Current recommendations [10, 12–14] are mostly based on the Suppression of Ovarian Function Trial (SOFT) and Tamoxifen and Exemestane Trial (TEXT) (Fig. 11.1) study results [16, 17]. TEXT was designed to evaluate 5 years of exemestane plus the gonadotropin-releasing hormone agonist (GnRHa) triptorelin versus tamoxifen plus triptorelin. SOFT was designed to evaluate 5 years of exemestane plus OFS versus tamoxifen plus OFS versus tamoxifen alone. In TEXT-SOFT duration of both oral ET and OFS was 5 years [18].

Treatment decisions in the individual patient should therefore accurately weigh benefits against side effects: absolute outcome improvements from different ETs may better assist clinicians to select the optimal strategy. A continuous, composite measure of recurrence risk (incorporating age, nodal status, tumor size and grade, HR and Ki67 expression levels) was developed in the TEXT-SOFT HER2- population (4891 women) [19]. Differential treatment effects on the 5-year breast cancer-free interval (BCFI) emerged according to the composite risk level. The 5-year BCFI in the overall population was 90.8% but ranged from 98.6% to 77.5% among patients with lowest and highest composite risk, respectively. In the lowest-risk group, patients did well with all treatments, whereas patients in the highest risk group experienced a 15% improvement by escalating ET.

Adjuvant chemotherapy may also exert an indirect endocrine effect in HR+ breast cancer through the induction of OFS. A recent meta-analysis demonstrated that chemotherapy-induced amenorrhea (CIA) is associated with improved DFS in HR+ patients [relative risk (RR), 0.73; 95% CI, 0.61–0.88; $P = 0.001$] and OS (RR, 0.60; 95% CI, 0.50–0.72; $P < 0.001$), irrespective of nodal status, type of chemotherapy, and ET [20].

In SOFT-TEXT patients with HER2+ tumors, according to local pathology, were a minority of the enrolled population (12% and 14.0%, respectively). HER2-targeted therapy was given in 54% of HER2+ women; its timing was after

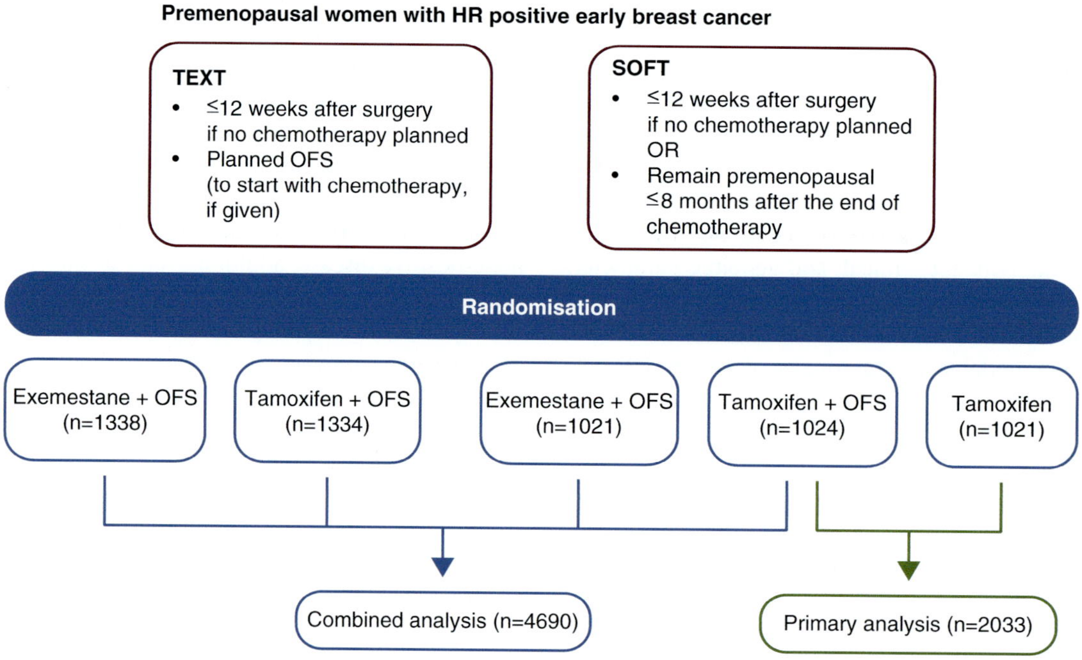

Fig. 11.1 SOFT and TEXT study designs

Table 11.1 Clinical risk of relapse

Low-risk	pT1a-b, pN0, G1 and/or low Ki67 (≤20%), high receptors
Intermediate-risk	pT1c-pT2, pN1a, G1-2 and/or intermediate Ki67 (20–30%), high-intermediate receptors
High-risk	pT3-pT4, pN2-pN3, G3 and/or high Ki67 (>30%), intermediate to low receptors

Table 11.2 8-year absolute disease improvements in SOFT low-risk HER2 patients

	No chemotherapy	% of absolute improvement
DFS		
T + OFS	90.6%	3.2
T	87.4%	
BCFI		
T + OFS	93.3%	1.3
T	92.0%	
DRFI		
T + OFS	98.0%	0.1
T	97.9%	
OS		
T + OFS	98.4%	−0.7
T	99.1%	

randomization in TEXT, whereas most SOFT patients completed it before randomization. Further investigation is therefore required (e.g., after central assessment of HER2 status) before HER2 status is used for selection of ET.

This chapter will illustrate and discuss the different ETs according to a pragmatic definition of the risk of relapse (Table 11.1), in particular indications and side effects of escalating ET from tamoxifen to tamoxifen-OFS, AIs-OFS, and extended ET. The outcomes in the HER2+ population are briefly discussed separately.

11.2 Patients at Low-Risk of Relapse

Tamoxifen alone is still considered the standard of care in patients at low-risk of relapse (Table 11.1). In the Early Breast Cancer Trialists' Collaborative Group (EBCTCG) 2011 meta-analysis [11], 5 years of tamoxifen compared to no ET was associated with an absolute 15-year risk reduction of 13.2% in breast cancer recurrence and of 9.2% in breast cancer mortality, regardless of age, the use of chemotherapy, and nodal status. The 5-year results of the SOFT trial [16] (*n* = 3066) showed that escalating ET by adding OFS to tamoxifen did not provide a significant benefit in the overall study population. In particular, among low-risk patients, in whom chemotherapy was not deemed indicated, the 5-year BCFI was >95% with either treatment, with few distant recurrences. The updated results, after a median follow-up of 8 years, show, in the overall population, a significant 4.4% absolute improvement in disease-free survival (DFS) by the addition of OFS to tamoxifen (83.2% versus 78.8%, hazard ratio (HR) 0.76; 95% CI, 0.62 to

0.93; *P* = 0.009) [21]. Among low-risk HER2-patients who did not receive chemotherapy, the absolute improvements in disease outcomes are summarized in Table 11.2. In particular, the BCFI was improved by 1.3% in patients receiving tamoxifen-OFS compared to tamoxifen alone (93.3% and 92.0%, respectively). There have been few distant recurrences in these low-risk patients and >98% were alive in each treatment group (Figs. 11.2 and 11.3).

The small Eastern Cooperative Oncology Group (ECOG) trial 3193 (*n* = 345) also compared tamoxifen and tamoxifen-OFS for 5 years in women with small (<3 cm) node-negative tumors who did not receive adjuvant chemotherapy [22]. With a median follow-up of 9.9 years, there was no significant difference between arms for both the 5-year DFS (87.9% *v* 89.7%; log-rank *P* = 0.62) and OS (95.2% versus 97.6%; log-rank *P* = 0.67).

Tamoxifen alone should therefore continue to be the preferred ET choice in low-risk women.

11.3 Patients at Intermediate-Risk of Relapse

The definition of clinical intermediate-risk of relapse (Table 11.1) is challenging and arbitrary. Overall, for these women, the benefit of exemestane-OFS over tamoxifen with/without OFS was moderate, approximately 5% at 5 years, requiring an individualized and balanced discus-

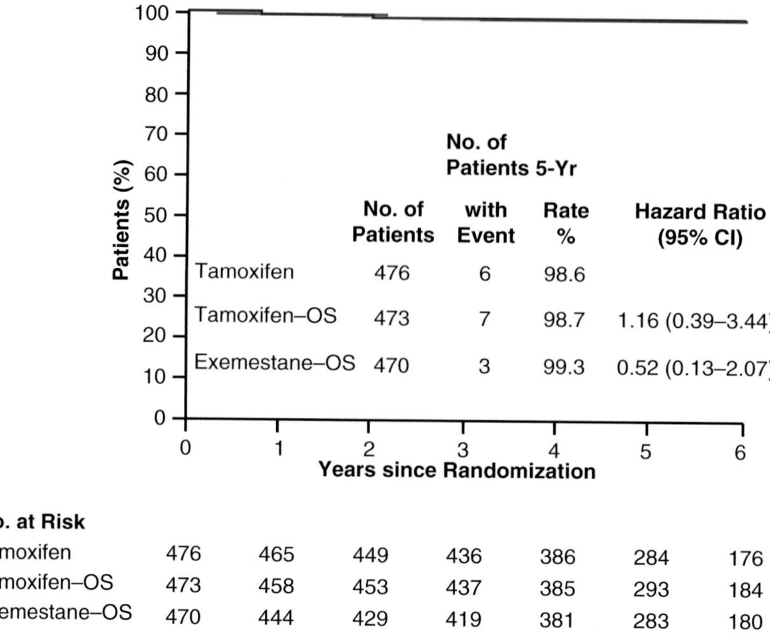

Fig. 11.2 5-year freedom from distant recurrence in SOFT patients not receiving chemotherapy

Fig. 11.3 8-year overall survival in SOFT patients not receiving chemotherapy

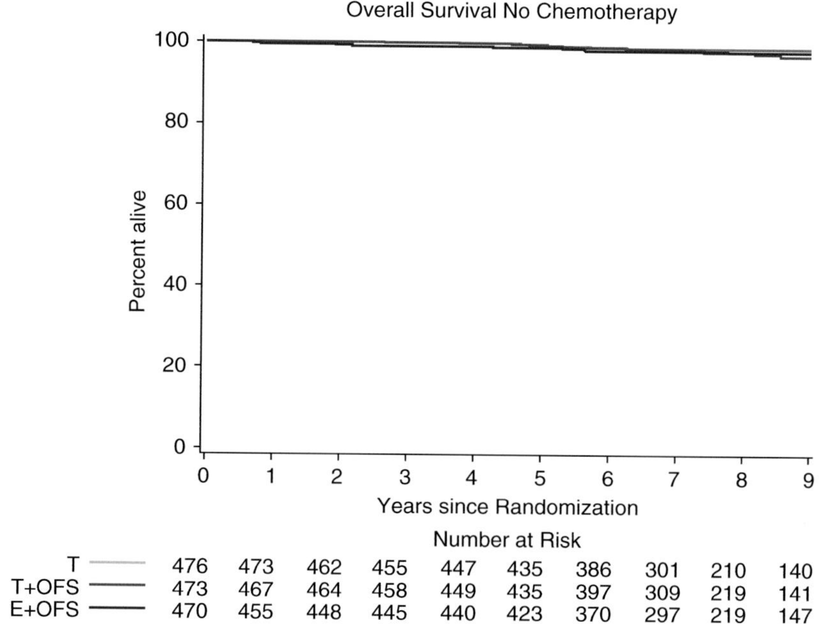

sion of benefits and adverse effects. Of note, women with the higher composite risk in this cohort who did not receive chemotherapy experienced an absolute benefit of approximately 10% with exemestane-OFS versus tamoxifen-OFS with a 5-year BCFI >95% [19], questioning the universal addition of adjuvant chemotherapy when effective combined ET is given. The outcomes in patients with intermediate-risk scores (11 to 25) randomized to receive ET alone or chemotherapy plus ET in the TAILORx study seem to differ according to age [23]. While in the overall group there was no benefit of adding chemotherapy to ET alone, an unplanned subgroup analysis showed a 6.5% improvement in distant recurrence rates at 9 years for patients <50 years who had a recurrence score between 21 and 25 and were randomized to receive chemotherapy, with no difference in OS. These results need to be interpreted with caution, considering in particular the post hoc unplanned nature of the analysis and that almost every premenopausal woman in the trial received tamoxifen alone (13% only received OFS). The results of the RxPONDER trial (NCT01272037), randomizing women with pN1a disease and a recurrence score <25 to ET alone or chemotherapy plus ET, will help better clarifying the role of adjuvant chemotherapy in addition to modern ET.

11.4 Patients at High-Risk of Relapse

Treatment escalation in patients at high-risk of relapse (Table 11.1) has been the subject of several studies [24], and the role of OFS in addition to oral ET has been debated for decades [25]. The proper identification of women most likely to benefit from treatment escalation is still challenging [26]. In SOFT, the absolute 8-year improvements in disease outcomes in HER2- high-risk patients ($n = 2.586$) are summarized in Table 11.3. In particular, DFS was improved by 11.2% among those treated with exemestane-OFS (83.1%) versus those under tamoxifen alone (71.9%) and DRFI by 6.0% (86.8% and 80.8%, respectively) [21]. In TEXT-SOFT, the absolute 8-year improvements in disease outcomes in HER2-patients ($n = 4035$) are summarized in Table 11.4. The analysis confirmed sustained benefits of exemestane-OFS; the DFS rate was improved by 5.4% (88.1% and 82.7%, respectively) and DRFI by2.1% (91.8% and 89.7%, respectively) in women who received exemestane-OFS compared to tamoxifen-OFS [21] (Table 11.4). Distant relapse has a great impact on breast cancer outcomes: a retrospective cohort study showed median time to all-cause mortality was significantly longer in women with locoregional recurrence than in those with distant metastases (6.4 versus 3.4 years, respectively)

Table 11.3 8-year absolute disease improvements in SOFT high-risk HER2- patients

	Chemotherapy cohort	% of absolute improvement versus T
8-y DFS		
E + OFS	83.1%	**11.2**
T + OFS	73.9%	**2.0**
T	71.9%	
8-y BCFI		
E + OFS	84.8%	**10.1**
T + OFS	76.3%	**1.6**
T	74.7%	
8-y DRFI		
E + OFS	86.8%	**6.0**
T + OFS	79.8%	**−1**
T	80.8%	
8-y OS		
E + OFS	88.7%	**3.5**
T + OFS	87.7%	**2.5**
T	85.2%	

Table 11.4 8-year absolute disease improvements in TEXT-SOFT HER2- patients

	Overall population	% of absolute improvement
DFS		
E + OFS	88.1%	**5.4**
T + OFS	82.7%	
BCFI		
E + OFS	90.1	**5**
T + OFS	85.1	
DRFI		
E + OFS	91.8%	**2.1**
T + OFS	89.7%	
OS		
E + OFS	94.0%	**1.0**
T + OFS	93.0%	

[27]. In addition, 10-year survival of women with local recurrence was 56%, compared with 9% in those with distant recurrence [28]. Distant recurrence in a premenopausal woman influences her QoL, family, and personal fulfillments and is associated with significant health-economic burden [29]. In the HER2-chemotherapy cohort in SOFT, OS at 8 years was improved by 3.5% in the exemestane-OFS group (88.7%) and by 2.5% in the tamoxifen-OFS group (87.7), compared to the tamoxifen group (85.2%) (Table 11.3). In the HER2-chemotherapy cohort in TEXT-SOFT, the 8-year DRFI was improved by 5.0% (TEXT)

and 7.0% (SOFT) among women assigned to exemestane-OFS compared to tamoxifen-OFS (Fig. 11.4). Knowing all patients would receive OFS in TEXT, whereas in SOFT OFS was administered by random assignment, possibly influenced patient selection for chemotherapy. For instance, more young patients (<40 years) (47.8% and 28.4%, respectively) and patients with node-negative disease (41.5% and 31.4%, respectively) received chemotherapy in SOFT than in TEXT, whereas over 20% of patients who received ET alone in TEXT had 1–3 positive nodes. The higher risk characteristics of women receiving adjuvant chemotherapy in SOFT can partly explain the slightly different absolute improvements compared to TEXT.

OS was 94.1% (95%CI, 92.9% to 95.1%) among patients assigned to exemestane-OFS and 93.4% (95%CI, 92.1% to 94.5%) among those receiving tamoxifen-OFS (HR 0.86; 95%CI, 0.68 to 1.10). SOFT-TEXT OS results differ from those of the Austrian Breast and Colorectal Cancer Study Group (ABCSG) 12 trial, which randomized 1803 premenopausal patients to 3 years of goserelin plus tamoxifen or anastrozole [30]. After 94.4 months of median follow-up, no DFS difference between treatments was reported, but a higher risk of death for anastrozole-treated patients was observed (HR = 1.63; 95% CI 1.05–1.45; p = 0.03). In SOFT-TEXT in contrast, no overall difference has emerged in the 8-year OS rate between study arms (HR 0.98; 95%CI, 0.79 to 1.22). ABCSG-12 and SOFT-TEXT have several differences which can potentially explain these results: in particular, in the Austrian trial,

the statistical power was lower (half the number of events), lower risk patients were enrolled (75% T1, 65% N0, only 10% received chemotherapy) and treatment duration was only 3 years, which is not the current standard of care for oral ET.

Very young women (<35 years) have historically poor outcomes, with increased rates of both local and distant recurrence [1, 5]. In high-risk HER2- <35 years old patients enrolled in SOFT (n = 240), the 5-year BCFI was improved by 8.8% in patients receiving tamoxifen-OFS (75.9%) and by 16.1% in women receiving exemestane-OFS (83.2%), compared to tamoxifen alone (67.1%). In TEXT HER2- patients (n = 145), 5-year BCFI was improved by 2.4% in patients treated with exemestane (81.6%) compared to tamoxifen (79.2%) [31]. Overall, in SOFT the updated 8-year DRFI was substantially improved in very young patients by escalating ET from tamoxifen (73.8%) to tamoxifen-OFS (77.5%) and exemestane-OFS (82.4%). In SOFT-TEXT HER2- patients <35 years, a 7.6% absolute improvement in DRFI with exemestane-OFS was achieved, which translated into a 4.0% OS improvement (Fig. 11.3).

The timing of OFS and chemotherapy, when given, differed in TEXT-SOFT, being concurrent in TEXT and sequential in SOFT. To address theoretical concerns about the concurrent use of ET with chemotherapy and the best timing for initiating OFS, the BCFI beginning 1 year after the final dose of chemotherapy was compared in 1872 HER2- patients enrolled in the 2 trials with about 5 years of median follow-up [32]. Neither detrimental nor beneficial effect of concurrent

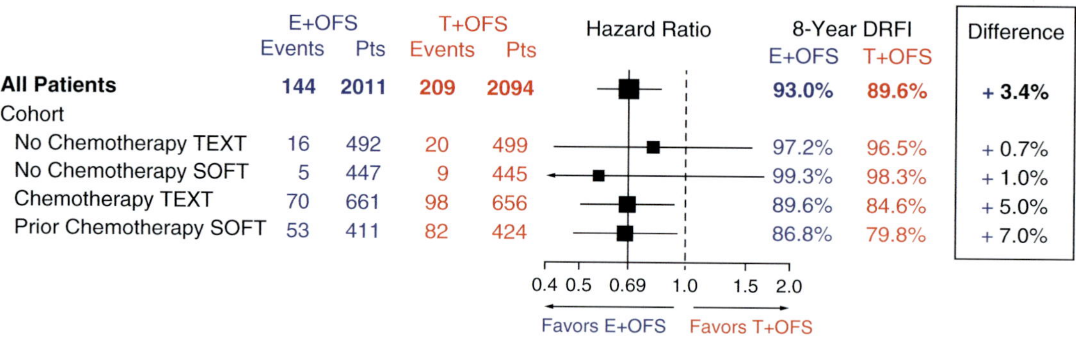

Fig. 11.4 8-year freedom from distant recurrence in SOFT-TEXT HER2- patients

OFS with chemotherapy was detected in the overall population (89% 4-year BCFI in both groups, HR = 1.11; 95% CI 0.72–1.72; $P = 0.72$) and in the small subgroup of 692 women<40 years at diagnosis, who are less likely to develop CIA (HR = 1.13; 95% CI 0.69–1.84). Clinicians can therefore select the most adequate individual strategy, taking also into account the potential protective effect of concomitant OFS on permanent CIA [33].

Conflicting evidence has questioned the benefit of AIs in overweight/obese patients: the increased body aromatization in fat tissue may potentially decrease the suppression of estrogen production by AIs. In overweight (BMI ≥ 25 kg/m^2) patients treated with anastrozole in the ABCSG-12 trial, the risks of recurrence and death were significantly higher (HR 1.49; 95% CI 0.93–2.38; $p = 0.08$ and HR 3.03; 95% CI 1.35–6.82; $p = 0.004$, respectively) than in patients treated with tamoxifen [34]. While waiting for the BMI data from TEXT-SOFT, there is no definitive data suggesting not prescribing AIs in overweight patients, if indicated.

Women with HR+ tumors show no plateau for both recurrence and death, with a low but continuous risk of late relapse and death [35]: the annual rate for late recurrences exceeds 2% for at least 15 years, even after 5 years of tamoxifen therapy. The analysis of 111,993 patients, diagnosed between 1990 and 2003 and included in the SEER database, showed different hazards of breast cancer-specific mortality (BCSM) according to HR expression. In the first 5 years BCSM was higher among patients with HR- tumors (HR 1.94; 95% CI 1.85–2.05 at years 2–5), whereas 5–10 years after diagnosis, patients with HR+ disease have an increased risk of BCSM compared with HR- patients (HR 0.71; 95% CI 0.66–0.76). In addition, young patients experience a significant higher hazard of BCSM at 5–10 years after diagnosis (HR, 0.43; 95% CI, 0.35 to 0.52), irrespective of nodal status [36]. Several clinico-pathological parameters (e.g., nodal status and tumor size) are also associated with an increased risk of late recurrence. Altogether these data may help clinicians select which patients are the best candidates for extended ET. None of the available gene expression signatures have been specifically developed and tested for the prediction of late (distant) recurrence [6, 37]. In particular, none of these tests can clarify if patients at higher risk of relapse substantially benefit from extended adjuvant ET. Further research is therefore needed to detect individual biomarkers or signatures for the identification of women at high risk of late recurrence, particularly in node-negative disease.

The only randomized data to support extended adjuvant ET in premenopausal women derive from the ATLAS [38] ($n = 15,244$) and aTTom (HR+ $n = $ ~6100) trials which explored the benefit of 10 versus 5 years of tamoxifen. In the ATLAS trial, 10 years of tamoxifen reduced the risk of breast cancer recurrence in HR+ disease by 3.7% (relative risk (RR) 0.84, CI 95% 0.76–0.94) after a median follow-up of 7.6 years. The extended therapy also significantly reduced breast cancer mortality (by 2.8%) during years 5–14 (12.2% versus 15.0%), overall mortality, and the incidence of contralateral breast cancer at 10 years. The protective effect on breast cancer outcomes extends well over the 10 years' treatment period (RR 0.90; 95% CI, 0.79–1.02 during years 5–9 and 0.70; 95% CI, 0.62–0.90 during subsequent years), regardless of nodal status. Premenopausal patients constituted a minority of the study population (19% <45 years), and statistical significance was not reached in this subgroup, likely because of the much smaller number of events. In the aTTom trial, even though HR status was untested in 60% of patients, the longer treatment group had fewer breast cancer recurrences compared with the 5-year treatment group (16.7% versus 19.3%; $P = 0.003$). The RR was time dependent, from 0.99 (0.86–1.15) during years 5–6 to 0.75 (0.66–0.86) in later years. Longer treatment also reduced breast cancer mortality by 3% (21% versus 24%; $P = 0.06$) in a time-dependent manner (RR 1.03 during years 5–9 and 0.77 subsequently) and overall mortality (849 versus 910 deaths, $p = 0.1$, RR 1.05 during years 5–9 and 0.86 later on). These results have been adopted by the most recent guidelines [10, 13, 14], all supporting discussing tamoxifen for 10 years in premenopausal women at high risk of disease recurrence. Non-breast cancer mortality was little affected by extended therapy in both trials: in the ATLAS trial, a higher risk for pulmonary embolism (RR 1.87, $p = 0.01$, CI 95%, 1–13-3.07), without an increased incidence of stroke (RR 1.06), was reported.

In the NCIC CTG MA.17/BIG 1–97 study [39], patients receiving 5 years of letrozole after 5 years of tamoxifen experienced, overall, an improved DFS, but a significant OS benefit was evident only in patients with node-positive disease. The best DFS benefit (HR 0.25; 95% CI 0.12–0.51) was achieved by premenopausal women at diagnosis who became definitively postmenopausal at the time of randomization, providing a new treatment option in this subgroup of patients, if clinically indicated.

The optimal duration of adjuvant GnRHa has not been established. In different trials, GnRHa were given for 2, 3, or 5 years, with no direct comparisons. The 2015 ESMO guidelines suggest at least 2 years of treatment [14]. The excellent outcome of patients treated for 3 years in the ABCSG-12 trial [30] suggests this can be reasonable, especially in low-risk women or reporting severe side effects. In TEXT-SOFT duration of OFS was 5 years. To date, there are no data on GnRHa extension beyond 5 years. A phase II single-arm trial evaluated, after at least 4.5 years of adjuvant tamoxifen, 2 years of OFS in combination with the AI letrozole [40]. The study closed after only 16 patients enrolled over 3.5 years, suggesting young women may not be highly motivated to extended OFS and challenging the feasibility of future studies.

The recent results of the randomized phase III ASTRRA study showed that adding 2 years of OFS to tamoxifen significantly improved the 5-year DFS, compared to tamoxifen alone, also in women with late (within 2 years) resumption of ovarian function after chemotherapy (3.6% absolute improvement, HR 0.686; 95% CI 0.483–0.972; $P = 0.033$) [41]. This new treatment possibility is of particular interest for older premenopausal women who are at higher risk of developing CIA.

11.5 HER2+ Population

In SOFT, at 8-year median follow-up, a greater DFS benefit of tamoxifen-OFS, as compared with tamoxifen alone, was suggested (HR 0.41; 95% CI 0.22–0.75). In TEXT, HER2+ women did not appear to derive an advantage from exemestane as compared with tamoxifen (HR 1.17; 95% CI 0.80– 1.71). A closer analysis is planned taking into account that adjuvant HER2-targeted therapy began during trial conduct and was therefore not received by all HER2+ patients, the differences in patients' characteristics as well as in chemotherapy regimens and OFS initiation (sequentially or concurrently with chemotherapy) in SOFT and TEXT.

11.6 Side Effects of Endocrine Therapy

ET is associated with several physical and psychosocial acute and late side effects, specific of the drugs used and their duration. Accurate evaluation of potential contraindications to specific compounds and strategies to manage the most common toxicities should be part of everyday clinical care. In particular, health professionals should routinely assess and encourage adherence to ET [42] and address specific side effects to reduce symptom burden and potentially improve adherence [43]. Patient-reported outcome measures (PROMs) have been reported to improve symptom/function monitoring, accuracy of symptom reporting, and detection of unrecognized problems [44] in cancer patients but not to impact patient management or improve health outcomes [45]. Particularly in young women, scientifically validated, innovative, and structured communication and supportive tools (e.g., online programs, Web-based interventions) would help to overcome barriers to accessing support, such as child and family care, work timetables, and geographical distance from healthcare services [10]. Electronic tools (e-PROs) might facilitate young patients to report adverse events from home, thus increasing safety of cancer treatments and standardizing toxicity documentation [46, 47]. As ET side effects derive from suppression of estrogen production or ER blockade, it has been questioned whether the development of side effects caused by estrogen deprivation might be related to ET benefit. A number of unplanned retrospective analyses evaluated the general association between ET-related side effects and breast cancer outcome. Most but not all analyses identified a positive association between musculoskeletal toxicity and improved DFS and OS. Associations between vasomotor symptoms and improved outcomes have also been reported. These data have major limitations (e.g., physician-graded adverse events instead of PROs, no consistent definition for musculoskeletal symptoms across studies, exclusion of symptomatic patients at baseline) which make difficult to apply these findings in clinical practice [48].

11.6.1 Tamoxifen

The most common side effects of tamoxifen include menopausal symptoms (e.g., hot flashes, weight gain, sleep disturbance, sexual dysfunction, and gynecologic complications) which may negatively impact QoL: rare but serious toxicities include increased risks of endometrial cancer and thromboembolism. In premenopausal women there is little uterine cancer risk or excess risk of fatal pulmonary embolism [11]. The incidence of endometrial cancer and thromboembolism is very low even with longer therapy duration (3.1% versus 1.6% endometrial cancers for tamoxifen- versus placebo-treated women and 1.87 relative risk of pulmonary embolism in the ATLAS trial) [38].

As opposed to menopausal women, tamoxifen may decrease bone mineral density (BMD) in premenopausal women, likely because its estrogen-like effect in the bones is weaker compared to the endogenous estrogens it is blocking. In the ZIPP (Zoladex in Premenopausal Patients) trial, comparing different adjuvant treatments (6 cycles of CMF ± 2 years of goserelin, goserelin plus tamoxifen, or tamoxifen), a significant decline in BMD was seen after 2 years of treat-

ment in patients receiving tamoxifen alone [49]. Tamoxifen was associated with bone loss in 111 Finnish premenopausal women who continued to menstruate after adjuvant chemotherapy and prevented bone loss in those who developed CIA [50]. BMD has therefore to be regularly checked and adequate intake of calcium and vitamin D through diet or supplements (1000 mg/day and 800–1000 UI/day, respectively) encouraged [10]. Treatment-related bone loss should be managed according to standard recommendations.

The decrease of low-density lipoproteins and total cholesterol reported in menopausal women is not evident in premenopausal patients [51].

The impact of tamoxifen on ovarian function is not well understood. A retrospective study in 250 US premenopausal women with ductal carcinoma in situ or EBC who did not receive chemotherapy showed that amenorrhea was more frequent in women taking tamoxifen compared to those who did not (22% versus 3%, $p < 0.001$) [52]. Young women should be informed of the possibility of getting pregnant while on tamoxifen, despite developing amenorrhea: the relatively high frequency of severe congenital abnormalities mandates a reliable nonhormonal contraception [53]. Tamoxifen may exert opposite effects on estrogen levels. Hypoestrogenism with consequent hyperandrogenism can induce side effects like hair loss, whereas the interference with the normal negative pituitary feedback results in FSH rise and ovarian steroidogenesis with increased incidence of ovarian cysts [54].

Tamoxifen may adversely affect cognition in menopausal women, affecting in particular verbal memory, executive functioning, and narrative writing [55, 56], but few specific investigations have been conducted in premenopausal women. In the ZIPP trial, neither endocrine treatment nor chemotherapy (CMF) affected the patients' self-evaluation of memory and concentration [57]. Cognitive function has been prospectively investigated in patients participating in the CO-SOFT sub-study [58]: despite the small sample size (86 participants), no differences in global cognitive function emerged in patients treated with tamoxifen alone versus those receiving OFS plus oral

ET, the latter complaining of greater deterioration in self-reported cognitive function. A recent meta-analysis of 14 studies (911 breast cancer patients on AIs or tamoxifen and 911 controls, i.e., non-cancer and breast cancer patients not using ET) [59] showed verbal learning/memory was the only domain where ET patients performed worse than both controls. Tamoxifen and AI patients did not differ overall from one another. Additional studies assessing change from pre-treatment performance and potential differences between steroidal and nonsteroidal AIs are warranted.

Genetic polymorphisms may classify low or extensive tamoxifen metabolizers, via the CYP2D6 enzyme, resulting in different plasma concentrations of endoxifen, a clinically active metabolite of tamoxifen. In menopausal women many attempts have been undertaken to explore the impact of tamoxifen metabolism on toxicity and outcome with discordant results, preventing so far the utilization of pharmacogenomics data to inform clinical decision-making [60, 61]. The simultaneous administration of drugs that inhibit CYP2D6 may lead to reduced concentrations of endoxifen. Therefore, during treatment with tamoxifen, potent CYP2D6 inhibitors (e.g., paroxetine, fluoxetine, quinidine, cinacalcet, or bupropion) should be avoided, if possible.

11.6.2 Ovarian Function Suppression

The addition of OFS to oral ET is associated with greater menopausal symptoms, anxiety, and depression [12]: in women who develop severe side effects, the risk-benefit ratio should be discussed according to the individual risk of relapse and OFS interruption proposed.

Side effects [16] and quality of life (QoL) [62] have been extensively analyzed in SOFT. Overall, OFS added to tamoxifen resulted in worse endocrine symptoms and sexual functioning, depression, musculoskeletal symptoms, hypertension, and diabetes. With all women beyond the 5-year treatment period, no new toxicity signal has emerged [21]: osteoporosis (T-score < −2.5) was doubled in patients receiving OFS compared to those under tamoxifen. Global QoL was

impacted during the first 2 years of treatment, but changes from baseline were small and similar between treatments. The short-term differences in symptom-specific QoL, treatment burden, and coping effort measured by the PACIS (Perceived Adjustment to Chronic Illness Scale) [63] were less pronounced for patients with prior chemotherapy, the cohort that benefits most from OFS in terms of disease control.

Hormone levels should be regularly checked (e.g., every 6 months) under OFS, especially if there are concerns that ovarian function is not suppressed and if the patient is receiving an AI [10], as amenorrhea per se is not a reliable indicator of effective OFS [15]. Available assays are not standardized, and their accuracy and interpretation can be problematic in presence of very low levels of estradiol [64]. In the SOFT-EST sub-study, optimal estrogen suppression was not achieved in up to 17% of patients after 12 months of treatment [65].

The efficacy and safety of 3-monthly versus monthly administration of GnRHa has not been properly investigated. Masuda and colleagues showed that 3-monthly goserelin is not inferior to monthly administration in terms of estradiol suppression, safety, and tolerability [66]. In clinical practice, the quarterly administration may not efficiently suppress estradiol levels in women <40 years and monthly formulations should therefore be preferred [10]. In case of proven inadequate suppression with either formulation, a switch to tamoxifen alone or bilateral oophorectomy should be individually discussed, according to the patient's age and disease characteristics.

Bilateral oophorectomy and ovarian function ablation through pelvic radiotherapy are reasonable alternatives to GnRHa in countries where cost and availability are problematic, but pharmacological OFS should be preferred whenever possible in order to avoid premature menopause and allow for pregnancy planning, if desired.

11.6.3 Aromatase Inhibitors

In TEXT, the adverse event profile of exemestane-OFS was similar to that seen with AIs in postmenopausal women: musculoskeletal symptoms and sexual dysfunction were the most frequent side effects [17]. At 8-year median follow-up, toxicities did not differ from earlier evaluation [21]: in particular, the rates of osteoporosis (T-score < -2.5) and fractures did not increase substantially with longer follow-up (14.8% and 7.7%, respectively). Overall, over the 5 years, changes in global QoL from baseline were small and not substantially different between tamoxifen-OFS and exemestane-OFS [67]. From a QoL perspective, no strong indication to favor either treatment emerged, suggesting the distinct side effects of the two treatments need to be addressed with patients individually.

The CYP19A1 gene encodes for the enzyme aromatase: genetic variations of this gene may result in increased or decreased aromatase activity and influence levels of circulating estrogens. A recent review and meta-analysis analyzed the influence of common CYP19A1 polymorphisms in postmenopausal patients treated with AIs [68], indicating heterogeneity between studies. In SOFT-TEXT, the CYP19A1 rs10046 variant T/T favors lower incidence of hot flashes/sweating under exemestane-OFS when compared to patients with the C/T or C/C variants [69]. Additional research and evidence are needed before genetic polymorphisms can be used to guide AI treatment in individual patients.

11.7 Adherence

ET adherence and persistence are relevant and may affect disease outcomes [70, 71]. Young age is a known risk factor for nonadherence (i.e., not to take the correct dosage at the prescribed frequency) and non-persistence (i.e., discontinue therapy) to ET [72], but the reasons why young women are less likely to take ET as prescribed are poorly understood. In 515 premenopausal patients, <45 years with HR+ disease for whom tamoxifen was recommended, 71.1% persisted with treatment, 13.4% declined initiation, and 15.5% stopped tamoxifen prior to 5 years [73]. Main patients' reasons for noninitiation included concerns about side effects (36%) and fertility (34%). Fertility concerns were second to side effects as the most common reported reason also

for discontinuation. In addition, no longer fearing cancer relapse, lack of social support and no opportunity to ask questions at diagnosis can also affect tamoxifen interruption over time [74].

In SOFT, after a median follow-up of 8 years, early discontinuation of oral ET occurred in 22.5% of the tamoxifen group, 18.5% of the tamoxifen-OFS group, and 27.8% of the exemestane-OFS group. Early cessation of GnRHa injections, without substitution of ovarian ablation, was similar between treatment groups (~20%). In SOFT-TEXT, overall, after a median follow-up of 8 years, 21.5% of the patients stopped oral ET early, more frequently among the patients assigned to exemestane (23.7%) than those in the tamoxifen group (19.3%). Early cessation of triptorelin, without substitution of ovarian ablation, occurred in 14% and 19% of the patients, respectively [21]. Overall, 19.8% of women <35 years in SOFT-TEXT [31] stopped all protocol-assigned therapy early. Nonadherence with assigned oral ET was higher in women <35 years ($P = 0.01$) than in women ≥ 35 years (25% and 21% at 4 years after initiation, respectively). Nonadherence with medical OFS was also significantly higher among patients <35 years ($P = 0.009$) than in older premenopausal patients (23% and 17% at 4 years after initiation, respectively). In individual patients, health professionals should carefully weigh side effects and impact on QoL associated with escalating ET against the risk of recurrence and the expected absolute improvement in disease outcome. According to the latest guidelines [10], clinics specifically dedicated to the assessment and management of early and late treatment side effects should be implemented in order to improve both adherence and persistence.

11.8 Future Perspectives and Challenges

Despite substantial outcome improvements in young women with HR+ breast cancer receiving modern adjuvant ET, both healthcare professionals and patients still face several challenges. Endocrine resistance may in fact develop and induce disease relapse. Several potentially targetable mechanisms of endocrine resistance have been identified, such as upregulation of alternative growth pathways (e.g., mTOR and CDK4/6) [75]. Several studies, open also to premenopausal patients, are evaluating the efficacy and safety of adding CDK4/6 inhibitors to standard adjuvant ET: PALLAS (NCT02513394) is investigating the addition of palbociclib; MonarchE (NCT03155997) is evaluating abemaciclib in patients with high-risk, node-positive disease; earLEE-1 (NCT03078751) and earLEE-2 (NCT03081234) will evaluate ribociclib in patients with high- and intermediate-risk, respectively. The mTOR inhibitor everolimus is being evaluated in patients with high-risk disease (NCT01674140).

11.9 Conclusions

To further improve the management of young women with HR+ early breast cancer, clinicians need to learn how to best incorporate the information collected by modern randomized clinical trials into the individual patient care. The oncologist is therefore challenged to precisely assess the risk of recurrence according to currently available predictive and prognostic factors in order to identify patients for whom escalating ET from tamoxifen to tamoxifen-OFS and exemestane-OFS justifies the additional side effects. Treatment planning should always be discussed and agreed in a multidisciplinary context.

Tamoxifen remains the standard of care in low-risk patients or in case of intolerance to combined treatment with pharmacological OFS or AIs. Combination treatment is indicated in intermediate-high risk disease. Improving QoL and reducing side effects are also pivotal in order to best exploit available treatments. The patient should always be considered an active partner in the treatment decision process, to improve treatment motivation and adherence. Finally, the therapeutic choice should take into account drug availability and pharmaco-economic issues, which unfortunately still prevent, in many low-income countries, the provision of many effective treatments.

References

1. Azim HA Jr, et al. Elucidating prognosis and biology of breast cancer arising in young women using gene expression profiling. Clin Cancer Res. 2012;18(5):1341–51.
2. Keegan TH, et al. Occurrence of breast cancer subtypes in adolescent and young adult women. Breast Cancer Res. 2012;14(2):R55.
3. Swain SM, et al. Quantitative gene expression by recurrence score in ER-positive breast Cancer, by age. Adv Ther. 2015;32(12):1222–36.
4. Chollet-Hinton L, et al. Breast cancer biologic and etiologic heterogeneity by young age and menopausal status in the Carolina breast cancer study: a case-control study. Breast Cancer Res. 2016;18(1):79.
5. Partridge AH, et al. Subtype-dependent relationship between young age at diagnosis and breast cancer survival. J Clin Oncol. 2016;34(27):3308–14.
6. Sestak I, Cuzick J. Markers for the identification of late breast cancer recurrence. Breast Cancer Res. 2015;17:10.
7. Paik S, et al. A multigene assay to predict recurrence of tamoxifen-treated, node-negative breast cancer. N Engl J Med. 2004;351(27):2817–26.
8. Sparano JA, et al. Prospective validation of a 21-gene expression assay in breast cancer. N Engl J Med. 2015;373(21):2005–14.
9. Cardoso F, et al. 70-gene signature as an aid to treatment decisions in early-stage breast cancer. N Engl J Med. 2016;375(8):717–29.
10. Paluch-Shimon S, et al. ESO-ESMO 3rd international consensus guidelines for breast cancer in young women (BCY3). Breast. 2017;35:203–17.
11. Early Breast Cancer Trialists' Collaborative Group (EBCTCG), et al. Relevance of breast cancer hormone receptors and other factors to the efficacy of adjuvant tamoxifen: patient-level meta-analysis of randomised trials. Lancet. 2011;378(9793):771–84.
12. Burstein HJ, et al. Adjuvant endocrine therapy for women with hormone receptor-positive breast cancer: American Society of Clinical Oncology clinical practice guideline update on ovarian suppression. J Clin Oncol. 2016;34(14):1689–701.
13. Curigliano G, et al. De-escalating and escalating treatments for early-stage breast cancer: the St. Gallen international expert consensus conference on the primary therapy of early breast Cancer 2017. Ann Oncol. 2017;28(8):1700–12.
14. Senkus E, et al. Primary breast cancer: ESMO clinical practice guidelines for diagnosis, treatment and follow-up. Ann Oncol. 2015;26(Suppl 5):v8–30.
15. Dowsett M, et al. The biology of steroid hormones and endocrine treatment of breast cancer. Breast. 2005;14(6):452–7.
16. Francis PA, et al. Adjuvant ovarian suppression in premenopausal breast cancer. N Engl J Med. 2015;372(5):436–46.

17. Pagani O, et al. Adjuvant exemestane with ovarian suppression in premenopausal breast cancer. N Engl J Med. 2014;371(2):107–18.

18. Regan MM, et al. Adjuvant treatment of premenopausal women with endocrine-responsive early breast cancer: design of the TEXT and SOFT trials. Breast. 2013;22(6):1094–100.

19. Regan MM, et al. Absolute benefit of adjuvant endocrine therapies for premenopausal women with hormone receptor-positive, human epidermal growth factor receptor 2-negative early breast Cancer: TEXT and SOFT trials. J Clin Oncol. 2016;34(19):2221–31.

20. Zhou Q, et al. Prognostic impact of chemotherapy-induced amenorrhea on premenopausal breast cancer: a meta-analysis of the literature. Menopause. 2015;22(10):1091–7.

21. Francis PA, et al. Tailoring adjuvant endocrine therapy for premenopausal breast cancer. N Engl J Med. 2018;379(2):122–37.

22. Tevaarwerk AJ, et al. Phase III comparison of tamoxifen versus tamoxifen plus ovarian function suppression in premenopausal women with node-negative, hormone receptor-positive breast cancer (E-3193, INT-0142): a trial of the eastern cooperative oncology group. J Clin Oncol. 2014;32(35):3948–58.

23. Sparano JA, et al. Adjuvant chemotherapy guided by a 21-gene expression assay in breast Cancer. N Engl J Med. 2018;379(2):111–21.

24. Francis PA. Adjuvant endocrine therapy for premenopausal women: type and duration. Breast. 2017;34(Suppl 1):S108–11.

25. Rossi L, Pagani O. The role of gonadotropin-releasing-hormone analogues in the treatment of breast Cancer. J Women's Health (Larchmt). 2018;27(4):466–75.

26. Pagani O, Regan MM, Francis PA. Are SOFT and TEXT results practice changing and how? Breast. 2016;27:122–5.

27. Lamerato L, et al. Breast cancer recurrence and related mortality in U.S. pts with early breast cancer. J Clin Oncol. 2005;23(Suppl 16):738.

28. Le MG, et al. Prognostic factors for death after an isolated local recurrence in patients with early-stage breast carcinoma. Cancer. 2002;94(11):2813–20.

29. Sorensen SV, et al. Incidence-based cost-of-illness model for metastatic breast cancer in the United States. Int J Technol Assess Health Care. 2012;28(1):12–21.

30. Gnant M, et al. Zoledronic acid combined with adjuvant endocrine therapy of tamoxifen versus anastrozol plus ovarian function suppression in premenopausal early breast cancer: final analysis of the Austrian breast and colorectal Cancer study group trial 12. Ann Oncol. 2015;26(2):313–20.

31. Saha P, et al. Treatment efficacy, adherence, and quality of life among women younger than 35 years in the international breast Cancer study group TEXT and SOFT adjuvant endocrine therapy trials. J Clin Oncol. 2017;35(27):3113–22.

32. Regan MM, et al. Concurrent and sequential initiation of ovarian function suppression with chemotherapy in premenopausal women with endocrine-responsive early breast cancer: an exploratory analysis of TEXT and SOFT. Ann Oncol. 2017;28(9):2225–32.

33. Lambertini M, et al. Gonadotropin-releasing hormone agonists during chemotherapy for preservation of ovarian function and fertility in premenopausal patients with early breast cancer: a systematic review and meta-analysis of individual patient-level data. J Clin Oncol. 2018;36(19):1981–90.

34. Pfeiler G, et al. Impact of body mass index on the efficacy of endocrine therapy in premenopausal patients with breast cancer: an analysis of the prospective ABCSG-12 trial. J Clin Oncol. 2011;29(19):2653–9.

35. Jatoi I, et al. Breast cancer adjuvant therapy: time to consider its time-dependent effects. J Clin Oncol. 2011;29(17):2301–4.

36. Yu KD, et al. Hazard of breast cancer-specific mortality among women with estrogen receptor-positive breast cancer after five years from diagnosis: implication for extended endocrine therapy. J Clin Endocrinol Metab. 2012;97(12):E2201–9.

37. Wimmer K, et al. Optimal duration of adjuvant endocrine therapy: how to apply the newest data. Ther Adv Med Oncol. 2017;9(11):679–92.

38. Davies C, et al. Long-term effects of continuing adjuvant tamoxifen to 10 years versus stopping at 5 years after diagnosis of oestrogen receptor-positive breast cancer: ATLAS, a randomised trial. Lancet. 2013;381(9869):805–16.

39. Goss PE, et al. Impact of premenopausal status at breast cancer diagnosis in women entered on the placebo-controlled NCIC CTG MA17 trial of extended adjuvant letrozole. Ann Oncol. 2013;24(2):355–61.

40. Ruddy KJ, et al. Extended therapy with letrozole and ovarian suppression in premenopausal patients with breast cancer after tamoxifen. Clin Breast Cancer. 2014;14(6):413–6.

41. Noh WC, et al. Role of adding ovarian function suppression to tamoxifen in young women with hormone-sensitive breast cancer who remain premenopausal or resume menstruation after chemotherapy: the ASTRRA study. J Clin Oncol. 2018;36(Suppl 15):502.

42. Runowicz CD, et al. American Cancer Society/American Society of Clinical Oncology breast Cancer survivorship care guideline. J Clin Oncol. 2016;34(6):611–35.

43. Rosenberg SM, et al. Symptoms and symptom attribution among women on endocrine therapy for breast Cancer. Oncologist. 2015;20(6):598–604.

44. Takeuchi EE, et al. Impact of patient-reported outcomes in oncology: a longitudinal analysis of patient-physician communication. J Clin Oncol. 2011;29(21):2910–7.

45. Chen J, Ou L, Hollis SJ. A systematic review of the impact of routine collection of patient reported outcome measures on patients, providers and health organisations in an oncologic setting. BMC Health Serv Res. 2013;13:211.

46. Absolom K, et al. Electronic patient self-reporting of adverse-events: patient information and aDvice

(eRAPID): a randomised controlled trial in systemic cancer treatment. BMC Cancer. 2017;17(1):318.

47. Holch P, et al. Development of an integrated electronic platform for patient self-report and management of adverse events during cancer treatment. Ann Oncol. 2017;28(9):2305–11.

48. Henry, NL. Endocrine therapy toxicity: management options. Am Soc Clin Oncol Educ Book. 2014:e25–30.

49. Sverrisdottir A, et al. Bone mineral density among premenopausal women with early breast cancer in a randomized trial of adjuvant endocrine therapy. J Clin Oncol. 2004;22(18):3694–9.

50. Vehmanen L, et al. Tamoxifen treatment after adjuvant chemotherapy has opposite effects on bone mineral density in premenopausal patients depending on menstrual status. J Clin Oncol. 2006;24(4):675–80.

51. Rossi L, Pagani O. The modern landscape of endocrine therapy for premenopausal women with breast Cancer. Breast Care (Basel). 2015;10(5):312–5.

52. Chien AJ, et al. Association of tamoxifen use and ovarian function in patients with invasive or pre-invasive breast cancer. Breast Cancer Res Treat. 2015;153(1):173–81.

53. Braems G, et al. Use of tamoxifen before and during pregnancy. Oncologist. 2011;16(11):1547–51.

54. Christinat A, Di Lascio S, Pagani O. Hormonal therapies in young breast cancer patients: when, what and for how long? J Thorac Dis. 2013;5(Suppl 1):S36–46.

55. Paganini-Hill A, Clark LJ. Preliminary assessment of cognitive function in breast cancer patients treated with tamoxifen. Breast Cancer Res Treat. 2000;64(2):165–76.

56. Schilder CM, et al. Effects of tamoxifen and exemestane on cognitive functioning of postmenopausal patients with breast cancer: results from the neuropsychological side study of the tamoxifen and exemestane adjuvant multinational trial. J Clin Oncol. 2010;28(8):1294–300.

57. Nystedt M, et al. Side effects of adjuvant endocrine treatment in premenopausal breast cancer patients: a prospective randomized study. J Clin Oncol. 2003;21(9):1836–44.

58. Phillips KA, et al. Adjuvant ovarian function suppression and cognitive function in women with breast cancer. Br J Cancer. 2016;114(9):956–64.

59. Underwood EA, et al. Cognitive sequelae of endocrine therapy in women treated for breast cancer: a meta-analysis. Breast Cancer Res Treat. 2018;168(2):299–310.

60. Kelly CM, Pritchard KI. CYP2D6 genotype as a marker for benefit of adjuvant tamoxifen in post-menopausal women: lessons learned. J Natl Cancer Inst. 2012;104(6):427–8.

61. Sacco K, Grech G. Actionable pharmacogenetic markers for prediction and prognosis in breast cancer. EPMA J. 2015;6(1):15.

62. Ribi K, et al. Adjuvant Tamoxifen plus ovarian function suppression versus Tamoxifen alone in premenopausal women with early breast Cancer: patient-reported outcomes in the suppression of ovarian function trial. J Clin Oncol. 2016;34(14):1601–10.

63. Hurny C, et al. The Perceived Adjustment to Chronic Illness Scale (PACIS): a global indicator of coping for operable breast cancer patients in clinical trials. Swiss Group for Clinical Cancer Research (SAKK) and the International Breast Cancer Study Group (IBCSG). Support Care Cancer. 1993;1(4):200–8.

64. Dowsett M, Folkerd E. Deficits in plasma oestradiol measurement in studies and management of breast cancer. Breast Cancer Res. 2005;7(1):1–4.

65. Bellet M, et al. Twelve-month estrogen levels in premenopausal women with hormone receptor-positive breast Cancer receiving adjuvant Triptorelin plus Exemestane or Tamoxifen in the suppression of ovarian function trial (SOFT): the SOFT-EST substudy. J Clin Oncol. 2016;34(14):1584–93.

66. Masuda N, et al. Monthly versus 3-monthly goserelin acetate treatment in pre-menopausal patients with estrogen receptor-positive early breast cancer. Breast Cancer Res Treat. 2011;126(2):443–51.

67. Bernhard J, et al. Patient-reported outcomes with adjuvant exemestane versus tamoxifen in premenopausal women with early breast cancer undergoing ovarian suppression (TEXT and SOFT): a combined analysis of two phase 3 randomised trials. Lancet Oncol. 2015;16(7):848–58.

68. Artigalas O, et al. Influence of CYP19A1 polymorphisms on the treatment of breast cancer with aromatase inhibitors: a systematic review and meta-analysis. BMC Med. 2015;13:139.

69. Johansson H, et al. Impact of CYP19A1 and ESR1 variants on early-onset side effects during combined endocrine therapy in the TEXT trial. Breast Cancer Res. 2016;18(1):110.

70. Pagani O, et al. Impact of SERM adherence on treatment effect: international breast Cancer study group trials 13-93 and 14-93. Breast Cancer Res Treat. 2013;142(2):455–9.

71. Hershman DL, et al. Early discontinuation and nonadherence to adjuvant hormonal therapy are associated with increased mortality in women with breast cancer. Breast Cancer Res Treat. 2011;126(2):529–37.

72. Murphy CC, et al. Adherence to adjuvant hormonal therapy among breast cancer survivors in clinical practice: a systematic review. Breast Cancer Res Treat. 2012;134(2):459–78.

73. Llarena NC, et al. Impact of fertility concerns on Tamoxifen initiation and persistence. J Natl Cancer Inst. 2015;107(10):djv202.

74. Cluze C, et al. Adjuvant endocrine therapy with tamoxifen in young women with breast cancer: determinants of interruptions vary over time. Ann Oncol. 2012;23(4):882–90.

75. Brufsky AM, Dickler MN. Estrogen receptor-positive breast Cancer: exploiting signaling pathways implicated in endocrine resistance. Oncologist. 2018;23:528.

Management of Advanced Breast Cancer in Young Women: What's New in Systemic Treatment

12

Simona Volovat[$], Joana Mourato Ribeiro[$], Assia Konsoulova[$], Shani Paluch-Shimon, and Fatima Cardoso

12.1 Introduction

Although breast cancer (BC) in young women is a rare disease, with fewer than 5% occurring in women <40 years old [1], it is still the leading cause of cancer death among women 20–39 years old [1]. In 1983, the median survival time for premenopausal women with advanced breast cancer (ABC) was 35 months, with only 28% still alive at 5 years [2]. Mortality rates from ABC have remained stable; in the 1975–2014 SEER report, the overall 5-year relative survival rate was 27% for stage IV BC [3], although the absolute number of deaths is rising with an estimated 43% increase in BC deaths by 2030 [4].

In the last decade, advances in treatment of ABC and incremental benefits have been achieved in some BC subsets, namely, in HER2+ BC. We must underline that only modest improvements in outcomes have occurred in hormone-dependent BC and little to no improvements have occurred in TNBC, which together represent more than 80% of patients [4].

Compared with women aged >45, those ≤45 years are slightly less likely to be estrogen receptor positive (ER+); ER positivity may decrease to approximately 55% in women aged 20–39 years [5].

There are few clinical trials that have focused on the treatment of young women with ABC, and current guideline recommendations for this age group are predominantly based on retrospective data or extrapolated from current recommendations for postmenopausal women.

In ER+ ABC, several endocrine therapy (ET) options have proven to be effective, including selective estrogen receptor modulators [SERMs]—such as tamoxifen -, aromatase inhibitors [AI]—such as anastrozole, letrozole, exemestane -, ovarian function suppression/ablation [OFS/OA] ± tamoxifen or an AI, selective ER downregulators [SERDs]—fulvestrant -, progestational agents -megestrol acetate - [6, 7].

The recently approved combinations of endocrine agents with CDK inhibitors (CDKi) or mTOR inhibitors (mTORi) have gained an important role in the management of luminal ABC in both pre- and postmenopausal patients.

[$]Simona Volovat, Joana Mourato Ribeiro, and Assia Konsoulova contributed equally to this work.

S. Volovat · J. M. Ribeiro (✉) · F. Cardoso
Breast Unit, Champalimaud Clinical Center/
Champalimaud Foundation, Lisbon, Portugal
e-mail: joana.ribeiro@fundacaochampalimaud.pt;
fatimacardoso@fundacaochampalimaud.pt

A. Konsoulova
Medical Oncology Clinic, University Hospital Sveta Marina, Varna, Bulgaria

S. Paluch-Shimon
Breast Oncology Unit, Shaare Zedek Medical Centre, Jerusalem, Israel
e-mail: shanips@szmc.org.il

© Springer Nature Switzerland AG 2020
O. Gentilini et al. (eds.), *Breast Cancer in Young Women*,
https://doi.org/10.1007/978-3-030-24762-1_12

12.2 Systemic Therapy in ER+ ABC

12.2.1 Endocrine Therapy

There is a paucity of data on the management of ER+ premenopausal women with ABC because these patients traditionally were not included in clinical trials evaluating endocrine therapies with or without targeted agents, particularly in the first-line setting.

Unless there is a visceral crisis/life-threatening disease or a highly symptomatic patient, ET must be the preferred option among young women with ABC. ET after discontinuation of chemotherapy (maintenance ET) to maintain achieved benefit should be considered, although this modality has not been evaluated in randomized trials [7].

So far and despite intensive research, the only biomarkers predictive of response to ET are the hormonal receptor expression and their level of positivity. No biomarker exists to help choose among different ET agents or to identify patients who could benefit the most from combinations of ET and targeted agents.

The most recent ESO-ESMO ABC guidelines recommend that young women with ER+ ABC have adequate OFS/OA and then be treated in the same way as postmenopausal women, i.e., with ET with or without targeted therapies [7, 8].

12.2.1.1 Ovarian Suppression/ Ablation

Use of gonadotropin-releasing hormone agonists (GnRHa) to downregulate GnRH production by the hypothalamus effectively produces a "medical ablation" of the ovaries and is an alternative to surgical or irradiation-induced ablation. The effectiveness of GnRHa in patients with ABC was first published using buserelin [9] and goserelin [10]. Other compounds of this class include leuprorelin and triptorelin. Goserelin is the most extensively investigated GnRHa. No comparisons between the different GnRHa have been reported. On the contrary, comparisons between "medical" and "surgical" ablation have been performed. In a randomized trial, patients with ER+ and/or PR tumors were assigned to receive goserelin depot ($n = 69$) or surgical oophorectomy ($n = 67$) [11].

The two treatment arms showed comparable objective response rates (ORR) (goserelin 31%; oophorectomy 27%) and stable disease (goserelin 28%; oophorectomy 26%). Overall survival and progression-free survival (PFS) were similar for both goserelin and oophorectomy. Surgical OFS is a more cost-effective procedure and induces permanent estrogen suppression and contraception, leading to definitive menopause in young patients with ABC and potentially avoiding the "flare syndrome" sometimes seen with GnRHa. However, its permanent characteristic is often psychologically difficult to accept for young women. In all cases, the best modality should be discussed and decided with the patient [12, 13].

Goserelin monotherapy effectiveness in the treatment of ABC in pre- and perimenopausal women was evaluated in several phase II studies with response rates ranging from 14 to 70% [14], with degree of hormone receptor expression strongly predictive of response. A combined analysis of 29 phase II studies, enrolling 333 patients with histologically confirmed stage III or IV BC between 1982 and 1988 [15], reported the following outcomes for patients receiving monthly goserelin: median survival of 26.5 months (range, 0.8–69 months), 33.1 months in ER+ vs. 15.9 months in ER- patients [16]; ORR was 36% (83/228 patients), 44% in ER+ vs. 31% in ER-patients, and the median duration of response was 44 weeks. In general, OFS alone is not a recommended approach but may be acceptable under special circumstances or when combined ET is intolerable.

Radiation-induced OA remains a cost-effective option for premenopausal patients who need to be rendered menopausal, although its use is decreasing. A meta-analysis [17] that included 3317 patients showed similar efficacy of OFS/OA independently from the method used to achieve it (medical, surgical, or RT) in terms of overall survival (OS) ($p = 0.37$) without significant adverse effects. In these trials the majority of patients were treated with large field sizes with parallel-opposed anteroposterior and posteroanterior pelvic fields. Radiotherapy doses of 1500 cGy in five fractions, 1500 cGy in four fractions, 1600 cGy in four fractions, and 2000 cGy in ten fractions were delivered [17]. Occasional long-term complications have been described, such as longer time to achieve castrate levels of estradiol and unreliable long-term suppression making it the least preferred option in most guidelines [7, 18].

Young women with ABC are more likely to suffer from psychosocial distress and anxiety compared to older patients [19]. In addition, for many young women, the idea of oophorectomy, especially at ABC diagnosis, is devastating. In these cases oophorectomy should be offered again later [20].

12.2.1.2 Ovarian Suppression/ Ablation with or Without Tamoxifen

After its development in the 1970s, tamoxifen has become the preferred therapeutic option in premenopausal women with ABC because of the ease of its oral administration and the fact that it does not require OFS/OA. Several randomized trials in the past decades have compared tamoxifen to OFS/OA as first-line ET for premenopausal women with ABC. Despite several limitations (small populations, uncertainty regarding hormone receptor status), they suggested similar outcomes between the two approaches [21–23]. In 1997, a meta-analysis of 4 studies in more than 200 evaluable patients found no significant difference in ORR, disease progression, or mortality between the two treatment modalities [24].

Several studies, including a meta-analysis comparing GnRHa ± tamoxifen, demonstrated significantly superior outcomes in patients who received the combination of OFS and ET [25]. All major international and national guidelines [7, 8, 18, 26, 27] state that for premenopausal women OFS/OA combined with additional ET is the first choice (LoE:1A). Tamoxifen alone can also be considered, although available data suggest improved outcomes when OFS is also used.

Three randomized trials have compared combined ET with tamoxifen and a GnRHa to endocrine monotherapy (GnRH analogue in all but one of the trials) in premenopausal women with ABC [28–30]. A meta-analysis of these trials, evaluating 506 patients with a median follow-up of 6.8 years, has been published [31]. The

results suggest that combination ET is superior to monotherapy. Patients who underwent combination ET had superior OS (hazard ratio [HR] 0.78; $p = 0.02$) and PFS (HR 0.70; $p = 0.0003$). Rate of objective clinical response (39 vs. 30%) and duration of response (DoR) (19.4 vs. 11.3 months) also favored the combination arm [31]. Quality of life (QoL) and toxicity data were not routinely collected when these trials were performed.

12.2.1.3 Scheduling Considerations of Ovarian Suppression

The pharmacodynamics of goserelin in BC was examined in the 1980s, and studies started with the use of daily subcutaneous injections [10] followed by the monthly depot formulation (3.6 mg) that is now used in clinical practice. The effectiveness of the monthly goserelin administration to suppress serum concentrations of FSH, LH, and estradiol was also established in a study of 118 pre- and perimenopausal patients with ABC in whom mean serum estradiol values fell into the postmenopausal range (i.e., <30 pg/ml) 2–3 weeks after treatment [32].

The development of a longer-acting goserelin formulation (3-monthly, 10.8 mg) can represent an advantage since such a formulation would require fewer clinic visits and could potentially be more convenient for the patient. However, issues, including efficacy and safety of goserelin every 3 months vs. monthly in premenopausal women, have been raised. To address this, a randomized trial compared these two schedules of administration in a Japanese population consisting of premenopausal women with ER + early BC ($n = 170$) [33]. Primary endpoint was a non-inferiority analysis (10.8/3.6 mg) of the area under the concentration–time curve (AUC) of estradiol (E2) over the first 24 weeks. The analysis demonstrated that the E2 suppression with 3-monthly goserelin was non-inferior to monthly goserelin. No clinically important differences in safety and tolerability were observed between the two groups. Another study assessed the non-inferiority of a 6-month depot formulation, TAP-144-SR 22.5 mg to the 3-month depot formulation and TAP-144-SR 11.25 mg regarding its suppressive effect on serum estradiol

(E2) in premenopausal patients with hormone receptor-positive early breast cancer. The primary endpoint was suppression rate of serum E2 to the menopausal level ($\leq$30 pg/mL). In this phase III trial, 167 patients were randomized, and overall, 150 patients (75 patients in each treatment group) completed the 96-week study treatment. The suppression rate of serum E2 to the menopausal level ($\leq$30 pg/mL) was 97.6% (95% CI 91.6–99.7) in the 6 months group and 96.4% (95% CI 89.9–99.3) in the 3 months group supporting the non-inferiority of the 6-monthly administration [34]. In spite of long-acting formulations availability data comparing their efficacy is scarce. Monthly administrations is recommended according to the guidelines [7, 18] but further research needed.

12.2.1.4 Aromatase Inhibitors

Clinical data regarding AIs in premenopausal patients with ABC have been increasing due to the available evidence from recent phase III studies, comparing ET vs. ET plus targeted agents that allowed inclusion of premenopausal patients. The initial data, however, came from several small studies, evaluating the combination of AIs and GnRHa [35–37]. These studies demonstrated a benefit for AIs in combination with OFS/OA. The use of these agents in combination with targeted therapies will be discussed in the next paragraphs.

When an AI is considered in premenopausal patients, it is important to achieve ovarian suppression before initiating the AI. In clinical practice, oral ET is to be started 6–8 weeks after the initiation of the GnRHa, to allow the decline in ovarian estrogen production or as soon as suppression is confirmed by hormonal levels. These levels must be rechecked at least once after the start of the AI due to the stimulating nature of AIs in premenopausal women. In the SOFT-EST substudy [34], up to 17% of patients had estrogen levels greater than the threshold, supporting the indication of ovarian function monitoring. In the same study, LH, FSH, and serum estrogens levels were measured every 3 months in the first 6 months and then every 6 months for the first 2 years and afterward annually. In light of this, routine monitoring of hormonal levels should be performed [38].

12.2.1.5 Selective Estrogen Receptor Downregulators (SERDs)

Fulvestrant may be used in the first- or advanced line settings as monotherapy or in combination with CDK4/6 inhibitors or everolimus. Unfortunately, the question of whether efficacy of SERDs requires concurrent OFS/OA has never been addressed in a clinical trial, and thus current guidelines recommend the addition of OFS/OA to fulvestrant [7, 18, 26]. Fulvestrant is known to compete with estradiol for the ER and its clinical activity is related to its plasma concentration. As premenopausal women have higher levels of estradiol, it has been hypothesized that higher concentrations of fulvestrant may induce a better clinical response in this subset of patients.

A phase II study [39] compared a high-dose of 750 mg of fulvestrant to tamoxifen in 60 premenopausal women with early BC. Both drugs significantly decreased Ki-67 and ER expression ($p < 0.0001$), and a more significant reduction in PR expression was seen with fulvestrant ($p < 0.0001$). This suggests that fulvestrant has antitumor activity in premenopausal patients. Further clinical trials are needed to confirm these findings. Another study that included 26 patients, pretreated with TAM and AIs in combination with goserelin, demonstrated a clinical benefit rate of 58% with fulvestrant plus goserelin, with a median time to progression of 6 months and OS of 32 months [40].

The FALCON study [41], a phase III trial that compared fulvestrant 500 mg to anastrozole in first-line metastatic setting, included postmenopausal women as young as 38 years in the fulvestrant arm. The study that required women to be rendered postmenopausal for inclusion showed that fulvestrant was associated with a statistically significant improvement in PFS (HR 0.79; 95% confidence interval [CI], 0.63–0.99; $p = 0.0486$) being the median PFS 16.6 months (95% CI 13.8–20.9) with fulvestrant vs. 13.8 months (95% CI 11.99–16.59) with anastrozole (difference in medians of 2.8 months) [41].

12.2.1.6 Other Hormonal Therapies

Megestrol acetate and medroxyprogesterone acetate are progestational anticancer agents inhibiting aromatase activity or increasing estrogen turnover in ABC. Several studies, which mainly focused on postmenopausal women, showed response rates of approximately 25% and acceptable tolerability with these agents [42, 43]. More recently, a phase II trial evaluated the antitumor activity and toxicity of megestrol acetate in postmenopausal women with ER ABC who had experienced disease progression on a third-generation nonsteroidal AI [44]. The clinical benefit rate (CBR) was 40% (95% CI 25–55%), and the median duration of clinical benefit was 10.0 (95% CI 8.0–14.2) months. The median PFS was 3.9 (95% CI 3.0–4.8) months. These agents are an acceptable option in later line settings [7].

12.2.2 Combined Biological and Endocrine Therapies

12.2.2.1 mTOR Inhibitors

The PI3K/AKT/mTOR pathway is activated in various cancers, playing a role in treatment resistance. Activation of the PI3K/AKT/mTOR signaling pathway is the most frequently mutated pathway in BC [45]. There is growing evidence suggesting a close interaction between the mTOR pathway and ER signaling, leading to resistance in ER+ BC. Targeting this pathway with various drugs has proved efficacious in terms of objective responses and PFS [46]. Everolimus, a selective mTOR inhibitor, has been widely studied in combination with ET in ER + ABC. The BOLERO-2 trial [47] included 724 postmenopausal patients aged between 28 and 93 years old that were randomized to everolimus and exemestane vs. exemestane alone. The median OS in patients receiving the combination of everolimus and exemestane was 31.0 months compared with 26.6 months in patients receiving placebo and exemestane (HR 0.89; 95% CI 0.73–1.10; $P = 0.14$). Median PFS was prolonged from 3.2 months with exemestane to 7.8 months with everolimus and exemestane (HR = 0.45; $p < 0.0001$). Everolimus is currently approved in combination with exemestane in ABC. Two phase II ongoing trials (NCT02313051, NCT02344550) are currently investigating the efficacy of everolimus in combination with an aromatase inhibitor and a GnRHa in premenopausal patients after progression on tamoxifen and the combination of everolimus with fulvestrant in ABC patients resistant to AI (PrE0102).

Adequate prevention, close monitoring, and proactive treatment of adverse events are needed when using everolimus, due to the increased incidence of toxic deaths reported in the BOLERO-2 trial (LoE/GoR: I/B) [47].

12.2.2.2 CDK4/6 Inhibitors

CDK-Rb pathway aberrations have been documented in BC, with CCDN1 overexpression found in almost 50% of breast tumors [48]. Consequently, this tumor cell regulatory mechanism has become a therapeutic target and various CDK4/6 inhibitors (CDK4/6i) have been tested in clinical trials. Currently, CDK4/6i in association with an AI or with fulvestrant are approved in the metastatic setting as first or latter lines of treatment in pre- and postmenopausal patients. Efficacy data of these agents in premenopausal patients with advanced disease are more limited than in postmenopausal because not all studies have allowed inclusion of these patients. The main body of evidence comes from the MONALEESA-7 trial [49] where CDK4/6i were used as first or latter line of treatment for ABC.

The MONALEESA-7 trial (NCT02278120) is a phase III randomized clinical trial, designed to evaluate the efficacy (primary endpoint PFS) of ribociclib in combination with ET (tamoxifen or an AI) and goserelin, exclusively in pre- or perimenopausal patients with ABC. All patients ($n = 672$) received OFS with GnRHa making them all postmenopausal. In this study 40% of patients presented with de novo metastatic disease. The first results reported at a median follow-up of 19.2 months have shown a significant improvement in DFS with the addition of ribociclib (23.8 vs. 13.0 months; HR 0.55; $P = 9.83 \times 10^{-8}$). The improvement was consistent across all subgroups and no difference between the AI or tamoxifen was seen. The toxicity profile was similar to what has been described in other CDK4/6i trials with neutropenia being the most frequently reported adverse event. The Febrile neutropenia rate in ribociclib arm was low (2.1%). QTc prolongation is a distinctive side effect of this agent (6.9% in ribociclib arm vs. 1.2% in placebo arm). Additional medication with potential interactions should be taken into account. QoL outcomes were reported and showed both improvement in pain score and delayed time to QoL deterioration within the ribociclib arm [49].

Other trials addressing the use of CDK4/6i in first line that allowed enrollment of young ABC patients if rendered postmenopausal include MONALEESA-2 and MONARCH-3.

The MONALEESA-2 study [50] evaluated the combination of letrozole with or without ribociclib among postmenopausal women in first-line metastatic setting. The study enrolled 668 patients aged between 23 and 91 years old. After a median follow-up of 26.4 months, the PFS 25.3 months (95% CI 23.0–30.3) vs. 16.0 months (95% CI 13.4–18.2) and ORR 42.5% vs. 28.7% ($P = 9.18 \times 10^{-5}$;OS (HR 0.746; 95% CI 0.517–1.078; $p = 0.059$) favored the combination arm. OS data remain immature in this second interim analysis [51].

The other phase III trial in first-line setting is the MONARCH-3 study [52], which explored the efficacy of an AI combined with abemaciclib in 493 postmenopausal patients with age between 38 and 87 years. The trial also showed a benefit in PFS with the combination (HR 0.543; $p = 0.000021$) after a median follow-up of 17.8 months.

The use of CDK4/6i as second or latter lines of treatment of young women with ABC was addressed in PALOMA-3 and MONARCH-2. PALOMA-3 [53] is the first phase III study that provided data regarding the clinical efficacy of CDK4/6i in ABC; the study randomly assigned 521 metastatic patients who progressed on previous endocrine therapy to either fulvestrant and palbociclib or fulvestrant and placebo. Pre- and perimenopausal women receiving monthly goserelin were eligible to participate in the trial. In this cohort, 21% of patients were pre- or peri-

menopausal. Median PFS was 11.2 months in the fulvestrant plus palbociclib group compared to 4.6 months in the fulvestrant plus placebo group (HR:0.5; 95% CI 0.40–0.62; $p < 0.000001$). Overall survival, a secondary endpoint, was 34.9 months (95% confidence interval [CI], 28.8 to 40.0) in the palbociclib–fulvestrant group and 28.0 months (95% CI, 23.6 to 34.6) in the placebo–fulvestrant group (hazard ratio for death, 0.81; 95% CI, 0.64 to 1.03; $P = 0.09$; absolute difference, 6.9 months), but unfortunately the difference did not reach statistical significance [54]. However in the pre-specified analysis according to sensitivity to previous endocrine therapy, the median OS was 39.7 months (95% CI, 34.8 to 45.7) in the palbociclib–fulvestrant group and 29.7 months (95% CI, 23.8 to 37.9) in the placebo–fulvestrant group (hazard ratio, 0.72; 95% CI, 0.55 to 0.94). This translates in a 10-month absolute survival benefit in this patient population [54].

The MONARCH-2 study [55] evaluated the role of abemaciclib in patients progressing after ET. The study enrolled 669 patients randomized to abemaciclib and fulvestrant vs. fulvestrant alone. In the overall study population, there was a PFS benefit in favor of the combination treatment (16.4 vs. 9.3 months; HR 0.553; 95% CI 0.449–0.681; $P = 0.001$). The study included 114 women as young as 32 years, who had been rendered postmenopausal; their median PFS was not reached for the combination arm and was 10.5 months for fulvestrant + GnRHa (HR 0.446, 95% CI 0.264–0.754; $p = 0.002$); the ORR was also higher for the combination with abemaciclib (60.8 vs. 28.6% ($p = 0.006$) [56]).

CDK4/6i are emerging as a drug class with consistently positive and similar results across several well-powered, phase III randomized clinical trials. This suggests a clear class effect leaving toxicity and accessibility as major considerations to the choice between the different agents. Trials comparing the use of ET + CDK4/6i with chemotherapy are currently ongoing.

The ESO-ESMO ABC 4 guidelines recommend that premenopausal women with luminal ABC receive OFS/OA and be treated with the same options as postmenopausal women. They also strongly recommend that these patients should not be excluded from clinical trials addressing new treatment strategies in ABC [7].

12.2.2.3 PI3K Inhibitors

The Cancer Genome Atlas Network profiled 825 BC using next-generation sequencing and demonstrated that the most frequently observed somatic mutation in patients with luminal BC occurs in the *PIK3CA* gene [45]. Upstream inhibition of the PI3K/AKT/mTOR pathway involving targets such as PI3K and AKT becomes a significant promise as a treatment strategy. The phase II FERGI trial [57] randomized 168 patients who progressed to prior AI treatment to pictilisib and fulvestrant vs. fulvestrant alone. The study also evaluated the efficacy of PI3K inhibitors in patients with or without *PI3K* mutations. The study included young women rendered postmenopausal. The addition of pictilisib to fulvestrant was associated with a PFS increase from 5.1 to 6.6 months (HR 0.74; $p = 0.096$). Mutation in *PI3K* was not predictive of treatment benefit in this study.

The efficacy of PI3K inhibitors such as buparlisib in combination with fulvestrant has been studied in postmenopausal women with ABC [58, 59]. The BELLE-2 randomized phase III trial included 1147 patients that were randomized to fulvestrant plus buparlisib or placebo. The median PFS was only minimally different between arms (6.9 vs. 5 months; HR 0.78, 95% CI 0.67–0.89; $p = 0.00021$), both in the PI3K muted and the wild-type subgroups. The toxicity profile included elevated liver enzymes (18–25 vs. 1–3%), hyperglycemia (15 vs. 1%), and rash (8% vs. none) [58]. The BELLE-3 randomized phase III trial evaluated the efficacy of buparlisib vs. placebo in patients with ABC who have progressed on or after ET and mTOR inhibitors. 432 patients were randomized to buparlisib and fulvestrant ($n = 289$) or placebo and fulvestrant ($n = 143$). The median PFS was dismal in both arms and only minimally different (3.9 vs. 1.8 months, HR 0.67, 95% CI 0.53–0.84; $p = 0.0003$), with similar side effects as in BELLE-2 trial and serious adverse events in 22% of patients compared to fulvestrant alone (16% of

patients) [59]. Based on these results, the development of buparlisib has been stopped. Other important studies are currently ongoing regarding more specific PI3K inhibitors.

We must underline the increased number of potential toxicities of these agents that may eventually limit their use, such as hyperglycemia or rash (common to several PI3K/AKT/mTOR signaling pathway inhibitors) and others like neutropenia, gastrointestinal toxicity, and mood disorders which have been observed in clinical trials of pan-PI3K inhibitors. Recognition of the toxicities associated with these agents is essential to develop best practices for patient management and education.

12.2.2.4 Bevacizumab

Studies evaluating the efficacy of bevacizumab combined with endocrine or chemotherapy treatments in ABC failed to show an OS benefit. Younger patients were included in the trials in combination with chemotherapy, if rendered postmenopausal, and with ET.

The CALGB 40503 study [60] comparing ET with or without bevacizumab in 350 postmenopausal women with ABC showed a PFS benefit of 5 months (20.2 vs. 15.6 months, HR 0.75; 95% CI 0.59–0.96 $p = 0.016$), with significant grade 3 and 4 treatment-related toxicity.

Another study [61] included 374 postmenopausal patients with ABC and evaluated the efficacy of bevacizumab and ET (fulvestrant or letrozole) vs. ET alone. The study failed to show PFS benefit with the combination treatment (median PFS of 19.3 vs. 14.4 months, HR 0.83; 95% CI 0.65–1.06; $p = 0.126$).

In first-line setting, the combination of bevacizumab with taxanes (ECOG 2100 and AVADO studies) showed a moderate benefit in PFS, but no impact in OS. As a second line, in combination with capecitabine (AVF2119g), neither PFS nor OS was improved.

The ECOG 2100 study [62, 63] comparing first-line weekly paclitaxel with or without bevacizumab in 722 women (age 29–84 years) with ABC showed a PFS benefit of 5.4 months in the total population (11.4 vs. 5.8 months, HR

0.42; 95% CI 0.34–0.52; $p < 0.001$), with significant grade 3 and 4 bevacizumab-related toxicity. Thirty percent of all patients ($N = 220$) were premenopausal women (27–49 years): overall, in the subgroup analysis, their PFS benefit was even greater, 7.0 months (12.5 vs. 5.5 months HR 0.50; 95% CI 0.38–0.67; $p < 0.001$) [63], but only 8% of these patients were young (27–40 years, $N = 59$), and their benefit in PFS was not statistically significant (HR 0.54; 95% CI 0.26–1.09) [62].

The AVADO study [64] included 736 patients with ABC (age 29–83 years) and studied the efficacy of two different doses of bevacizumab (7.5 and 15 mg/kg), added to 3-weekly docetaxel. The proportion of younger patients was not reported. PFS was improved in both bevacizumab containing arms: 0.9 months for the dose of 7.5 mg/kg (9.0 vs. 8.1 months, HR 0.8, 95% CI 0.65–1.0; $p = 0.045$) and 1.9 months for 15 mg/kg (10.0 vs. 8.1 months, HR 0.67, 95% CI 0.54–0.83; $p < 0.001$). Subgroup analyses for age below and above 65 were done, whereas there was no analysis according to menopausal status or younger age below 40–45 years.

In AVF2119g study [65], capecitabine was studied in combination with or without bevacizumab as second line in 462 patients with ABC (age 29–78 years). The addition of bevacizumab to capecitabine did not improve neither median PFS (4.86 vs. 4.17 months; $P = 0.857$) nor median OS (15.1 vs. 14.5 months; $p = 0.63$). There was no subgroup analysis according to age or menopausal status and the proportion of younger patients was not reported.

12.3 Optimal Sequencing of Endocrine and Biological Therapies

The optimal sequence of endocrine-based therapy is uncertain. It depends on which agents have been previously used (in the (neo)adjuvant or advanced settings), the burden of disease, patient's preference, costs, and availability. Available options include AI, tamoxifen, fulvestrant, AI/fulvestrant + CDK4/6i, and AI/tamoxifen/fulvestrant + everolimus. In later lines also megestrol acetate and estradiol, as well as repetition of previously used agents, may be used [7]. At this moment evidence is lacking regarding how the different combinations of endocrine plus targeted agents compare with each other and with single-agent chemotherapy. Trials are ongoing to answer these questions.

For premenopausal women who already progressed after tamoxifen in the adjuvant setting, the addition of OFS/OA to an AI with a CDK4/6i is one of the preferred options in the first-line metastatic setting [7]. For patients with relapse after adjuvant ET with tamoxifen or AI in combination with OFS, there are limited data regarding the optimal management; however, OFS/OFA is still recommended, combined with a different ET agent than the one used in the adjuvant setting [7].

12.4 Systemic Chemotherapy

Physicians often treat young women more aggressively and give preference to chemotherapy despite the presence of ER+ disease.

A Cochrane systematic review and several randomized trials show that neither survival nor QoL is improved by treating patients with chemotherapy when ET has a reasonable chance of providing disease control [66]. Additionally, clinical trials have established that ET in the first-line setting provided similar duration of disease control regardless of visceral organ involvement, in the absence of visceral crisis/life-threatening disease [7]. For all these reasons, chemotherapy should only be the initial option in cases of immediately life-threatening disease or highly symptomatic patients. This holds true as well for premenopausal patients. International guidelines have reiterated that age alone is not a reason to give chemotherapy or to treat young patients more aggressively [7, 18].

Chemotherapy is a valid option in case of multidrug endocrine resistance or in case of exhaustion of all available endocrine treatments. As in postmenopausal women, the choice of agent depends on the previous exposure and the response obtained. Similarly, preference is given to sequential monotherapy and combination regimens are reserved for patients with rapid clinical progression, life-threatening visceral metastases, or need for rapid symptom and/or disease control [7].

12.5 HER2-Positive ABC

Treatment of HER2-positive young patients with ABC does not differ substantially from postmenopausal women, and anti-HER2-directed therapies should be the mainstay of the treatment [7]. As there are no validated predictive markers for specific targeted therapies, the choice of anti-HER2 treatment should take into account previous use of trastuzumab in the adjuvant setting, treatment-free interval, and availability of new agents. The duration of anti-HER2 treatment in patients with an optimal response should be individualized, as there are no prospective data regarding treatment duration [7]. The optimal sequence of agents is currently unknown, but it should not differ from postmenopausal patients. If all anti-HER2 agents are available, international guidelines recommend the use of dual blockade (trastuzumab + pertuzumab) with chemotherapy as first-line therapy and T-DM1 as second or beyond line. Additional options are also other chemotherapy agents with trastuzumab or with lapatinib + trastuzumab. For HER2-positive ER+ ABC, combinations of ET + anti-HER2 agents are also an available option [7, 26].

12.6 Triple-Negative ABC

Triple-negative (TN) ABC is more frequent in younger women and is a distinct BC subtype for which the mainstay of treatment is chemotherapy. TN ABC is also characterized by shorter time to disease progression and death [67]. There have been only few advances in the management of non-BRCA-associated TN ABC, and the systemic treatment does not depend on age or menopausal status of the patient. Both combination chemotherapy and sequential single-agent chemotherapy are valid options, but the preferred choice is sequential monotherapy.

Age alone should not lead to preference of combination chemotherapy regimens which should rather be considered for patients with rapid clinical progression, life-threatening disease, and/or need for rapid symptom control [7]. The main difference of TN ABC (regardless of BRCA status) is its sensitivity to platinum compounds which makes them an important treatment option if anthracyclines ± taxanes were used in (neo)adjuvant setting [7, 27]. Capecitabine and vinorelbine are also effective as first or subsequent treatment options, especially if avoiding alopecia is important. Reuse of taxanes or anthracyclines is a possible option (if not used or if progression occurred more than 12 months after (neo)adjuvant taxanes); eribulin and gemcitabine monotherapy are available for further lines. Thus, besides the role of platinum compounds, the treatment of TN ABC follows the recommendations for chemotherapy in HER2-negative ABC.

The randomized phase III TNT trial [68] compared efficacy of single-agent carboplatin vs. docetaxel in 376 women (age 48–63 years) with TN ABC (97% of the patients) or any ER/PR/HER2 ABC with known *BRCA1/2* mutations. Crossover between treatment arms was permitted upon disease progression. In the overall population as well as in the non-BRCA1/2 mutated subgroup, ORR was similar between the two treatment groups (31.4 for carboplatin vs. 35.6% for docetaxel; $p = 0.44$) [69].

Immunotherapy agents and combinations are currently under investigation in TN ABC. The phase III randomized trial IMpassion 130 [70] compared the efficacy of the addition of atezolizumab or placebo to first-line nab-paclitaxel in 902 patients. At a median follow-up of 12.9 months, there was a small increase in PFS from 5.5 months to 7.2 months (HR 0.80, 95% CI 0.69–0.92; $p = 0.0025$). In the subgroup of patients with tumors with PD-L expression >1%, the addition of atezolizumab to chemotherapy prolonged PFS from 5.0 to 7.5 months and initial (still immature) OS data seem to indicate an important 10-month benefit (15.5 vs. 25.0 months; HR 0.62, 95% CI 0.45–0.86; $p = 0.0035$).

The ongoing characterization of different subgroups within the TN ABC subtype may lead to development of specific therapies for each of the subgroups: PI3K/AKT/mTOR inhibitors, immune checkpoint inhibitors, or antibody-drug conjugates are such examples. Antiandrogens including bicalutamide [71], abiraterone [72], or enzalutamide [73] are also under investigation as there are data for androgen receptor (AR) enriched subset of TN ABC (luminal AR subtype). Despite the early efficacy signals, these agents should not be routinely used in clinical practice as data is still limited.

The treatment of BRCA-related TN ABC will be discussed below.

12.7 Metronomic Systemic Therapy

Preclinical and clinical studies have established a new strategy for the treatment of ABC metronomic chemotherapy. It refers to the frequent administration of chemotherapy agent(s) at biologically optimized doses, which are far below the maximum tolerated dose (MTD) with no prolonged drug-free breaks. This results into maintenance of low blood concentrations of the drug without significant toxic side effects [74]. Thus, rather than a direct antitumor effect, metronomic chemotherapy mainly exerts indirect effects on tumor cells, their stroma, and microenvironment via inhibition of tumor angiogenesis and stimulation of anticancer immune response [75]. The most well-studied regimens are combination of cyclophosphamide and methotrexate (CM), capecitabine, and vinorelbine as monotherapy in different doses and schedules. Oral agents are typically preferred as there is a potential for long-term use. Data come predominantly from phase II studies with ORRs of about 19–50% and PFS of about 7 months [76, 77]. There are ongoing phase III trials with metronomic chemotherapy, as well as phase III trials in the early setting [78], and this approach is adopted by current guidelines, being recommended until disease progression or unacceptable toxicity [7].

12.8 Hereditary Breast Cancer and Genetic Testing

Genetic counseling should be considered as early as possible in young patients with HER2-negative ABC as it might have therapeutic implications. The genes to be tested depend on the personal and family history, taking into account that at present, only germline mutations in BRCA1/2 have proven clinical therapeutic significance with the use of anti-poly(ADP-ribose)polymerase inhibitors (PARPi). If a mutation in BRCA1/2 has not been identified but there is suspicion of a hereditary cancer syndrome, multigene panel testing may be considered [18].

Assessment of the precise role of PARPi in germlineBRCA1/2 mutant carriers is still ongoing. In two trials, OlympiAD and EMBRACA, the use of PARPi, olaparib and talazoparib, respectively, increased PFS of about 3 months in platinum-sensitive HER2-negative disease, associated with improved QoL.

In the OlympiAD phase III trial [79], olaparib monotherapy up to third line was compared to standard single-agent chemotherapy as per physician's choice (capecitabine, eribulin, or vinorelbine) in 302 patients with HER-2 negative ABC and a germline BRCA mutation. Patients included in the trial did not receive previous platinum agents in the adjuvant or metastatic setting. Monotherapy with olaparib prolonged the median PFS of 2.8 months (7.0 vs. 4.2 months; HR 0.58; 95% CI 0.43–0.80; $p < 0.001$). The toxicity profile and the QoL were better in the olaparib arm as compared to chemotherapy. In the prespecified final OS data, 192/302 deaths had occurred (64% maturity). HR for OS in the olaparib vs. TPC group was 0.90 (95% CI 0.66, 1.23; $P = NS$; median 19.3 months [mo] vs. 17.1 months). Although median OS was 2.2 months longer for olaparib monotherapy vs. standard single-agent chemotherapy in the overall population, this difference was not statistically significant [80].

The EMBRACA phase III trial [81] compared another PARP inhibitor – talazoparib – to physician's choice of mono-chemotherapy (capecitabine, eribulin, vinorelbine, or gemcitabine) in 431 patients with ABC and a germline

BRCA mutation. At a median follow-up time of 11.2 months, PFS was 3 months longer in the talazoparib arm (8.6 vs. 5.6 months; HR 0.54; 95% CI 0.41–0.71; $p < 0.0001$) and OS at interim analysis was 22.3 vs. 19.5 months (HR 0.76; $p = 0.11$) [81]; QoL was also significantly better in the PARPi arm as compared to single-agent chemotherapy.

As described above, the phase III TNT trial [68] compared the efficacy of single-agent carboplatin vs. docetaxel in 376 women (age 48–63 years) with TN ABC or any ER/PR/HER2 ABC with known *BRCA1/2* mutations. 7.5% of the patients had BRCA1/2-associated tumors and carboplatin induced significantly higher ORR compared to docetaxel (68.0 vs. 33.3%; $p = 0.03$) in this subgroup [69]. Thus the use of carboplatin in BRCA1/2-associated TN ABC is recommended by the international guidelines [7], and in some of them, this recommendation is even with a higher level of evidence than for non-BRCA1-/2-mutated TN ABC [27].

12.9 ABC and Pregnancy Considerations

If ABC is diagnosed during pregnancy, several dilemmas must be addressed and careful discussion with the patient and her family about the overall prognosis of advanced disease is crucial so that the final decision concerning pregnancy is taken. Termination of pregnancy might not improve maternal outcome as long as appropriate systemic chemotherapy is deliverable; still, literature about treatment of ABC during pregnancy is scarce and is limited to a very small number of patients [82, 83]. Chemotherapy (anthracycline or taxanes) [84, 85] as well as vinca alkaloids and alkylating agents [86, 87] may be administered during second and third trimester with close monitoring of the pregnancy until delivery. Both ET and anti-HER2 agents are contraindicated during pregnancy due to their teratogenicity risk. Tamoxifen may cause congenital anomalies, most frequently maxillofacial or urogenital malformations [88]. Anti-HER2 agents (trastuzumab or pertuzumab) may lead to long-term

sequelae for the fetus or development of oligo- or anhydramnios during pregnancy. Since the early use of anti-HER2 agents substantially improves survival, delaying these agents until after delivery may negatively impact maternal prognosis. Systemic administration of antiangiogenic agents such as bevacizumab is also contraindicated in pregnant patients with ABC as angiogenesis is crucial for embryogenesis and for the fetal development [89].

There is a risk of pregnancy despite amenorrhea while on chemotherapy, endocrine therapy, or anti-HER2 therapy for ABC. This must be discussed with young patients with ABC, and they should be counseled for the need of adequate nonhormonal contraception, if sexually active [18].

12.10 Future Directions

With the aim to overcome endocrine resistance, novel treatment options are currently being investigated in clinical trials. Studies evaluating the efficacy of combined ET and targeted therapies should always include premenopausal women with ABC. Advances in our understanding of how tumors evolve under ET have identified changes in gene expression (ESR1, PIK3CA mutational status, HDAC enzyme expression, and acetylation levels) and mutational profiles that have the potential to improve the prediction of which specific patients will respond to ET and allow unraveling of mechanisms of resistance which will lead to the development of novel drugs.

PI3K mutations are detected in almost 40% of BC [45]. The BELLE-2 study showed a modest PFS improvement in postmenopausal ABC patients with buparlisib in combination with fulvestrant, also in PI3K mutated patients. However, considerable toxicity has been reported with these agents. PI3KCA mutational status as a biomarker of endocrine sensitivity/resistance is still controversial. Further studies with new PI3K inhibitors allowing the inclusion of premenopausal patients should be considered.

Specific mutations in the ER (*ESR1*) gene, namely, in the ER ligand-binding domain, appear to be associated with acquired resistance to AI. Such mutations are rare in primary breast cancers but are found in 10–40% of recurrent/metastatic disease, especially after long-term ET that includes AIs [90, 91]. Some of these mutations may lead to relative resistance to tamoxifen and fulvestrant and may require higher doses of fulvestrant [92]. Several ongoing trials are exploring higher doses of fulvestrant in (NCT01823835) or testing new SERDs, namely, AZD9496 (NCT02248090).

Despite all research efforts, no biomarkers exist apart from ER/PR, to select patients for specific endocrine-based approaches, and further research is necessary. In particular, age alone is not a reason to give preference to chemotherapy over ET and to treat young patients with ABC more aggressively.

Besides standard systemic treatment, metronomic anticancer therapy is becoming more widely used in patients with ABC. Future research would identify the best "metronomic" agents and define the biologically optimal dose of each agent, used either alone or in combination, as well as the timing of drug administration. Combinations of metronomic with radiotherapy and/or targeted therapy are also under evaluation.

12.11 Conclusions

ET with or without biological therapies is the preferred treatment for advanced ER + ABC, except for highly symptomatic patients, with visceral crisis or life-threatening disease in which rapid disease control is needed.

Young women have specific medical and psychosocial concerns that need to be addressed in a multidisciplinary setting.

Premenopausal patients should not be excluded from clinical trials of endocrine-based approaches, as long as they are rendered postmenopausal by OFS/OA, and should be treated with the same options available for postmenopausal patients with regular monitoring of LH, FSH, and serum estrogens, ensuring adequate OFS/OA in initially premenopausal women.

For HER2-positive ABC, the early use of anti-HER2 agents, the use of trastuzumab beyond progression, and the availability of the different anti-HER2 agents have changed the control and the evolution of this ABC subtype. There are no specific recommendations for younger patients with HER2-positive ABC.

For TN ABC, chemotherapy is the mainstay of the treatment, and there are also no specific recommendations for young patients. Combination chemotherapy should be reserved for life-threatening disease or highly symptomatic patients and should not be preferred in younger patients. Several new agents are also under intense research, aiming to optimize the management of TN ABC.

References

1. Siegel RL, Miller KD, Jemal A. Cancer statistics, 2018. CA Cancer J Clin. 2018;68(1):7–30. https://doi.org/10.3322/caac.21442.
2. Falkson G, Holcroft C, Gelman RS, Tormey DC, Wolter JM, Cummings FJ. Ten-year follow-up study of premenopausal women with metastatic breast cancer: an Eastern Cooperative Oncology Group Study. J Clin Oncol. 1995;13(6):1453–8.
3. Howlader N, Noone A, Krapcho M, Miller D, Bishop K, Kosary C, et al. SEER cancer statistics review, 1975–2014. Bethesda, MD: Natl Cancer Institute; 2017.
4. Cardoso F, Beishon M, Cardoso MJ, Corneliussen-James D, Gralow J, Mertz S, et al. Global status of advanced/metastatic breast cancer (ABC/mBC): a decade report 2005–2015. Eur J Cancer. 2016;57:S5–6.
5. Li HC, Wen XF, Hou YF, Shen KW, Wu J, Lu JS, et al. Addition of adjuvant tamoxifen to cyclophosphamide, methotrexate and 5-fluorouracil for premenopausal women with oestrogen receptor-positive breast cancer. Asian J Surg. 2003;26(3):163–8.
6. NCCN. NCCN Clinical Guidelines Version 1.2018: Genetic/familial high-risk assessment: breast and ovarian. 2018.
7. Cardoso F, Senkus E, Costa A, Papadopoulos E, Aapro M, André F, Harbeck N, Lopez BA, Barrios CH, Bergh J, Biganzoli L, Boers-Doets CB, Cardoso MJ, Carey LA, Cortés J, Curigliano G, Diéras V, El Saghir NS, Eniu A, Fallowfield L, Francis PA, et al. 4th ESO-ESMO International Consensus Guidelines for Advanced Breast Cancer (ABC 4). Ann Oncol. 2018;29(8):1634–57.

8. NCCN. NCCN Clinical Practice Guidelines in Oncology (NCCN Guidelines). Breast cancer. Version 1.2018 [Internet]. 2018. https://www.nccn.org/professionals/physician_gls/pdf/breast.pdf

9. Klijn JGM, De Jong FH. Treatment with a luteinising-hormone-releasing analogue (Buserelin) in premenopausal patients with metastatic breast cancer. Lancet. 1982;319(8283):1213–6.

10. Williams MR, Walker KJ, Turkes A, Blamey RW, Nicholson RI. The use of an LH-RH agonist (ICI 118630, Zoladex) in advanced premenopausal breast cancer. Br J Cancer. 1986;53(5):629–36.

11. Taylor CW, Green S, Dalton WS, Martino S, Rector D, Ingle JN, et al. Multicenter randomized clinical trial of goserelin versus surgical ovariectomy in premenopausal patients with receptor-positive metastatic breast cancer: an intergroup study. J Clin Oncol. 1998;16(3):994–9.

12. Horton S, Gauvreau CL. Cancer in low- and middle-income countries: an economic overview. In: Disease control priorities, Cancer, vol. 3. 3rd ed. Bethesda, MD: NCBI; 2015.

13. Prinja S, Nandi A, Horton S, Levin C, Laxminarayan R. Costs, effectiveness, and cost-effectiveness of selected surgical procedures and platforms. In: Disease control priorities, Essential surgery, vol. 1. 3rd ed. Washington, DC: The World Bank; 2015.

14. Robertson JF, Blamey RW. The use of gonadotrophin-releasing hormone (GnRH) agonists in early and advanced breast cancer in pre- and perimenopausal women. Eur J Cancer. 2003;39(7):861–9. http://www.ncbi.nlm.nih.gov/entrez/query.fcgi?cmd=Retrieve&db=PubMed&dopt=Citation&list_uids=12706354%5CnF:%5CDocuments%5CEpapers%5CRobertson

15. Blamey RW, Jonat W, Kaufmann M, Raffaele Bianco A, Namer M. Goserelin depot in the treatment of premenopausal advanced breast cancer. Eur J Cancer. 1992;28(4–5):810–4.

16. Blamey RW, Jonat W, Kaufmann M, Bianco ARNM. Survival data relating to the use of goserelin depot in the treatment of premenopausal advanced breast cancer. Eur J Cancer. 1993;29A(10):1498.

17. Al Asiri M, Tunio MA, Abdulmoniem R. Is radiation-induced ovarian ablation in breast cancer an obsolete procedure? Results of a meta-analysis. Breast Cancer Targets Ther. 2016;8:109–16.

18. Paluch-Shimon S, Pagani O, Partridge AH, Abulkhair O, Cardoso M-J, Dent RA, et al. ESO-ESMO 3rd international consensus guidelines for breast cancer in young women (BCY3). Breast. 2017;35:203–17.

19. Freedman RA, Partridge AH. Management of breast cancer in very young women. The Breast [Internet]. 2013;22:S176–9. http://linkinghub.elsevier.com/retrieve/pii/S0960977613001690

20. Havrilesky LJ, Moss HA, Chino J, Myers ER, Kauff ND. Mortality reduction and cost-effectiveness of performing hysterectomy at the time of risk-reducing salpingo-oophorectomy for prophylaxis against serous/serous-like uterine cancers in BRCA1 mutation carriers. Gynecol Oncol. 2017;145(3):549–54.

21. Buchanan RB, Blamey RW, Durrant KR, Howell A, Paterson AG, Preece PE, et al. A randomized comparison of tamoxifen with surgical oophorectomy in premenopausal patients with advanced breast cancer. J Clin Oncol. 1986;4(9):1326–30.

22. Ingle JN, Krook JE, Green SJ, Kubista TP, Everson LK, Ahmann DL, et al. Randomized trial of bilateral oophorectomy versus tamoxifen in premenopausal women with metastatic breast cancer. J Clin Oncol. 1986;4(2):178–85. http://www.ncbi.nlm.nih.gov/pubmed/3511184

23. Sawka CA, Pritchard KI, Shelley W, DeBoer G, Paterson AHG, Meakin JW, et al. A randomized crossover trial of tamoxifen versus ovarian ablation for metastatic breast cancer in premenopausal women: a report of the National Cancer Institute of Canada Clinical Trials Group (NCIC CTG) trial MA.1. Breast Cancer Res Treat. 1997;44(3):211–5.

24. Crump M, Sawka CA, DeBoer G, Buchanan RB, Ingle JN, Forbes J, et al. An individual patient-based meta-analysis of tamoxifen versus ovarian ablation as first line endocrine therapy for premenopausal women with metastatic breast cancer. Breast Cancer Res Treat. 1997;44(3):201–10.

25. Michaud LB, Jones KL, Buzdar AU. Combination endocrine therapy in the management of breast cancer. Oncologist. 2001;6(1083–7159 SB–IM):538–46.

26. Rugo HS, Rumble RB, Macrae E, Barton DL, Connolly HK, Dickler MN, et al. Endocrine therapy for hormone receptor-positive metastatic breast cancer: American society of clinical oncology guideline. J Clin Oncol. 2016;34(25):3069–103.

27. Thill M, Liedtke C. AGO recommendations for the diagnosis and treatment of patients with advanced and metastatic breast cancer: update 2016. Breast Care. 2016;11(3):216–22.

28. Boccardo F, Rubagotti A, Perrotta A, Amoroso D, Balestrero M, De Matteis A, et al. Ovarian ablation versus goserelin with or without tamoxifen in pre-perimenopausal patients with advanced breast cancer: results of a multicentric Italian study. Ann Oncol. 1994;5(4):337–42.

29. Jonat W, Kaufmann M, Blamey RW, Howell A, Collins JP, Coates A, et al. A randomised study to compare the effect of the luteinising hormone releasing hormone (LHRH) analogue goserelin with or without tamoxifen in pre- and perimenopausal patients with advanced breast cancer. Eur J Cancer. 1995;31(2):137–42.

30. Klijn JGM, Beex LVAM, Mauriac L, Van Zijl JA, Veyret C, Wildiers J, et al. Combined treatment with buserelin and tamoxifen in premenopausal metastatic breast cancer: a randomized study. J Natl Cancer Inst. 2000;92(11):903–11. http://www.scopus.com/inward/record.url?eid=2-s2.0-0034616656&partnerID=40&md5=ffdbe2e42f10044c14cd0dafabaed9bb

31. Klijn JG, Blamey RW, Boccardo F, Tominaga T, Duchateau L, Sylvester R. Combined tamoxifen and

luteinizing hormone-releasing hormone (LHRH) agonist versus LHRH agonist alone in premenopausal advanced breast cancer: a meta-analysis of four randomized trials. J Clin Oncol. 2001;19:343–53. http://www.ncbi.nlm.nih.gov/entrez/query.fcgi?cmd=Retrieve&db=PubMed&dopt=Citation&list_uids=11208825

32. Kaufmann M, Jonat W, Kleeberg U, Eiermann W, Jänicke F, Hilfrich J, et al. Goserelin, a depot gonadotrophin-releasing hormone agonist in the treatment of premenopausal patients with metastatic breast cancer. German Zoladex Trial Group. J Clin Oncol. 1989;7(8):1113–9. http://www.ncbi.nlm.nih.gov/pubmed/2526863

33. Masuda N, Iwata H, Rai Y, Anan K, Takeuchi T, Kohno N, et al. Monthly versus 3-monthly goserelin acetate treatment in pre-menopausal patients with estrogen receptor-positive early breast cancer. Breast Cancer Res Treat. 2011;126(2):443–51.

34. Bellet M, Gray KP, Francis PA, Láng I, Ciruelos E, Lluch A, et al. Twelve-month estrogen levels in premenopausal women with hormone receptor-positive breast cancer receiving adjuvant triptorelin plus exemestane or tamoxifen in the suppression of ovarian function trial (SOFT): the SOFT-EST substudy. J Clin Oncol. 2016;34(14):1584–93.

35. Nishimura R, Anan K, Yamamoto Y, Higaki K, Tanaka M, Shibuta K, et al. Efficacy of goserelin plus anastrozole in premenopausal women with advanced or recurrent breast cancer refractory to an LH-RH analogue with tamoxifen: results of the JMTO BC08-01 phase II trial. Oncol Rep. 2013;29(5):1707–13.

36. Carlson RW, Theriault R, Schurman CM, Rivera E, Chung CT, Phan SC, et al. Phase II trial of anastrozole plus goserelin in the treatment of hormone receptor-positive, metastatic carcinoma of the breast in premenopausal women. J Clin Oncol. 2010;28(25):3917–21.

37. Cheung KL, Agrawal A, Folkerd EJ, Dowsett M, JFR R, Winterbottom L. Suppression of ovarian function in combination with an aromatase inhibitor as treatment for advanced breast cancer in pre-menopausal women. Eur J Cancer. 2010;46(16):2936–42. http://www.ncbi.nlm.nih.gov/pubmed/20832294

38. Kurebayashi J, Toyama T, Sumino S, Miyajima E, Fujimoto T. Efficacy and safety of leuprorelin acetate 6-month depot, TAP-144-SR (6M), in combination with tamoxifen in postoperative, premenopausal patients with hormone receptor-positive breast cancer: a phase III, randomized, open-label, parallel-group comparative. Breast Cancer. 2017;24(1):161–70.

39. Young OE, Renshaw L, Macaskill EJ, White S, Faratian D, Thomas JSJ, et al. Effects of fulvestrant 750mg in premenopausal women with oestrogen-receptor-positive primary breast cancer. Eur J Cancer. 2008(44, 3):391–9. http://www.ncbi.nlm.nih.gov/pubmed/18083023

40. Bartsch R, Bago-Horvath Z, Berghoff A, Devries C, Pluschnig U, Dubsky P, et al. Ovarian function suppression and fulvestrant as endocrine therapy in pre-menopausal women with metastatic breast cancer. Eur J Cancer. 2012;48(13):1932–8.

41. Robertson JFR, Bondarenko IM, Trishkina E, Dvorkin M, Panasci L, Manikhas A, et al. Fulvestrant 500 mg versus anastrozole 1 mg for hormone receptor-positive advanced breast cancer (FALCON): an international, randomised, double-blind, phase 3 trial. Lancet [Internet]. 2016;388(10063):2997–3005. http://linkinghub.elsevier.com/retrieve/pii/S0140673616323893

42. Buzdar A, Jonat W, Howell A, Jones SE, Blomqvist C, Vogel CL, et al. Anastrozole, a potent and selective aromatase inhibitor, versus megestrol acetate in postmenopausal women with advanced breast cancer: results of overview analysis of two phase III trials. J Clin Oncol. 1996;14(7):2000–11.

43. Willemse PH, van der Ploeg E, Sleijfer DT, Tjabbes T, van Veelen H. A randomized comparison of megestrol acetate (MA) and medroxyprogesterone acetate (MPA) in patients with advanced breast cancer. Eur J Cancer. 1990;26(3):337–43.

44. Bines J, Dienstmann R, Obadia RM, Branco LGP, Quintella DC, Castro TM, et al. Activity of megestrol acetate in postmenopausal women with advanced breast cancer after nonsteroidal aromatase inhibitor failure: a phase II trial. Ann Oncol. 2014;25(4):831–6. http://www.ncbi.nlm.nih.gov/pubmed/24615412

45. Koboldt DC, Fulton RS, McLellan MD, Schmidt H, Kalicki-Veizer J, McMichael JF, et al. Comprehensive molecular portraits of human breast tumours. Nature. 2012;490(7418):61–70.

46. Dhillon S. Everolimus in combination with exemestane: a review of its use in the treatment of patients with postmenopausal hormone receptor-positive, her2-negative advanced breast cancer. Drugs. 2013;73(5):475–85.

47. Baselga J, Campone M, Piccart M, Burris HA, Rugo HS, Sahmoud T, et al. Everolimus in postmenopausal hormone-receptor–positive advanced breast cancer. N Engl J Med. 2012;366(6):520–9. https://doi.org/10.1056/NEJMoa1109653.

48. Barnes DM, Gillett CE. Cyclin D1 in breast cancer. Breast Cancer Res Treat. 1998;52(1–3):1–15. http://www.ncbi.nlm.nih.gov/htbin-post/Entrez/query?db=m&form=6&dopt=r&uid=10066068

49. Tripathy D, Im SA, Colleoni M, Franke F, Bardia A, Harbeck N, et al. Ribociclib plus endocrine therapy for premenopausal women with hormone-receptor-positive, advanced breast cancer (MONALEESA-7): a randomised phase 3 trial. Lancet Oncol. 2018;19(7):904–15.

50. Hortobagyi GN, Stemmer SM, Burris HA, Yap Y-S, Sonke GS, Paluch-Shimon S, et al. Ribociclib as first-line therapy for HR-positive, advanced breast Cancer. N Engl J Med. 2016;375(18):1738–48. https://doi.org/10.1056/NEJMoa1609709.

51. Hortobagyi GN, Stemmer SM, Burris HA, Yap YS, Sonke GS, Paluch-Shimon S, et al. Updated results from MONALEESA-2, a phase III trial of first-line ribociclib plus letrozole versus placebo plus letro-

zole in hormone receptor-positive, HER2-negative advanced breast cancer. Ann Oncol. 2018;29:1541–7.

52. Goetz MP, Toi M, Campone M, Sohn J, Paluch-Shimon S, Huober J, et al. MONARCH 3: Abemaciclib as initial therapy for advanced breast cancer. J Clin Oncol. 2017;35(32):3638–46. https://doi.org/10.1200/JCO.2017.75.6155. http://www.ncbi.nlm.nih.gov/pubmed/28968163

53. Cristofanilli M, Turner NC, Bondarenko I, Ro J, Im SA, Masuda N, et al. Fulvestrant plus palbociclib versus fulvestrant plus placebo for treatment of hormone-receptor-positive, HER2-negative metastatic breast cancer that progressed on previous endocrine therapy (PALOMA-3): final analysis of the multicentre, double-blind, phase. Lancet Oncol. 2016;17(4):425–39.

54. Turner NC, Slamon DJ, Ro J, Bondarenko I, Im S-A, Masuda N, Colleoni M, DeMichele A, Loi S, Verma S, Iwata H, Harbeck N, Loibl S, André F, Theall KP, Huang X, Carla G, Colleoni M. Overall survival with palbociclib and fulvestrant in advanced breast cancer. N Engl J Med. 2018;379(20):1926–36.

55. Sledge GW, Toi M, Neven P, Sohn J, Inoue K, Pivot X, et al. MONARCH 2: Abemaciclib in combination with fulvestrant in women with HR+/HER2-advanced breast cancer who had progressed while receiving endocrine therapy. J Clin Oncol. 2017;35(25):2875–84.

56. Neven P, Rugo HS, Tolaney SM, Iwata H, Toi M, Goetz MP, Kaufman PA, Barriga S, GWS YL. Abstract 1002: Abemaciclib for pre/perimenopausal women with HR+, HER2− advanced breast cancer. J Clin Oncol. 2018;36:1002.

57. Krop IE, Mayer IA, Ganju V, Dickler M, Johnston S, Morales S, et al. Pictilisib for oestrogen receptor-positive, aromatase inhibitor-resistant, advanced or metastatic breast cancer (FERGI): a randomised, double-blind, placebo-controlled, phase 2 trial. Lancet Oncol. 2016;17(6):811–21.

58. Baselga J, Im SA, Iwata H, Cortés J, De Laurentiis M, Jiang Z, et al. Buparlisib plus fulvestrant versus placebo plus fulvestrant in postmenopausal, hormone receptor-positive, HER2-negative, advanced breast cancer (BELLE-2): a randomised, double-blind, placebo-controlled, phase 3 trial. Lancet Oncol. 2017;18(7):904–16.

59. Di Leo A, Johnston S, Lee KS, Ciruelos E, Lønning PE, Janni W, et al. Buparlisib plus fulvestrant in postmenopausal women with hormone-receptor-positive, HER2-negative, advanced breast cancer progressing on or after mTOR inhibition (BELLE-3): a randomised, double-blind, placebo-controlled, phase 3 trial. Lancet Oncol. 2018;19(1):87–100.

60. Dickler MN, Barry WT, Cirrincione CT, Ellis MJ, Moynahan ME, Innocenti F, et al. Phase III trial evaluating letrozole as first-line endocrine therapy with or without bevacizumab for the treatment of postmenopausal women with hormone receptor-positive advanced-stage breast cancer: CALGB 40503 (Alliance). J Clin Oncol. 2016;34(22):2602–9.

61. Martin M, Loibl S, von Minckwitz G, Morales S, Martinez N, Guerrero A, et al. Phase III trial evaluating the addition of bevacizumab to endocrine therapy as first-line treatment for advanced breast cancer: the letrozole/fulvestrant and avastin (LEA) study. J Clin Oncol. 2015;33(9):1045–52. http://www.ncbi.nlm.nih.gov/pubmed/25691671

62. Gray R, Bhattacharya S, Bowden C, Miller K, Comis RL. Independent review of E2100: a phase III trial of bevacizumab plus paclitaxel versus paclitaxel in women with metastatic breast cancer. J Clin Oncol. 2009;27(30):4966–72. http://jco.ascopubs.org/content/27/30/4966.long

63. Miller K, Wang M, Gralow J, Dickler M, Cobleigh M, Perez E, et al. Paclitaxel plus bevacizumab versus paclitaxel alone for metastatic breast cancer. N Engl J Med. 2007;357(26):2666–76. http://www.pubmedcentral.nih.gov/articlerender.fcgi?artid=3684040&tool=pmcentrez&rendertype=abstract

64. Miles DW, Chan A, Dirix LY, Cortés J, Pivot X, Tomczak P, et al. Phase III study of bevacizumab plus docetaxel compared with placebo plus docetaxel for the first-line treatment of human epidermal growth factor receptor 2-negative metastatic breast cancer. J Clin Oncol. 2010;28(20):3239–47. http://www.ncbi.nlm.nih.gov/pubmed/20498403

65. Miller KD, Chap LI, Holmes FA, Cobleigh MA, Marcom PK, Fehrenbacher L, et al. Randomized phase III trial of capecitabine compared with bevacizumab plus capecitabine in patients with previously treated metastatic breast cancer. J Clin Oncol. 2005;23(4):792–9.

66. Wilcken N, Hornbuckle J, Ghersi D. Chemotherapy alone versus endocrine therapy alone for metastatic breast cancer. Cochrane Database Syst Rev. 2003;2:CD002747.

67. Kim H, Choi DH, Park W, Huh SJ, Nam SJ, Lee JE, et al. Prognostic factors for survivals from first relapse in breast cancer patients: analysis of deceased patients. Radiat Oncol J. 2013;31(4):222–7.

68. Tutt A, Tovey H, Cheang MCU, Kernaghan S, Kilburn L, Gazinska P, et al. Carboplatin in BRCA1/2-mutated and triple-negative breast cancer BRCAness subgroups: the TNT trial. Nat Med. 2018;24(5):628–37.

69. Tutt A, Ellis P, Kilburn L, Gilett C, Pinder S, Abraham J, Barrett S, Barrett-Lee P, Chan S, Cheang M, Dowsett M, Fox L, Gazinska P, Grigoriadis A, Gutin A, Harper-Wynne C, Hatton M, Kernaghan S, Harries M, Bliss J. Abstract S3-01: The TNT trial: A randomized phase III trial of carboplatin (C) compared with docetaxel (D) for patients with metastatic or recurrent locally advanced triple negative or BRCA1/2 breast cancer (CRUK/07/012). Cancer Res. 2015;75(9):Abstract S3-01.

70. Schmid P, Adams S, Rugo HS, Schneeweiss A, Barrios CH, Iwata H, Dieras V, Hegg R, Im S-A, Wright GS, Henschel V, Molinero L, Chui SY, Funke R, Husain A, Winer EP, Loi S, Emens LA. Abstract LBA1_PR: IMpassion130: Results from a global, randomised, double-blind, phase 3 study of atezolizumab

(atezo) + nab-paclitaxel (nab-P) vs placebo + nab-P in treatment-naive, locally advanced or metastatic triple-negative breast cancer (mTNBC). Ann Oncol. 2018;29(Suppl_8):LBA1_PR.

71. Gucalp A, Tolaney S, Isakoff SJ, Ingle JN, Liu MC, Carey LA, et al. Phase II trial of bicalutamide in patients with androgen receptor-positive, estrogen receptor-negative metastatic breast cancer. Clin Cancer Res. 2013;19(19):5505–12.

72. Bonnefoi H, Grellety T, Tredan O, Saghatchian M, Dalenc F, Mailliez A, et al. A phase II trial of abiraterone acetate plus prednisone in patients with triple-negative androgen receptor positive locally advanced or metastatic breast cancer (UCBG 12-1). Ann Oncol. 2016;27(5):812–8.

73. Lyons T, Gucalp A, Arumov A, Patil S, Edelweiss M, Gorsky M, et al. Abstract 531: Safety and tolerability of adjuvant enzalutamide for the treatment of early stage androgen receptor positive (AR+) triple negative breast cancer. J Clin Oncol. 2018;38:Abstract 531.

74. Kerbel RS, Kamen BA. The anti-angiogenic basis of metronomic chemotherapy. Nat Rev Cancer. 2004;4(6):423–36. http://www.nature.com/doifinder/10.1038/nrc1369

75. André N, Carré M, Pasquier E. Metronomics: towards personalized chemotherapy? Nat Rev Clin Oncol. 2014;11(7):413–31.

76. Cazzaniga ME, Dionisio MR, Riva F. Metronomic chemotherapy for advanced breast cancer patients. Cancer Lett. 2017;400:252–8.

77. Lien K, Georgsdottir S, Sivanathan L, Chan K, Emmenegger U. Low-dose metronomic chemotherapy: a systematic literature analysis. Eur J Cancer. 2013;49(16):3387–95.

78. Colleoni M, Gray KP, Gelber S, Láng I, Thürlimann B, Gianni L, et al. Low-dose Oral cyclophosphamide and methotrexate maintenance for hormone receptor-negative early breast cancer: international breast Cancer study group trial 22-00. J Clin Oncol. 2016;34(28):3400–8.

79. Robson M, Im S-A, Senkus E, Xu B, Domchek SM, Masuda N, et al. Olaparib for metastatic breast cancer in patients with a Germline *BRCA* mutation. N Engl J Med. 2017;377(6):523–33. Available from: https://doi.org/10.1056/NEJMoa1706450.

80. Tung NM, Im S-A, Senkus-Konefka E, Xu B, Domchek SM, Masuda N, Li W, Armstrong AC, Conte PF, Wu W, Goessl CD, MER SR. Abstract 1052: Olaparib versus chemotherapy treatment of physician's choice in patients with a germline BRCA mutation and HER2-negative metastatic breast cancer (OlympiAD): efficacy in patients with visceral metastases. J Clin Oncol. 2018;36(15):1052.

81. Litton JK, Rugo HS, Ettl J, Hurvitz SA, Gonçalves A, Lee K-H, et al. Talazoparib in patients with advanced breast cancer and a germline BRCA mutation. N Engl J Med. 2018;379(8):753–63.

82. Cardonick E, Dougherty R, Grana G, Gilmandyar D, Ghaffar S, Usmani A. Breast cancer during pregnancy: maternal and fetal outcomes. Cancer J. 2010;16(1):76–82. https://doi.org/10.1097/PPO.0b013e3181ce46f9.

83. Azim HA Jr, Peccatori FA. Treatment of metastatic breast cancer during pregnancy: we need to talk! Breast. 2008;17:426–8.

84. Loibl S, Schmidt A, Gentilini O, Kaufman B, Kuhl C, Denkert C, et al. Breast cancer diagnosed during pregnancy adapting recent advances in breast cancer care for pregnant patients. JAMA Oncol. 2015;1(8):1145–53.

85. Peccatori FA, Azim HA, Orecchia R, Hoekstra HJ, Pavlidis N, Kesic V. G. Pentheroudakis on behalf of the EGWG. Cancer, pregnancy and fertility: ESMO Clinical Practice Guidelines for diagnosis, treatment and follow-up. Ann Oncol. 2013;24(6):160–70. https://doi.org/10.1093/annonc/mdt199.

86. Azim HA, Peccatori FA, Pavlidis N. Treatment of the pregnant mother with cancer: a systematic review on the use of cytotoxic, endocrine, targeted agents and immunotherapy during pregnancy. Part I: solid tumors. Cancer Treat Rev. 2010;36(2):101–9.

87. Cuvier C, Espie M, Extra JM, Marty M. Vinorelbine in pregnancy. Eur J Cancer Part A. 1997;33(1):168–9.

88. Braems G, Denys H, De Wever O, Cocquyt V, Van den Broecke R. Use of tamoxifen before and during pregnancy. Oncologist. 2011;16(11):1574–51.

89. Azim HA, Azim H, Peccatori FA. Treatment of cancer during pregnancy with monoclonal antibodies: a real challenge. Expert Rev Clin Immunol. 2010;6(6):821–6.

90. Toy W, Shen Y, Won H, Green B, Sakr RA, Will M, et al. ESR1 ligand-binding domain mutations in hormone-resistant breast cancer. Nat Genet. 2013;45(12):1439–45.

91. Jeselsohn R, Buchwalter G, De Angelis C, Brown M, Schiff R. ESR1 mutations-a mechanism for acquired endocrine resistance in breast cancer. Nat Rev Clin Oncol. 2015;12(10):573–83.

92. Toy W, Weir H, Razavi P, Lawson M, Goeppert AU, Mazzola AM, et al. Activating ESR1 mutations differentially affect the efficacy of ER antagonists. Cancer Discov. 2017;7(3):277–87.

Sibylle Loibl and Sabine Seiler

13.1   Introduction

Cancer is the second leading cause of death during the reproductive years and complicates between 1:1000 and 2000 pregnancies [1]. The most frequent cancers in women of childbearing age are breast and cervical cancer, leukemia, lymphoma, and malignant melanoma. Although rare, breast cancer is one of the most common cancers diagnosed during pregnancy. The reported crude incidence rate varies from 1.3 to 7.9 per 100.000 births in population-based studies [2–5]. Allied to the upward trend of breast cancer occurrence and the current tendency to postpone childbearing to the later reproductive years, the incidence rate of pregnancy-associated breast cancer has been increasing during the last few decades [6–8].

Throughout the literature the definition of pregnancy-associated breast cancer varies from study to study and refers to breast cancer diagnosed during and up to few years subsequent to a delivery. The most common used specific definition of pregnancy-associated breast cancer is restricted to diagnosis of breast cancer during or within 1 year after delivery.

Delayed diagnosis and suboptimal therapy worsen prognosis. The general treatment concepts should adhere as much as possible to those of young nonpregnant female patients. This chapter summarizes the current therapeutic approaches of breast cancer during pregnancy with focus on systemic therapy, surgical management, and radiation therapy as well as on staging workup and aims to provide practical guidance on identifying the best treatment strategy.

13.2   Prognosis

Eighty percent of pregnancy-associated breast cancers are described to be nodal positive at time of first diagnosis. During pregnancy, hormone-induced physiological changes of glandular mammary tissue progressively complicate breast exam and may hinder detection of suspicious masses, resulting in more locally advanced diseases at the time of diagnosis compared with nonpregnant women [9]. However, histologic characteristics and breast cancer subtypes are comparable between pregnant and nonpregnant women. Breast cancers during pregnancy are almost exclusively invasive-ductal, 50% are hormone- receptor negative and in 75% of cases undifferentiated [10]. Data regarding maternal prognosis is in part contradictory, and

S. Loibl (✉)
German Breast Group, Neu-Isenburg, Germany

Centrum für Hämatologie und Onkologie Bethanien, Frankfurt am Main, Germany
e-mail: sibylle.loibl@gbg.de

S. Seiler
German Breast Group, Neu-Isenburg, Germany

© Springer Nature Switzerland AG 2020
O. Gentilini et al. (eds.), *Breast Cancer in Young Women*,
https://doi.org/10.1007/978-3-030-24762-1_13

heterogeneous patient cohorts as well as the use of outdated therapies complicate the comparability of published studies. This information is important when patients are counseled. Results from an international collaborative study show similar survival rates for patients diagnosed with breast cancer during pregnancy compared with nonpregnant patients [11]. This is in contrast to the results of a meta- analysis of 30 studies with 3628 pregnant and 37,100 nonpregnant women. Here, breast cancer-associated pregnancies are independently associated with poor survival, particularly those diagnosed shortly postpartum [12]. Findings of a more recent study reported by Callihan et al. also show that diagnosis of breast cancer during the first 5 years postpartum confers poorer maternal prognosis [13]. Thus, physiological and/or biological changes of the breast microenvironment during lactation may have a significant and so far unclear role in the pathobiology and prognosis of breast cancer-associated pregnancies.

13.3 Clinical Presentation and Diagnostic Evaluation

During pregnancy, hormone-induced proliferation and differentiation of glandular mammary tissue result in an increase of breast density, breast volume, and sometimes nipple discharges. These physiological changes progressively complicate the clinical breast exam during pregnancy. Therefore, a clinical breast examination by the doctor at the beginning of pregnancy is recommended. However, most breast cancers during pregnancy are diagnosed by the patients themselves.

Even if 80% of breast masses found during pregnancy are benign, it is important to note that delayed treatment of breast cancer during pregnancy by 1 month increases the risk of nodal involvement by 0.9–1.8%, whereas a delay of 6 months increases the risk by 5.1–10.2% [14, 15]. In consequence, any clinically suspicious and persistent breast or axillary mass as well as breast inflammation should be evaluated without delay via diagnostic imaging and investigated by imaging-guided core biopsy for histologi-

cal diagnosis. The pathologist must be informed about the pregnancy to avoid misinterpretation of pregnancy-related changes. Due to physiological hyperproliferative tissue changes during pregnancy, fine needle biopsy and aspiration cytology may give false-negative or false-positive results and are generally not recommended during pregnancy [16].

13.4 Imaging and Staging Workup

During pregnancy, it is important to balance the clinical needs and benefits of the mother with the potential risk for adverse effects to the child. Ionizing radiation exposure occurs with common imaging modalities and could cause significant harm to the fetus. In general, ionizing radiation exposure is affected by imaging technique, proper accomplishment, anatomic site, and gestational age. Therefore, imaging and staging workup for patients with breast cancer during pregnancy may deviate from existing guidelines and should be individualized in order to reduce the risk of fetal radiation exposure.

Deterministic effects do not occur below certain threshold doses but include teratogenic effects such as malformations, impaired mental and growth development, and fetal death due to damage of multiple cells. The threshold for harmful effects on the fetus is estimated to be approximately 100 mGy, with uncertainty between 50 and 100 Gy. However, the risk and severity increase with the given radiation dose [17]. Especially during organogenesis in the first trimester, exposure above the threshold may lead to clinically important and severe deterministic effects, whereas the risk of toxicity is decreasing in the second and third trimester.

Stochastic effects cause damage of single cells and may lead to carcinogenic effects like childhood cancer and leukemia. The risk of stochastic effects increases with escalating radiation dose and there is no threshold dose. Even if stochastic effects are thought to be small, they should be discussed with the patient.

Awareness of radiation doses of imaging modalities may contribute to reduction in the risk of fetal radiation exposure. Whenever possible, clinicians should choose an imaging modality during pregnancy that has little or no ionizing radiation. Ultrasound can be safely and effectively performed during the whole pregnancy. Due to lack of ionizing radiation, the possibility to discriminate between benign and malignant lesions, and its high sensitivity in the detection of breast cancer during pregnancy, ultrasound is the primary imaging technique and is generally recommended for the further evaluation of a pregnant patient presenting with a palpable breast/axillary mass [16, 18]. In addition, it can be used for abdominal staging, to guide core biopsies and to assess response during neoadjuvant systemic treatment.

Bilateral mammography should be performed in pregnant patients with already confirmed malignant disease or with unclear and highly suspicious masses. In this context, it must be remembered that the assessment of a mammography during pregnancy is more challenging due to the cumulative higher breast density in young women and the physiological changes induced by the pregnancy. Therefore, sensitivity of this imaging modality is reduced. Robbins et al. report a 78–100% for mammography compared with a 100% sensitivity for ultrasound [18]. As in nonpregnant women, mammography should always be performed bilateral in order to determine not only the extent of disease of the affected breast but also to evaluate the contralateral breast and to assess suspicious microcalcifications.

Due to a minimal ionizing radiation exposure to the uterus and fetus of less than 0.03 μGy, mammography can be performed safely during pregnancy with an extremely low risk to the fetus. Ionizing radiation exposure could be further decreased by adequate lead shielding techniques [18, 19].

Long-term safety of magnetic resonance imaging (MRI) during the first trimester as well as of gadolinium-based contrast agents during the whole pregnancy remains unclear. Gadolinium crosses the blood-placental barrier and is considered to be teratogenic [20].

In a retrospective Canadian cohort study, the exposure to MRI during the first trimester of pregnancy compared with non-exposure was not associated with increased risk of fetal harm, whereas gadolinium-based MRI at any time during pregnancy was associated with an increased risk for stillbirth or neonatal death and of rheumatological, inflammatory, or infiltrative skin conditions in childhood [21]. In addition, prospective clinical data concerning sensitivity and specificity of breast MRI during pregnancy are lacking. Therefore, contrast- enhanced MRI of the breast is not recommended during pregnancy, whereas non-contrast MRI is thought to be safe for the fetus in the second and third trimester and may be considered for staging procedures [22].

Staging procedures should be performed during pregnancy only if they will change the treatment plan. Unnecessary or less accurate procedures should be avoided. The following imaging procedures are considered to be safe and can be used to determine the extent of the disease:

- Chest X-ray with abdominal shielding
- Ultrasound of the liver

Bone scans, contrast-enhanced computed tomography (CT), and positron-emission tomography/CT (PET-CT) are generally not recommended during pregnancy. If indicated, a non-contrast MRI of the suspicious area could be considered. After delivery, staging procedures should be completed.

In theory, the placenta is an ideal environment for tumor cells due to the large surface and pronounced blood flow. However, only a few cases of placental metastases have been described in the global literature and documented maternal metastases to the child are exceptional, with only 17 cases described so far [23]. Despite this, histopathological evaluation of the placenta should be performed after delivery [16].

13.5 General Concepts on Treatment of Breast Cancer During Pregnancy

Most treatment options including surgery and chemotherapy can be performed during pregnancy depending on the gestational age at diagnosis. However, the selection and timing of local and systemic therapies must be adapted to ensure

Table 13.1 Therapeutic options for breast cancer during pregnancy

Therapeutic option	First trimester	Second trimester	Third trimester
Radiotherapy	Only in exceptional cases during the first and early second trimester[a]	Contraindicated	
Chemotherapy[b]	Contraindicated	Feasible[c]	
Endocrine therapies	Contraindicated		
Targeted therapies	Contraindicated		
Breast surgery	Feasible		
SNB	Feasible		

SNB Sentinel lymph node biopsy
[a]With careful consideration of possible fetal risks
[b]The use of standard regimes with anthracyclines, cyclophosphamide, and taxanes is widely accepted
[c]Chemotherapy should be stopped 3–4 weeks before delivery to prevent hematologic toxicity to mother and child during/after delivery

patient's wish and safety for both the fetus and the mother (Table 13.1). Therefore, treatment plan should be discussed by an experienced multidisciplinary team, including at least a neonatologist, perinatologist, obstetrician, oncologist, and a surgeon. The pregnant patient and her family should be clearly informed about maternal prognosis, treatment strategies, as well as the impact of those on pregnancy and delivery and should be involved in the decision-making progress regarding the planned treatment.

Clinicopathological tumor characteristics, genetic status, and patient's desires determine the appropriate treatment. Delayed as well as suboptimal therapy approaches impair the prognosis. In consequence, the general concepts concerning local and systemic treatment should adhere as much as possible to standardized protocols for young, nonpregnant patients. Postponement of therapy is generally not recommended and termination of pregnancy does not seem to improve prognosis of the patients [10]. However, termination of pregnancy can be considered during the first trimester in case of advanced breast cancer and poor maternal prognosis if desired by the patient and her family.

13.6 Surgical Considerations

Surgical recommendations for patients with breast cancer during pregnancy are similar to recommendations for nonpregnant patients. In general, surgical treatment can safely be done throughout the whole period of pregnancy with the highest possible safety for mother and child during the second trimester [24]. Table 13.2 summarizes the current key points for surgery of breast cancer during pregnancy.

If surgery of breast cancer is indicated during the first trimester, increased risk for an abortion should be discussed, whereas during the third trimester, there is an increased risk for intraoperative fetal hypoxia/asphyxia as well as for preterm labor and delivery.

Historically, mastectomy was the standard surgical treatment for patients with breast cancer during pregnancy [14]. It should be noted that mastectomy is not mandatory solely on the basis of pregnancy. Surgical planning depends on stage, genetic status, gestational age, and planned systemic treatment. Most routine operations such as breast-conserving surgery and mastectomy as well as sentinel node biopsy and/or axillary node dissection can safely be performed during pregnancy [25]. However, it should be taken into account that radiotherapy during pregnancy is generally contraindicated and delaying or postponing radiotherapy until after delivery might increase the risk for locoregional recurrence [26]. Radiotherapy might be safely applied during the first or early second trimester. For many patients with breast cancer during pregnancy, chemotherapy is indicated. Neoadjuvant chemotherapy can provide improved options for breast-conserving

Table 13.2 Key points for surgery of breast cancer during pregnancy

Trimester	Surgical considerations
I.	1. In general, operations are feasible but increased risk for an abortion 2. Depending on maternal prognosis and week of gestation, consider postponement of surgery until second trimester 3. Breast-conserving surgery or mastectomy, sentinel node biopsy, or axillary node dissection: indication as in nonpregnant women 4. Breast-conserving therapy → delay of radiotherapy might increase risk for locoregional recurrence
II.	1. Trimester of pregnancy with the highest possible safety for mother and child 2. Breast-conserving surgery or mastectomy, sentinel node biopsy, or axillary node dissection: indication as in nonpregnant women 3. Consider neoadjuvant chemotherapy to achieve improved options for breast-conserving surgery 4. In case of breast-conserving therapy → delay of radiotherapy has to be considered
III.	1. Increased risk for an intraoperative fetal hypoxia/asphyxia as well as for preterm labor and delivery 2. Consider surgery followed by adjuvant chemotherapy after delivery 3. Consider neoadjuvant chemotherapy to achieve improved options for breast-conserving surgery 4. Breast-conserving surgery or mastectomy, sentinel-node biopsy, or axillary node dissection: indication as in nonpregnant women

surgery due to reducing the size of cancer and will often postpone surgery until third trimester or delivery. In consequence, radiation therapy may then be performed postpartum without detrimental treatment delay.

Breast reconstruction after mastectomy is an important component in the treatment plan. For patients with breast cancer during pregnancy, unpredictable physiological changes of the breast during and after pregnancy as well as operation time must be considered. To date, available data concerning immediate breast reconstruction after mastectomy in patients with breast cancer during pregnancy is based on a single published experience. Lohsiriwat et al. reported a short operation time and excellent pregnancy outcomes without obstetrical or maternal complications after surgery in 78 patients who underwent immediate breast reconstruction with expander following mastectomy for breast cancer during pregnancy [27]. Hence, immediate breast reconstruction could be considered during pregnancy, whereas contralateral reshaping and definitive implants are not appropriate. Breast reconstruction by autologous tissue is generally not recommended during pregnancy due to the long duration of operations, increased risk of blood loss, and possible postoperative complications.

Sentinel lymph node biopsy (SNB) is an accepted standard of care in patients with localized, clinically node-negative disease. Due to radiation exposure in the context of lymphoscintigraphy with radiocolloid reagent, possible teratogenicity of blue dyes, as well as possible maternal anaphylaxis to blue dyes, concerns on SNB in patients with breast cancer during pregnancy have been numerous. In consequence, the role of SNB in pregnancy has been the subject of controversy, and historically, consensus panels recommended against SNB in pregnancy. Previously published data describe maternal and fetal outcomes following SNB during pregnancy, and despite concerns, it has been shown that SNB can be safely and effectively performed during pregnancy [28–30].

Fetal radiation exposure depends inter alia on dose and timepoint of radiocolloid injection and ranges from 1.14 µGy to 4.3 mGy—well below the threshold of concern for fetal harm [28, 31]. Therefore, the lowest possible radiocolloid dose should be injected on the same day of the operation. Tracer is excreted via the kidneys and insertion of a bladder catheter could further reduce the fetal radiation exposure.

Both isosulfan blue and methylene blue are pregnancy class C drugs, with an unknown potential for teratogenicity, and, in addition, isosulfan blue can cause maternal anaphylaxis. Therefore, lymphatic mapping with blue dyes is generally not recommended during pregnancy [16, 30].

13.7 Radiotherapy

Radiotherapy plays an important role in the treatment of breast cancer. However, pregnancy is considered one of the few radiotherapy contraindications because deterministic and stochastic effects on the developing fetus may induce malformations, spontaneous abortions, neurodevelopmental disorders, carcinogenic and even lethal effects [32]. In general, it is recommended to delay radiotherapy whenever possible until after delivery, but as already mentioned, postponing radiotherapy might lead to an increased risk for locoregional recurrence [26]. When radiotherapy during pregnancy is indicated, maternal risks of delaying radiotherapy and disadvantages for the fetus should be carefully weighed. Radiation dose received by the fetus depends on both gestational age and the distance between the uterus and the radiotherapy field and could be further decreased by adequate shielding techniques. During the first months of pregnancy, the uterus lies protected within the pelvis and the fetal dose will be 0.1–0.3% of the dose to the irradiated breast which is considered to carry low fetal risk [33]. To date, available data concerning radiotherapy during pregnancy is based only on case reports and low fetal doses have been shown to result in delivery of healthy babies. In consequence, radiotherapy might be considered during the first or early second trimester of pregnancy, if clinically strictly indicated.

13.8 Systemic Therapy

13.8.1 Chemotherapy

When chemotherapy is indicated for patients with breast cancer during pregnancy, gestational age at diagnosis must be considered. Due to organogenesis and the risk for major fetal malformations and abortions, chemotherapy is generally contraindicated during the first trimester of pregnancy. After completion of the first trimester, administration of chemotherapy in the neoadjuvant as well as the adjuvant setting is widely accepted [16].

Most of the available data on teratogenic risk of chemotherapy are based on case reports and retrospective series. The rates of fetal malformations have been shown to be approximately 3–5%, comparable with rates reported for the general population in the USA (3%) and to rates reported in a German registry study (6.9%) and in the registry of the International Network on Cancer, Infertility and Pregnancy (4%) [34–36].

In addition, German study results demonstrated that although more complications were reported for children exposed to systemic therapy during pregnancy, complications were more common among children after premature delivery, irrespective of exposure to systemic therapy during pregnancy [10].

In general, systemic treatment regimens should adhere as much as possible to standardized protocols for young, nonpregnant patients. Delayed as well as suboptimal therapy approaches might worsen prognosis. However, the selection of systemic therapies must be modified to ensure the safety of the fetus. Table 13.3 summarizes the current key points for chemotherapy during pregnancy.

Due to potential fetal toxicity, targeted agents like trastuzumab and pertuzumab should be avoided during pregnancy [37]. The use of standard chemotherapies for breast cancer such as anthracyclines, cyclophosphamide, and taxanes

Table 13.3 Key points for chemotherapy during pregnancy

1. Chemotherapy is generally contraindicated during the first trimester of pregnancy
2. Chemotherapy regimens should adhere as much as possible to standardized published protocols for young, nonpregnant patients. Neither decrease nor increase the dose or the treatment intervals
3. Anthracycline- and taxane-based chemotherapy regimens can be safely initiated in the second and third trimester. Anti-HER2 therapy is contraindicated and should be postponed until after delivery
4. Maintain dose intensity
5. In order to avoid underdosing, each dose of chemotherapy should be based on the actual body surface area (with exception of overweight women)
6. Chemotherapy should be stopped 3–4 weeks before delivery to prevent hematologic toxicity to mother and child during/after delivery

during the second and third trimester is widely accepted, and in consequence administration of standard combination therapies such as epirubicin in combination with cyclophosphamide followed by weekly paclitaxel (or the reverse sequence) can be used during pregnancy [38]. Anthracycline- or taxane-free regimens or 5-fluorouracil should be avoided because they are not considered to be the standard in young nonpregnant women. The use of carboplatin for the neoadjuvant treatment of nonpregnant women with triple-negative/BRCA-mutated breast cancer has been shown to increase the pathological complete response [39–41]. However, data concerning the long-term survival outcome are still limited, and there is an obvious transfer of platinum agents through the placental barrier [42]. de Haan et al. reported a possible relationship between platinum-based chemotherapy and small for gestational birth, but this is based on a limited number of patients with mainly non-breast cancers [35]. Therefore, risks to the fetus and benefits for the mother must be weighed carefully. The preferred platinum salt is carboplatin due to the lower overall toxicity [37].

In nonpregnant high-risk patients, dose-dense or intensified dose-dense adjuvant chemotherapy has improved survival outcomes compared with conventional treatment schedules every 3 weeks [43, 44]. While dose-dense chemotherapy seems to be an option during pregnancy, intensified dose-dense chemotherapy is associated with more hematotoxicity and data concerning the use of granulocyte colony-stimulating factor are still limited [45]. Nonetheless, intensified dose-dense chemotherapy can be considered after careful risk benefit analysis in high-risk primary breast cancer patients.

Pregnancy-related changes in maternal physiology such as changes in hepatic metabolism, renal clearance, and blood volume must be taken into account and can affect the optimal drug dosing in pregnant patients. Especially increased activity of major enzymes involved in the metabolism of taxanes and anthracyclines during the late trimester of pregnancy may result in decreased maternal drug exposure. A comparison of pregnant versus nonpregnant patients in terms of pharmacokinetics of taxanes and anthracyclines reported, especially for paclitaxel, significantly decreased serum levels in the pregnant cohort [46]. However, it remains unclear if chemotherapy doses should be increased during pregnancy. In general, increasing the dose is not recommended, but reevaluation of dosing based on current weight and body surface area should be performed prior to every cycle.

Unfortunately, data regarding supportive treatment for pregnant patients receiving chemotherapy is very limited and the optimal supportive treatment during pregnancy is not well established. Supportive treatment is necessary for the majority of chemotherapy regimens and should be applied whenever indicated to ensure optimal safety for the mother as well as the unborn [37].

13.8.2 Targeted Therapies

Based on published case studies, in utero exposure of trastuzumab has been shown to be associated with oligohydramnios and anhydramnios, renal insufficiency, skeletal abnormalities, pulmonary hypoplasia, and fetal death [47, 48]. Therefore, administration of anti-HER2 therapy is contraindicated during all trimesters of pregnancy. However, in case of accidental fetal exposure to trastuzumab, fetus as well as amniotic fluid should be closely monitored.

Use of pertuzumab, bevacizumab, everolimus, and palbociclib as well as bone-modifying therapies have not been studied during pregnancy and are strictly contraindicated.

13.8.3 Endocrine Therapy

Endocrine therapy is of major therapeutic value in patients with hormone receptor-positive tumors. Endocrine agents, such as the selective estrogen receptor modulator tamoxifen, aromatase inhibitors, and ovarian suppression, can disturb the hormonal environment and are contraindicated during pregnancy and lactation. Tamoxifen, the mainstay of endocrine therapy in premenopausal women, has the potential to induce fetal harm during pregnancy and is associated with birth defects including craniofacial malformations, ambiguous genitalia, and fetal death as well as vagina bleeding and miscarriage [49–51].

13.9 Treatment of Metastatic Breast Cancer

Among the pregnant breast cancer population, only a minority presents with stage IV disease [10, 35]. General concepts concerning oncological management should adhere as much as possible to those of nonpregnant patients with advanced disease. However, the use of systemic therapies in the palliative setting is a challenging situation due to potential side effects of drugs to the fetus which may require restrictions regarding endocrine and targeted therapies.

Pregnancy-preserving management should be considered for women with favorable therapeutic index and low-burden metastatic disease. Therefore, administration of chemotherapies with single agents to control disease and symptoms is considered to be the optimal systemic anticancer treatment after completion of the first trimester until delivery. Trastuzumab and endocrine therapies are generally not recommended during all trimesters of pregnancy. However, individual decisions may be taken in urgent situations of advanced disease [48, 50]. For those women for whom trastuzumab is deemed necessary, risk of oligohydramnios and anhydramnios needs to be considered. Therefore, close monitoring of amniotic fluid levels, fetal growth, and kidney function are required.

For pregnant patients with unfavorable therapeutic index and poor prognosis, termination of pregnancy may be discussed in the first trimester to avoid restrictions or delay in treatment.

13.10 Obstetrical Considerations

Timing is very important in treating patients with breast cancer during pregnancy. Therefore, the complex therapeutic strategies should be established in a multidisciplinary setting, incorporating a neonatologist, a perinatologist, and an obstetri-

cian. The morbidity and mortality risk is higher in preterm-delivered infants. Premature delivery increases the risk of neurodevelopmental impairment with a direct correlation between gestational age at birth and negative outcomes [52]. Therefore, premature delivery should be avoided, whenever possible. However, a high frequency of preterm deliveries in patients with cancer during pregnancy was shown. Investigators of a German registry described a rate of preterm delivery of 50% with a mean gestational age at delivery of 36–37 weeks [10]. The most recent cohort study reports an overall frequency of live birth <37 weeks of 43% [35]. In addition, antenatal chemotherapy has been shown to be associated with an increased risk of preterm rupture (3 vs. 0%) of membranes and preterm labor (6 vs. 2%) [10].

The available evidence on neonatal and long-term consequences of in utero exposure to systemic therapies is still based on small numbers with a short follow-up period and focus on morphologic observations made very close to the time of delivery. Data collected on children's long-term toxicity such as delayed effects of treatment on general development and cardiac development as well as on neurological, intellectual, and behavioral functioning are incomplete and are hampered by a lack of well-designed population-based studies. However, several cohort studies of children who were exposed to chemotherapy in utero showed no impairment of neurodevelopment and auditory, cardiac, or general health development as well as no increased rate of congenital abnormalities compared with general population standards. But prematurity was correlated with impaired cognitive outcome, independent of cancer treatments [53–56]. Intrauterine growth may be affected and needs close monitoring. While some studies found normal weights and heights according to gestational health, others reported an increased incidence of intrauterine growth restriction [10, 53].

In addition to standard prenatal care, regular ultrasound assessments of fetal growth and amniotic fluid in combination with Doppler measurements should be performed prior to the start of therapy and at least every 3 weeks in order to follow the course of pregnancy and the development of the fetus. Delivery should be planned as closely as possible to term. Regardless of therapy, obstetric requirements and patient's wish determine the mode of delivery. To allow recovery of maternal and fetal bone marrow in order to reduce the risk of perinatal hematologic toxicity, chemotherapy should be discontinued at approximately week 35–37 of gestation [37]. Depending on mode of delivery, systemic therapy could be restarted 2–3 weeks after birth.

13.11 Breastfeeding

Based on available data, it is not necessary to wean breastfeeding if the systemic therapy has been terminated 4 weeks prior to initiation of breastfeeding. However, if a further systemic therapy is indicated, the mother should be advised to wean after the delivery [57]. Of note, the decision to delay further systemic treatment in order to allow lactation should be based on individual risk. Effects of radiation on lactation have not been studied and should be avoided.

13.12 Conclusion

Treatment of breast cancer during pregnancy is an enormous challenge for the pregnant women, her family, as well as for the treatment team. Breast cancer during pregnancy can be treated closely to the standards for nonpregnant women. However, the selection and timing of local and systemic therapies must be modified to ensure safety to both the fetus and the mother and should be discussed by an experienced multidisciplinary team. Of course, the pregnant women and the family should be clearly informed about maternal prognosis, treatment strategies, as well as impact on pregnancy and delivery and should be involved in the decision-making progress concerning the planned treatment.

Further research is needed to provide all patients diagnosed with breast cancer during pregnancy with the best individualized treatment plan in order to optimize maternal and neonatal outcomes. Since there are no randomized studies feasible in patients with breast cancer during pregnancy, register studies need to be supported and international collaborations to be continued and expanded.

References

1. Pavlidis NA. Coexistence of pregnancy and malignancy. Oncologist. 2002;7(4):279–87.
2. Stensheim H, Moller B, van Dijk T, et al. Cause-specific survival for women diagnosed with cancer during pregnancy or lactation: a registry-based cohort study. J Clin Oncol. 2009;27(1):45–51.
3. Lee YY, Robets CL, Dobbins T, et al. Incidence and outcomes of pregnancy-associated cancer in Australia, 1994–2008: a population-based linkage study. BJOG. 2012;119(13):1572–82.
4. Haas JF. Pregnancy in association with newly diagnosed cancer: a population-based epidemiologic assessment. Int J Cancer. 1984;34(2):229–35.
5. Abenhaim HA, Azoulay L, Holcroft CA, et al. Incidence, risk factors, and obstetrical outcomes of women with breast cancer in pregnancy. Breast J. 2012;18(6):564–8.
6. Sobotka T. United Nations Department of economic and social affairs. Pathways to low fertility: European perspectives. Expert Paper No 2013/08.
7. Andersson TM, Johansson AL, Hsieh CC, et al. Increasing incidence of pregnancy-associated breast cancer in Sweden. Obstet Gynecol. 2009;114(3):568–72.
8. Koch-Institut R. (Hrsg) und die Gesellschaft der epidemiologischen Krebsregister in Deutschland e.V. (Hrsg). Krebs in Deutschland 2011/2012. 10. Ausgabe. Berlin, 2015.
9. Amant F, Loibl S, Neven P, et al. Breast cancer in pregnancy. Lancet. 2012;379(9815):570–9.
10. Loibl S, Han SN, von Minckwitz G, Bontenbal M, et al. Treatment of breast cancer during pregnancy: an observational study. Lancet Oncol. 2012;13(9):887–96.
11. Amant F, von Minckwitz G, Han SN, et al. Prognosis of women with primary breast cancer diagnosed during pregnancy: results from an international collaborative study. J Clin Oncol. 2013;31(20):2532–9.
12. Azim HA Jr, Santoro L, Russell-Edu W, et al. Prognosis of pregnancy-associated breast cancer: a meta-analysis of 30 studies. Cancer Treat Rev. 2012;38:834–42.
13. Callihan EB, Gao D, Jindal S, et al. Postpartum diagnosis demonstrates a high risk for metastasis and merits an expanded definition of pregnancy-associated breast cancer. Breast Cancer Res Treat. 2013;138(2):549–59.
14. Woo JC, Yu T, Hurd TC. Breast cancer in pregnancy: a literature review. Arch Surg. 2003;138(1):91–8.
15. Nettleton J, Long J, Kuban D, et al. Breast cancer during pregnancy: quantifying the risk of treatment delay. Obstet Gynecol. 1996;87:414–8.

16. Amant F, Deckers S, Van Calsteren K, et al. Breast cancer in pregnancy: recommendations of an international consensus meeting. Eur J Cancer. 2010;46(18):3158–68.

17. American College of Radiology. ACR–SPR practice parameter for imaging pregnant or potentially pregnant adolescents and women with ionizing radiation. In: Resolution, vol. 39. Reston, VA: ACR; 2014. https://www.acr.org/Search-Results#q=pregnant%20 patients. Accessed 12 Mar 2018.

18. Robbins J, Jeffries D, Roubidoux M, Helvie M. Accuracy of diagnostic mammography and breast ultrasound during pregnancy and lactation. AJR Am J Roentgenol. 2011;196(3):716–22.

19. Vashi R, Hooley R, Butler R, et al. Breast imaging of the pregnant and lactating patient: imaging modalities and pregnancy associated breast cancer. AJR Am J Roentgenol. 2013;200(2):321–8.

20. Nguyen CP, Goodman LH. Fetal risk in diagnostic radiology. Semin Ultrasound CT MR. 2012;33(1):4–10.

21. Ray JG, Vermeulen MJ, Bharatha A, et al. Association between MRI exposure during pregnancy and fetal and childhood outcomes. JAMA. 2016;316(9):952–61.

22. Patenaude Y, Pugash D, Lim K, et al. Diagnostic imaging committee; Society of Obstetricians and Gynaecologists of Canada. The use of magnetic resonance imaging in the obstetric patient. J Obstet Gynaecol Can. 2014;36(4):349–63.

23. Pavlidis N, Pentheroudakis G. Metastatic involvement of placenta and foetus in pregnant women with cancer. Recent Results Cancer Res. 2008;178:183–94.

24. Berry DL, Theriault RL, Holmes FA, et al. Management of breast cancer during pregnancy using a standardized protocol. J Clin Oncol. 1999;17(3):855–61.

25. Toesca A, Gentilini O, Peccatori F, et al. Locoregional treatment of breast cancer during pregnancy. Gynecol Surg. 2014;11(4):279–84.

26. Huang J, Barbera L, Brouwers M, et al. Does delay in starting treatment affect the outcomes of radiotherapy? A systematic review. J Clin Oncol. 2003;21(3):555–63.

27. Lohsiriwat V, Peccatori FA, Martella S, et al. Immediate breast reconstruction with expander in pregnant breast cancer patients. Breast. 2013;22(5):657–60.

28. Gentilini O, Cremonesi M, Toesca A, et al. Sentinel lymph node biopsy in pregnant patients with breast cancer. Eur J Nucl Med Mol Imaging. 2010;37(1):78–83.2.

29. Khera SY, Kiluk JV, Hasson DM, et al. Pregnancy-associated breast cancer patients can safely undergo lymphatic mapping. Breast J. 2008;14:250–4. 3

30. Gropper AB, Calvillo KZ, Dominici L, et al. Sentinel lymph node biopsy in pregnant women with breast cancer. Ann Surg Oncol. 2014;21:2506–11.

31. Pandit-Taskar N, Dauer LT, Montgomery L, St Germain J, Zanzonico PB, Divgi CR. Organ and fetal absorbed dose estimates from 99mTc-sulfur colloid lymphoscintigraphy and sentinel node localization in breast cancer patients. J Nucl Med. 2006;47:1202–8.

32. Otake M, Schull WJ, Lee S. Threshold for radiation-related severe mental retardation in prenatally exposed A-bomb survivors: a re-analysis. Int J Radiat Biol. 1996;70(6):755–63.

33. Kal HB, Struikmans H. Radiotherapy during pregnancy: fact and fiction. Lancet Oncol. 2005;6(5):328–33.

34. National Toxicology Program. NTP monograph: developmental effects and pregnancy outcomes associated with cancer chemotherapy use during pregnancy. NTP Monogr. 2013;2:i–214.

35. de Haan J, Verheecke M, Van Calsteren K, et al. International Network on Cancer and Infertility Pregnancy (INCIP). Oncological management and obstetric and neonatal outcomes for women diagnosed with cancer during pregnancy: a 20-year international cohort study of 1170 patients. Lancet Oncol. 2018;19(3):337–46.

36. Queisser-Luft A, Stolz G, Wiesel A, et al. Malformations in newborn: results based on 30,940 infants and fetuses from the Mainz congenital birth defect monitoring system (1990–1998). Arch Gynecol Obstet. 2002;266:163–7.

37. Loibl S, Schmidt A, Gentilini O, et al. Breast cancer diagnosed during pregnancy: adapting recent advances in breast cancer care for pregnant patients. JAMA Oncol. 2015;1(8):1145–53.

38. Bines J, Earl H, Buzaid AC, Saad ED. Anthracyclines and taxanes in the neo/adjuvant treatment of breast cancer: does the sequence matter? Ann Oncol. 2014;25(6):1079–85.

39. von Minckwitz G, Schneeweiss A, Loibl S, et al. Neoadjuvant carboplatin in patients with triple-negative and HER2-positive early breast cancer (GeparSixto; GBG 66): a randomised phase 2 trial. Lancet Oncol. 2014;15(7):747–56.

40. Loibl S, O'Shaughnessy J, Untch M, et al. Addition of the PARP inhibitor veliparib plus carboplatin or carboplatin alone to standard neoadjuvant chemotherapy in triple-negative breast cancer (BrighTNess): a randomised, phase 3 trial. Lancet Oncol. 2018;19(4):497–509. https://doi.org/10.1016/ S1470-2045(18)30111-6.

41. Sikov WM, Berry DA, Perou CM, et al. Impact of the addition of carboplatin and/or bevacizumab to neoadjuvant once-per-week paclitaxel followed by dose-dense doxorubicin and cyclophosphamide on pathologic complete response rates in stage II to III triple-negative breast cancer: CALGB 40603 (Alliance). J Clin Oncol. 2015;33(1):13–21.

42. Köhler C, Oppelt P, Favero G, et al. How much platinum passes the placental barrier? Analysis of platinum applications in 21 patients with cervical cancer during pregnancy. Am J Obstet Gynecol. 2015;213(2):206. e1–5.

43. Gray R, Bradley R, Braybrooke J, et al. Increasing the dose density of adjuvant chemotherapy by shortening intervals between courses or by sequential drug

administration significantly reduces both disease recurrence and breast cancer mortality: An EBCTCG meta-analysis of 21,000 women in 16 randomised trials [abstract]. San Antonio Breast Cancer Symposium 2017. Cancer Res. 2018;78(4 Suppl):GS1-01.

44. Moebus V, Jackisch C, Lueck HJ, et al. Intense dose-dense sequential chemotherapy with epirubicin, paclitaxel, and cyclophosphamide compared with conventionally scheduled chemotherapy in high-risk primary breast cancer: mature results of an AGO phase III study. J Clin Oncol. 2010;28(17):2874–80.

45. Cardonick E, Gilmandyar D, Somer RA. Maternal and neonatal outcomes of dose-dense chemotherapy for breast cancer in pregnancy. Obstet Gynecol. 2012;120(6):1267–72.

46. van Hasselt JG, van Calsteren K, Heyns L, et al. Optimizing anticancer drug treatment in pregnant cancer patients: pharmacokinetic analysis of gestation-induced changes for doxorubicin, epirubicin, docetaxel and paclitaxel. Ann Oncol. 2014;25(10):2059–65.

47. Gottschalk I, Berg C, Harbeck N, et al. Fetal renal insufficiency following trastuzumab treatment for breast cancer in pregnancy: case report and review of the current literature. Breast Care (Basel). 2011;6:475–8.

48. Zagouri F, Sergentanis TN, Chrysikos D, et al. Trastuzumab administration during pregnancy: a systematic review and meta-analysis. Breast Cancer Res Treat. 2013;137(2):349–57.

49. Barthelmes L, Davidson LA, Gaffney C, Gateley CA. Tamoxifen and pregnancy. Breast. 2004;13(6):446–51.

50. Isaacs RJ, Hunter W, Clark K. Tamoxifen as systemic treatment of advanced breast cancer during pregnancy—case report and literature review. Gynecol Oncol. 2001;80:405–8.

51. Tewari K, Bonebrake RG, Asrat T, et al. Ambiguous genitalia in infant exposed to tamoxifen in utero. Lancet. 1997;350:183.

52. Wang ML, Dorer DJ, Fleming MP, Catlin EA. Clinical outcomes of near-term infants. Pediatrics. 2004;114(2):372–6.

53. Avilés A, Neri N. Hematological malignancies and pregnancy: a final report of 84 children who received chemotherapy in utero. Clin Lymphoma. 2001;2(3):173–7.

54. Nulman I, Laslo D, Fried S, et al. Neurodevelopment of children exposed in utero to treatment of maternal malignancy. Br J Cancer. 2001;85(11):1611–8.

55. Amant F, Vandenbroucke T, Verheecke M, et al. Pediatric outcome after maternal Cancer diagnosed during pregnancy. International network on Cancer, infertility, and pregnancy (INCIP). N Engl J Med. 2015;373(19):1824–34.

56. Cardonick E, Dougherty R, Grana G, et al. Breast cancer during pregnancy: maternal and fetal outcomes. Cancer J. 2010;16:76–82.

57. Pistilli B, Bellettini G, Giovannetti E, et al. Chemotherapy, targeted agents, antiemetics and growth-factors in human milk: how should we counsel cancer patients about breastfeeding? Cancer Treat Rev. 2013;39(3):207–11.

Clara Hungr and Sharon Bober

14.1 Introduction

BC is currently the most commonly occurring cancer for women worldwide including cancers among younger, premenopausal women below age 50 [1]. Although new incident rates have remained relatively stable over the past decade [2], improvements in screening and treatment have resulted in steadily decreasing rates of mortality with up to 90% of newly diagnosed women becoming long-term survivors [3]. However, this significant increase in survivorship also has brought recognition of treatment-related side effects characterized by both physical and psychological difficulties.

Due to biological differences in younger, premenopausal BC patients compared to their older cohort, young women more often face cancers that are more aggressive and require more intensive treatments [4, 5]. These treatments typically involve full or partial surgical resection of the breast, chemotherapy, and radiation, and for women with estrogen receptor (ER)-positive cancers, anti-estrogen therapies [6]. Such intensive treatments also lead to a host of challenges, which are unique to this age group. In particular, younger women report having greater difficulty with sexual function including gynecological problems, as well as increased difficulties with body image and disruptions to relationship intimacy [7, 8]. Unfortunately, changes in sexual function and body image are often not addressed as part of standard clinical care [9, 10]. This chapter begins with a brief overview of the specific challenges that characterize young women's psychosexual development, followed by a review of the impact of BC treatment on a young body image and sexuality. We will also discuss how cultural context is interwoven with these experiences [11]. Finally, practical suggestions will be overviewed for effectively querying young BC survivors about these issues, and recommendations will be offered for addressing common problems.

14.2 Developmental Stage of Young Adulthood

To better understand the unique experience young BC survivors face with regard to body image and sexual function after BC, it is important to appreciate the developmental challenges that are relevant to this cohort. The period between adolescence and middle adulthood, which for women can typically be understood as the years before

C. Hungr
Cambridge Health Alliance, Cambridge, MA, USA
e-mail: chung@challiance.org

S. Bober (✉)
Dana–Farber Cancer Institute, Boston, MA, USA
e-mail: sharon_bober@dfci.harvard.edu

© Springer Nature Switzerland AG 2020
O. Gentilini et al. (eds.), *Breast Cancer in Young Women*,
https://doi.org/10.1007/978-3-030-24762-1_14

the onset of menopause, is a busy time of change and opportunity [12]. Developmental psychologists have longed described the period of young adulthood as a formative time for establishing the psychological and interpersonal makeup of the self. This is fertile period for individuals to develop their view of themselves as well as their roles in relationships and in the larger society [13, 14]. For a young woman, these years often represent a time of exploring femininity and sexuality, developing and maintaining intimate relationships, and the consideration of child-bearing and motherhood [15]. In addition to establishing confidence in ones' roles in society, this developmental phase can also be a period of intense vulnerability. When young women are experimenting with their expression of sexuality and femininity, there is not surprisingly a heightened awareness of the social norms on youth and beauty. It has been noted that this awareness of normative standards can certainly amplify the psychological impact of discrete body changes during this period of life for cancer survivors [16].

14.3 Self-Image/Body Image

Considering that a young woman's premenopausal years are often a foundational period for psychosexual and identity development, the disruptions caused by BC diagnosis, treatment, and the consequent after-effects can have broad and longstanding implications. Self-image is a multifaceted construct that can be understood as an embodied view of "me," which includes a familiar sense of the physical body, the psychological sense of self, and the self as a co-construction of social interaction. From this "me," an expectation develops of how the body will function and respond in certain situations. When this familiar definition of the self is interrupted by a dramatic change—such as a cancer diagnosis for a younger woman who expects a healthy and functional body—bodily experience and by extension the sense of self can cease to feel familiar and/or safe [17]. Disruption to a young survivor's self-image is not uncommon and is characterized

by an experience of disharmony between social assumptions which define [survivors] as women and their own interior definitions of what this means in the context of BC [18].

Body image can be defined as how a person perceives and evaluates the appearance and physical functioning of their body. This includes one's attitude about whether the body is functional, whole, healthy, and attractive [19]. Body perception is highly subjective and is composed of a woman's thoughts, perceptions, and feelings about what is considered "healthy" and "attractive" [20]. BC treatments result in a range of physical changes that can lead a woman to not only question the physical integrity of her body but to also feel self-conscious about how to adapt to and accept these changes. Body image issues secondary to BC treatment can stem from external, visible changes, such as the surgical loss of breast tissues and scarring, chemotherapy-induced hair loss and weight change, and radiation-induced skin damage and discoloration. Although visible alterations are an obvious source of body image distress, nonvisible changes such as loss of sensation in the breast, nipple, and surrounding skin and internal changes to a woman's sense of her femininity, sensuality, and level of attractiveness have potential to significantly disrupt body image [21, 22]. In addition, disruption of body image is correlated with other domains of psychological distress, including anxiety, depression, fatigue, and a fear of cancer recurrence [22].

Younger women, in particular, are at higher risk than older women for having body image concerns after BC treatment [23]. Body image research indicates that although *satisfaction* with one's physical body remains somewhat consistent across ages, *self-esteem* about one's body is more significantly impacted in younger women [24, 25]. That is, changes to a woman's body may be equally dissatisfying to a woman, regardless of age, but to younger women, these changes may have a greater impact on their current assessment of self-worth. One explanation is that as women age, there is an organic acceptance of the aging process which is inherently characterized by expected changes in the body. However, for a younger woman, dramatic alterations from the "body ideal" are unexpected, and because they depart from what is "natural," they can result in a greater negative impact on overall self-esteem. From a developmental perspective, a central feature of young adulthood is building self-confidence and developing a strong relationship with oneself and intimate others. When young BC survivors face significant distressing physical changes during this sensitive developmental period, there is often a notable sense of loss on one's physical functionality and attractiveness [26].

More broadly speaking, permanent and distressing physical changes to one's body can act as a persistent reminder of physical vulnerability. Cancer represents a breakdown of healthy physical boundaries; a body which typically feels manageable and predictable in its shape and function can feel permeable, exposed, and out of control after being subjected to cancer [17]. Consistent with this perspective, studies show that BC survivors with heightened physical symptoms experience more body image concerns [22, 27]. In this way, experiencing tangible physical reminders of one's diagnosis and treatment can act as a reflexive reminder of an ailing body, where strength and safety within one's body cannot be assumed. This doubt can compromise the subjective experience of intact body image.

Depending on the extent to which the cancer impacts the breast tissue, women face different levels of surgical intervention with some women undergoing full mastectomies and some women eligible for breast-conserving procedures [28, 29]. Despite equivalent survival rates shown for both mastectomy and lumpectomy, recent studies indicate that an increasing number of women are opting for prophylactic mastectomies in order to decrease the risk of a secondary cancer [30]. These numbers include prophylactic unilateral mastectomies in lieu of lumpectomies, as well as contralateral mastectomies of the second, noncancerous breast [31–34]. Although the annual risk of most women with unilateral cancer developing a second cancer in the contralateral breast is low (approximately 0.5%) [35], the frequency of prophylactic contralateral mastectomies is significant and garnering greater attention. With regard to body image, it has been suggested that the significant uptick in prophylactic surgeries may not only be due to women's risk perceptions of preventing secondary cancer but also a reflection of concern about cosmetic outcomes. For example, women may choose to preventatively remove the second breast in part to achieve a more symmetrical chest postsurgery [36].

The findings on how different surgical interventions impact body image for young women are inconsistent. Overall, the evidence indicates that body image is better for women who undergo surgery that conserves more of the breast tissue (e.g., lumpectomy) than those who have more tissue removed (e.g., mastectomy) [37, 38]. Similarly, studies indicate that women who do not pursue breast reconstruction after undergoing prophylactic mastectomies experience significantly more distress with their postsurgical appearance, feelings of femininity, and well-being in sexual relationships [36, 39]. Broadly speaking, these results seem to suggest that the physical loss of the breast negatively impacts body image, and that for some women, reconstruction can counter this effect.

However, the literature also reveals that some women experience no difference in well-being related to the extent of surgery and not all women who receive reconstruction show improved body image. The fact that not all women respond to surgical outcomes the same way highlights the importance of additional psychological factors that contribute to the experience of body image. One interesting finding from the literature to date is that the more women play an active role in their surgery decisions, the more empowered and satisfied they feel about the consequences of surgery, regardless of the surgery's physical outcome [40, 41]. More specifically, it has been observed that the context of active engagement in treatment decision-making promotes a woman's ability to integrate physical alterations into her sense of self, in contrast to conditions which lead to feeling that physical change have been imposed on her [42, 43]. Although these findings underscore the importance of offering women active involvement in treatment decision-making, it should be recognized that patients could understandably find treatment decision-making stressful if multiple choices are available which boast similar outcomes. For this reason, shared decision-making is often emphasized as being preferable [42].

Further, it is important to acknowledge the complexity of how women perceive meaning of the breast. One framework for exploring this variation is by Langellier and Sullivan who discuss four separate but closely related "breast concepts." The "medicalized breast" represents the part of the breast affected by the cancer; the "functional breast" represents the physical function of the breast, specifically as it relates to an infant; the "gendered breast" is the breast's representation of femininity, physical attractiveness, and beauty; and the "sexualized breast" represents the visual and tactile experience of the breast [44]. It is proposed that conflict on the decision to remove or reconstruct the breast in part depends on how a woman identifies with these various concepts. For example, there can be enormous relief in fully removing the diseased tissue ("medicalized breast") while at the same time experiencing a sense of loss over the healthy, feminizing, and "sexualized breast." Women who receive reconstruction may be pleased with regaining the appearance of the "gendered" breast, yet there is often enormous disappointment in the complete sensory loss that accompanies reconstruction of breast tissue ("sexualized breast") [45]. Depending on age, stage in life, and other individual differences, women may ascribe a varying sense of identification with each or any of these domains.

Moreover, although body image is a concern for many young survivors, there are other young women who adaptively cope with their treatments without significant disruption in body image. Evidence indicates that women who have a stronger body image prior to their cancer cope better with physical changes arising from their BC treatment [19]. Body image distress may additionally be buffered by certain protective factors such as having a foundation of positive self-regard and self-confidence. This parallels the observation of psychological distress in BC survivors, where lower anxiety and depression before the cancer diagnosis predicts lower overall psychological distress during survivorship [46]. Positive social support is another protective factor that has been identified in the literature. For example, women who are in supportive, communicative relationships tend to cope more easily with physical changes after treatment [47]. Partner support in particular is viewed as a strong buffer against emotional distress, predicting lower levels of depression and anxiety [48, 49], as well as better self-esteem and body satisfaction after treatment [47]. Such findings have important clinical implications with regard to the importance of helping women develop compensatory coping skills in order to build a more positive foundation around body image and self-identity.

14.4 Sexual Function

In addition to the impact on self-image and body image, the majority of young BC survivors also struggle with treatment-related sexual dysfunction [50]. Treatment for BC typically involves a combination of surgery, chemotherapy, radiation therapy, and/or endocrine therapy all of which have the potential to negatively impact young women's sexual health [51, 52]. In particular for young BC patients and survivors, treatments that interrupt, suppress, or permanently deplete hormonal function can have a profound impact on sexual function [53]. Unfortunately, distressing sexual problems in young BC survivors are not consistently identified by clinicians and may be overlooked entirely [9, 46].

Hypoestrogenism, resulting from either chemotherapy or hormone suppression treatments, has a direct negative impact on vulvar and vaginal health. Dramatic loss of estrogen to the genital tissue results in thinning of the epithelium, loss of rugosity, blood flow, and vaginal moisture. There is also increase in pH and genital tissue can become pale and fragile. Further, there may be a progressive loss of tissue elasticity related to loss of collagen, hyalinization, and elastin. This complex of symptoms, known as vulvovaginal atrophy, is often paralleled by a range of urogenital symptoms such as increased urinary urgency and stress-related urinary incontinence [54]. Hypoestrogenism is also frequently accompanied by decrease in libido and arousal as well as orgasmic function. Chemotherapy leads to premature ovarian failure in 30–96% of young, premenopausal women [55] with the highest risk for women who are over age 40 and for women exposed to alkylating agents such as cyclophosphamide [56]. For young BC survivors, it is notable that chemotherapy-induced ovarian failure can lead to more significant and extreme symptoms in contrast to women who undergo natural menopause [57].

More recently, the frequency and duration of treatments to suppress ovarian function in younger BC survivors are steadily increasing [53, 58]. Recently, the American Society of Clinical Oncology revised clinical practice guidelines and now recommends more extensive consideration of ovarian function suppression therapy for premenopausal estrogen receptor-positive BC survivors for at least 5 years following active treatment [59]. Recent evidence regarding endocrine therapy-related sexual dysfunction is very significant in young survivors [60] with rates of sexual dysfunction ranging from 65 to 90% which is up to tenfold higher than rates of sexual dysfunction in same age women in the general population (9–22%) [61, 62]. These negative sexual side effects have been consistently observed across multiple trials of ovarian suppression treatment, and these side effects have been characterized as being "very hard on young women" [63, 64]. Of note, distressing sexual and urogynecological side effects are the primary reason why young women prematurely discontinue ovarian suppression therapy [65]. In one of the largest ovarian suppression clinical trials with premenopausal breast cancer survivors to date, almost 22% of women prematurely discontinued OS treatment for these reasons [66].

Unfortunately, young women are often not prepared to manage the wide range of sexual and menopausal symptoms that have been described [57]. Moreover, vulvovaginal atrophy, loss of arousal and desire, and loss of sexual satisfaction also do not self-resolve over time [67]. For example, women on ovarian suppression therapy continue to report significant decrease in pleasure, sexual frequency, and increase in discomfort at both one [68] and 2 years following treatment end [69]. In a recent study, looking at women at a median of 5 years after stopping ovarian suppression, women still had a high frequency of severe sexual problems [70]. Recent evidence suggests that the debilitating sexual side effects of ovarian suppression may actually worsen with time [58, 60]. In addition to the physical side effects of estrogen deprivation, women who undergo hormonal disruption also report distress on decreased sense of intimacy and diminished partner function [51, 71–73]. Loss of sexual function and satisfaction with intimacy are also associated with poorer quality of life for BC survivors [74]. Although breast cancer survivors worry about the impact of treatment-related sexual problems on intimate relationships [75], there is also evidence to suggest that emotional support from an intimate partner can buffer some of these concerns and promote positive coping strategies [76]. Though there is limited data with regard to the experience of sexuality and intimacy with unpartnered survivors, it has been shown that unpartnered BC survivors place greater importance on physical appearance as a reflection of self-worth compared to partnered women [77]. This observation certainly raises concerns for unpartnered survivors who express various worries about dating including finding an accepting partner, being sexually desirable, and being rejected [78].

14.5 Cultural Considerations

Before considering how to address these concerns around body image and sexuality, it is important to acknowledge that perception of body image and the experience of sexuality are always experienced within a sociocultural context and may vary accordingly. The sections above reference largely Caucasian Western ideals of body, gender, and sexuality. Overall, evidence indicates that women across ethnicities report similar body image and sexual functioning concerns related to their BC treatment [46, 79, 80]. However, studies also reveal some distinct variations across broad ethnic groups. Variations might be explained in part by differences across ethnic groups in early detection and access to quality healthcare, and factors associated with receiving diagnoses at later stages and requiring more aggressive treatments causing more distressing side effects [81]. Differences may also be explained in part by ranging cultural beliefs about the female gender and perceptions about relationship intimacy and sex. Cultural beliefs can vary not only between cultural groups but also within groups; for instance, members of an ethnic minority may be more or less acculturated to the majority population, with some holding stronger traditional values or religious affiliations. For example, qualitative studies indicate that issues concerning open communication and awareness of one's body and sexual functioning are more common among recent immigrants and non-English monolingual individuals than in more educated and/or acculturated women [82]. In order to highlight the role of the sociocultural context regarding young women's experience of body image and sexuality after BC, we will briefly give examples relying on research with regard to three groups: African-American women, women with Latina/Hispanic heritage, and sexual minority women. It is essential for providers to have an awareness of cultural norms and values in order to facilitate communication that is culturally sensitive. The following examples are intended to illustrate the complexity of cultural issues with the understanding that interventions for sexual health are likely to be most effective if they are tailored appropriately to the particular cultural context.

14.5.1 African-American

Although African-American women have lower incidence rates of BC than other ethnic groups in the United States, they show higher mortality rates [81]. This statistic indicates a tendency to be diagnosed at later stages of the disease, which require more aggressive treatments. Such treatments can result in more severe side effects including sexual function and body image [83, 84]. Although studies indicate that concerns about sexual satisfaction and body image similarly exist among African-American women,

for some there may be a disinclination to raise these sensitive concerns with medical providers [83]. This tendency may be reflective of a long-standing mistrust of doctors and medical systems, as has been reported in surveys of the African-American community [85–88]. Some women may fear that sensitive information about their bodies and sexual habits would be misunderstood or invalidated in a clinical setting. African-American women have also reported concern over the stereotype of African-Americans being highly sexual [85], again understandably inhibiting open discussion of sexual problems. Further, within the African-American community, cancer holds a stigma which can prevent open discussion and support-seeking. In contrast, previous research has shown that peer-support counseling groups have successfully delivered education and support about sexual dysfunction, menopause, and distress on infertility after BC [85, 89].

14.5.2 Latina/Hispanic

Hispanic/Latina populations have lower incidence rates of BC, but similar mortality rates to Caucasian and Asian American populations [81]. Studies also reveal that Hispanic/Latina women are more likely than other cultures to report difficulties after treatment with issues of sexual function [79]. Traditional Hispanic/Latina perspective places emphasis on virginity and female sexual purity, while at the same time valuing a curvaceous body with breasts symbolizing femininity and fertility [90, 91]. On the other hand, it has been proposed that as younger generations of Hispanic/Latina women adopt body ideals from popular culture, including "thinness" [90, 92], it is important to recognize that body image concerns may differ among Hispanic/Latina survivors depending on the extent to which they do or do not adopt traditional cultural views [91]. With the loss of the breast, women may feel a loss in feminine power along with a diminished ability to attract a partner and feel attractive [93, 94]. Qualitative interviews have observed that more traditionally oriented Hispanic/Latina survivors worry about their male partner's reactions to their missing breast and their loss of sexual desire. However, these concerns may be buffered by good communication and perceived partner support [95, 96].

14.5.3 Sexual Minority Women

Although research focusing on quality-of-life outcomes among BC survivors posttreatment finds few differences between sexual minority and heterosexual women [97], there is evidence that lesbian and bisexual BC survivors experience a range of unmet needs for supportive care including the need for attention to treatment-related sexual health [98]. Parallel to heterosexual women, sexual minority women also report dramatic negative impact of hormone-blocking therapies on sexual function [98]. One area of potential disparity between heterosexual and sexual women minority women is with body image after BC. Previously, it has been reported that lesbians report fewer problems with body image and report feeling more comfortable with their body both before and after breast cancer [99]. In a recent study of sexual minority women, 25% chose to "go flat" (i.e., choose no reconstruction) [98]. There is now growing attention to the idea that there are various sexist and heterosexist assumptions around the need for breast reconstruction that may be particularly distressing for sexual minority women who may not be as interested in breast reconstruction as their heterosexual peers [100]. One implication is that providers must be educated about how to discuss women's range of options post-mastectomy that do not assume reconstruction is necessary in order for a woman to feel "whole" again.

14.6   Clinical Pointers

14.6.1 Inquiry/Assessment

The majority of young BC survivors struggle with some distressing aspect of sexual function without getting adequate support to manage these changes. It is our belief that all young women who are diagnosed and treated for BC should receive basic and straightforward information and support about sexual health and well-being as part of standard clinical care. One useful guide for clinicians is the 5 A's Framework, which refers to five fundamental aspects of care: *Ask, Advise, Assess, Assist,* and *Arrange* [101]. To begin, clinicians must *Ask* all young BC survivors about their sexual health. After the initial inquiry, clinicians must signal their intention to *Advise* as needed. In contrast to giving advice, *Advise* is meant as a cue to clinicians to validate the presence of sexual problems after BC and confirm that help is available. Next, clinicians need to adequately *Assess* what kind of help is needed in order to *Assist* the patient/survivor. Assistance may range from giving an educational handout to making a referral for active treatment. Finally, a provider must make sure that they *Arrange* to follow up with the young woman so that this need for care does not get lost. To clarify, we strongly suggest those clinicians who see young BC survivors have or develop a referral network of experts who can address potential common problems. We suggest having a referral network that includes a urologist, gynecologist, endocrinologist, pelvic floor physical therapist, and a psychologist or onco-sexologist.

It is important to acknowledge that clinicians are not likely to *Ask* or *Assist* unless they have straightforward strategies for doing so. Regarding asking, one example is to use a question such as "Many BC patients and survivors have some challenges with sexual health or body image after treatment; are you distressed or bothered about any of these kinds of changes?" Another option is to use a brief checklist in order to inquire about areas of concern (see Fig. 14.1). Recently, members of Scientific Network on Female Sexual Health and Cancer, a multidisciplinary group of experts working in the field of female sexual dysfunction after cancer [102], modified the Brief Sexual Symptom Checklist, a general inventory intended for use in primary care settings [41]. The Brief Sexual Symptom Checklist (Brief Sexual Symptom Checklist-Cancer (BSSC-C)) is intended specifically for use with female cancer survivors

Sexual Symptom Checklist for Women

Please answer the following questions about your overall sexual function:

1. Are you satisfied with your sexual function? ❑ Yes ❑ No
if no, please continue.

2. Do you experience any of the following sexual problems or concerns?
❑ Little or no interest in sex
❑ Decreased sensation (or loss of sensation)
❑ Decreased vaginal lubrication (dryness)
❑ Difficulty reaching orgasm
❑ Pain during sex
❑ Vaginal or vulvar pain or discomfort (not during sex)
❑ Anxiety about having sex
❑ Other Problem or Concern: _______________

> *TIP*: Some patients will respond that they are not having these problems or concerns because they stopped having sex altogether. The provider should reassure the patient, let her know that she is not alone, and ask if she can recall what kinds of problems or concerns she was having that led her to stop having sex.

3. Would you like more information, resources, and/or to speak with someone about these issue?
❑ Yes ❑ No

Fig. 14.1 Sexual Symptom Checklist

[103]. This brief checklist begins with a starter question asking about overall sexual satisfaction. If women endorse being satisfied with current function, no further questions are asked. If women are not satisfied, then a brief list of problems is reviewed.

Regarding *assistance*, we strongly encourage clinicians to familiarize themselves with a number of the "simple strategies" that have been effective in managing treatment-related sexual dysfunction in young BC survivors [103, 104]. As noted earlier in this chapter, a majority of young BC survivors struggle with vaginal dryness secondary to treatment-related hypoestrogenism. This condition can be extremely distressing because it leads to a range of consequences including chafing and burning, pain, and bleeding. Not surprisingly, women suffering from these symptoms also may find sexual activity to be extremely uncomfortable if not impossible, and in parallel, sexual desire understandably may diminish. We recommend that clinicians inform young women of the need to maintain vaginal health after BC including restoring moisture, elasticity, and blood flow to vaginal

mucosa as needed. Specifically, clinicians who work with young BC survivors should be familiar with first-line treatment including being able to explain the distinction between vaginal lubricants and moisturizers. Whereas vaginal lubricants provide topical lubrication and can help to prevent irritation and potentially avoid mucosal tears during sexual activity, vaginal moisturizers are formulated to hydrate the vaginal mucosa over time. Moisturizers are intended to be used consistently for overall vaginal comfort and not only on an as-needed basis. Evidence indicates that the benefit of vaginal moisturizers depends upon consistent use up to five times per week [104]. This type of regimen is particularly important for young survivors who are on ovarian suppression treatment. Similarly, other strategies to be aware of include the use of vaginal dilaters to help women regain tissue elasticity and pelvic floor physical therapy, a modality which is invaluable for young women who have symptoms of vulvovaginal atrophy and can gain enormous benefit from exercises designed to improve pelvic muscle floor strength and tone and vaginal elasticity [105].

14.7 Conclusions

Because most young BC survivors struggle at some point with a treatment-related change in sexual function and body image, it is imperative that clinicians feel prepared to inquire about these issues as part of routine clinical care. In general, it is our strong recommendation that inquiry is made about body image and sexual health in parallel with any other review of systems. Comparable to the way that women may be asked about pain, nausea, or fatigue, the checklist that we have provided offers a straightforward model for how to inquire and begin a conversation about these common, distressing problems that are often completely ignored. Inquiry is an important initial step as it opens the door to providing women who endorse difficulties with effective interventions, and it also validates an important aspect of reality that is regularly ignored. The range of experience women can feel after cancer is wide. It is not simply about the extremes of feeling that sexual function or body image is either "intact" or "not intact." To this end, raising these questions in a clinical setting also allows for a discussion about a woman's individual adjustment to her situation.

Because the issues of body image and sexual function are truly at the nexus of psychological, physical, and interpersonal factors, it is helpful for clinicians to identify individual counselors, social workers, and/or couples' therapists they can refer to in addition to having other providers such as gynecologists or pelvic floor physical therapists in their arsenal of ancillary providers. Finally, given that these issues are experienced with a developmental and sociocultural context, it is important that clinicians maintain an awareness that young women may be very much in a process of discovery and exploration on sexuality, intimacy, and relationships and that they maintain an attitude of cultural sensitivity. Although intervention research in sexual health is gaining greater attention, there is an enormous unmet need to evaluate effectiveness of strategies with low- to middle-income populations and with young women receiving community-based care. In addition, further research is called for to gain greater insight into cultural differences and to adapt current interventions across a variety of cultural contexts. As quality of life is a hallmark goal of cancer survivorship, it is essential that we optimize efforts to help young women repair and restore body image and sexual function as they seek to live full and satisfying lives long after their diagnosis of BR CA.

References

1. Nichols HB, Schoemaker MJ, Wright LB, McGowan C, Brook MN, McClain KM, et al. The premenopausal breast cancer collaboration: a pooling project of studies participating in the National Cancer Institute Cohort Consortium. Cancer Epidemiol Biomark Prev. 2017;26(9):1360–9.
2. Bloom JR, Stewart SL, Chang S, Banks PJ. Then and now: quality of life of young breast cancer survivors. Psychooncology. 2004;13(3):147–60.
3. Howlader N, Noone AM, Krapcho M, Miller D, Bishop K, Altekruse SF, et al. SEER Cancer statistics review, 1975–2013. Bethesda, MD: National Cancer Institute; 2016.
4. Anders CK, Fan C, Parker JS, Carey LA, Blackwell KL, Klauber-DeMore N, et al. Breast carcinomas arising at a young age: unique biology or a surrogate for aggressive intrinsic subtypes? J Clin Oncol. 2011;29(1):e18–20.
5. Shannon C, Smith IE. Breast cancer in adolescents and young women. Eur J Cancer. 2003;39(18):2632–42.
6. Anderson WF, Chatterjee N, Ershler WB, Brawley OW. Estrogen receptor breast cancer phenotypes in the surveillance, epidemiology, and end results database. Breast Cancer Res Treat. 2002; 76(1):27–36.
7. Thewes B, Butow P, Girgis A, Pendlebury S. The psychosocial needs of breast cancer survivors; a qualitative study of the shared and unique needs of younger versus older survivors. Psychooncology. 2004;13(3):177–89.
8. Avis NE, Crawford S, Manuel J. Quality of life among younger women with breast cancer. J Clin Oncol. 2005;23(15):3322–30.
9. Katz A. The sounds of silence: sexuality information for cancer patients. J Clin Oncol. 2005;23(1):238–41.
10. Flynn KE, Reese JB, Jeffery DD, Abernethy AP, Lin L, Shelby RA, et al. Patient experiences with communication about sex during and after treatment for cancer. Psychooncology. 2012;21(6):594–601.
11. Bober SL, Varela VS. Sexuality in adult cancer survivors: challenges and intervention. J Clin Oncol. 2012;30(30):3712–9.
12. Dunn J, Steginga SK. Young women's experience of breast cancer: defining young and identifying concerns. Psychooncology. 2000;9(2):137–46.

13. Erikson EH. Identity: youth and crisis. Oxford: Norton & Co; 1968.
14. Levinson DJ. The seasons of a man's life. New York, NY: Random House Digital, Inc.; 1978.
15. Arnett JJ. Emerging adulthood: a theory of development from the late teens through the twenties. Am Psychol. 2000;55(5):469–80.
16. Schover LR. Sexuality and body image in younger women with breast cancer. J Natl Cancer Inst Monogr. 1994;16:177–82.
17. Waskul DD, van der Riet P. The abject embodiment of cancer patients: dignity, selfhood, and the grotesque body. Symb Interact. 2002;25:487–513.
18. Kasper AS. A feminist, qualitative methodology: a study of women with breast cancer. Qual Sociol. 1994;17:263–81.
19. Han J, Grothuesmann D, Neises M, Hille U, Hillemanns P. Quality of life and satisfaction after breast cancer operation. Arch Gynecol Obstet. 2010;282(1):75–82.
20. White CA. Body image dimensions and cancer: a heuristic cognitive behavioural model. Psychooncology. 2000;9(3):183–92.
21. Liu J, Peh CX, Mahendran R. Body image and emotional distress in newly diagnosed cancer patients: the mediating role of dysfunctional attitudes and rumination. Body Image. 2016;20:58–64.
22. Przezdziecki A, Sherman KA, Baillie A, Taylor A, Foley E, Stalgis-Bilinski K. My changed body: breast cancer, body image, distress and self-compassion. Psychooncology. 2013;22(8):1872–9.
23. Bakht S, Najafi S. Body image and sexual dysfunctions: comparison between breast cancer patients and healthy women. Procedia Soc Behav Sci. 2010;5:1493–7.
24. Tiggemann M. Body image across the adult life span: stability and change. Body Image. 2004;1(1):29–41.
25. Miller CT, Downey KT. A meta-analysis of heavyweight and self-esteem. Personal Soc Psychol Rev. 1999;3(1):68–84.
26. Paterson CL, Lengacher CA, Donovan KA, Kip KE, Tofthagen CS. Body image in younger breast cancer survivors: asystematic review. Cancer Nurs. 2016;39(1):E39–58.
27. Miller SJ, Schnur JB, Weinberger-Litman SL, Montgomery GH. The relationship between body image, age, and distress in women facing breast cancer surgery. Palliat Support Care. 2014;12(5):363–7.
28. Fisher B, Anderson S, Bryant J, Margolese RG, Deutsch M, Fisher ER, et al. Twenty-year follow-up of a randomized trial comparing total mastectomy, lumpectomy, and lumpectomy plus irradiation for the treatment of invasive breast cancer. N Engl J Med. 2002;347(16):1233–41.
29. Veronesi U, Cascinelli N, Mariani L, Greco M, Saccozzi R, Luini A, et al. Twenty-year follow-up of a randomized study comparing breast-conserving surgery with radical mastectomy for early breast cancer. N Engl J Med. 2002;347(16):1227–32.
30. Morrow M, Jagsi R, Alderman AK, Griggs JJ, Hawley ST, Hamilton AS, et al. Surgeon recommendations and receipt of mastectomy for treatment of breast cancer. JAMA. 2009;302(14):1551–6.
31. Gomez SL, Lichtensztajn D, Kurian AW, Telli ML, Chang ET, Keegan TH, et al. Increasing mastectomy rates for early-stage breast cancer? Population-based trends from California. J Clin Oncol. 2010;28(10):e155–7. author reply e8
32. Mahmood U, Hanlon AL, Koshy M, Buras R, Chumsri S, Tkaczuk KH, et al. Increasing national mastectomy rates for the treatment of early stage breast cancer. Ann Surg Oncol. 2013;20(5):1436–43.
33. Katipamula R, Degnim AC, Hoskin T, Boughey JC, Loprinzi C, Grant CS, et al. Trends in mastectomy rates at the Mayo Clinic Rochester: effect of surgical year and preoperative magnetic resonance imaging. J Clin Oncol. 2009;27(25):4082–8.
34. Tuttle TM, Habermann EB, Grund EH, Morris TJ, Virnig BA. Increasing use of contralateral prophylactic mastectomy for breast cancer patients: a trend toward more aggressive surgical treatment. J Clin Oncol. 2007;25(33):5203–9.
35. Herrinton LJ, Barlow WE, Yu O, Geiger AM, Elmore JG, Barton MB, et al. Efficacy of prophylactic mastectomy in women with unilateral breast cancer: a cancer research network project. J Clin Oncol. 2005;23(19):4275–86.
36. Anderson C, Islam JY, Elizabeth Hodgson M, Sabatino SA, Rodriguez JL, Lee CN, et al. Long-term satisfaction and body image after contralateral prophylactic mastectomy. Ann Surg Oncol. 2017;29:e18–20.
37. Yurek D, Farrar W, Andersen BL. Breast cancer surgery: comparing surgical groups and determining individual differences in postoperative sexuality and body change stress. J Consult Clin Psychol. 2000;68(4):697–709.
38. Engel J, Kerr J, Schlesinger-Raab A, Sauer H, Holzel D. Quality of life following breast-conserving therapy or mastectomy: results of a 5-year prospective study. Breast J. 2004;10(3):223–31.
39. Frost MH, Schaid DJ, Sellers TA, Slezak JM, Arnold PG, Woods JE, et al. Long-term satisfaction and psychological and social function following bilateral prophylactic mastectomy. JAMA. 2000;284(3):319–24.
40. Pinto AC. Sexuality and breast cancer: prime time for young patients. J Thorac Dis. 2013;5(Suppl 1):S81–6.
41. Kedde H, van de Wiel HB, Weijmar Schultz WC, Wijsen C. Sexual dysfunction in young women with breast cancer. Support Care Cancer. 2013;21(1):271–80.
42. Rumsey N, Harcourt D. Body image and disfigurement: issues and interventions. Body Image. 2004;1(1):83–97.
43. Lansdown R, Rumsey N, Bradbury E, Carr T, Partridge J. Visibly different: coping with disfigurement. London: Hodder Arnold; 1997.
44. Langellier KM, Sullivan CF. Breast talk in breast cancer narratives. Qual Health Res. 1998;8(1):76–94.
45. Kwait RM, Pesek S, Onstad M, Edmonson D, Clark MA, Raker C, et al. Influential forces in breast can-

cer surgical decision making and the impact on body image and sexual function. Ann Surg Oncol. 2016;23(10):3403–11.

46. Fobair P, Stewart SL, Chang S, D'Onofrio C, Banks PJ, Bloom JR. Body image and sexual problems in young women with breast cancer. Psychooncology. 2006;15(7):579–94.

47. Helgeson VS, Cohen S. Social support and adjustment to cancer: reconciling descriptive, correlational, and intervention research. Health Psychol. 1996;15(2):135–48.

48. Manne S. Couples coping with cancer: research issues and recent findings. J Clin Psychol Med Settings. 1994;1(4):317–30.

49. Peters-Golden H. Breast cancer: varied perceptions of social support in the illness experience. Soc Sci Med. 1982;16(4):483–91.

50. Sadovsky R, Basson R, Krychman M, Morales AM, Schover L, Wang R, et al. Cancer and sexual problems. J Sex Med. 2010;7(1 Pt 2):349–73.

51. Katz A. Breast cancer and women's sexuality. Am J Nurs. 2011;111(4):63–7.

52. Bredart A, Dolbeault S, Savignoni A, Besancenet C, This P, Giami A, et al. Prevalence and associated factors of sexual problems after early-stage breast cancer treatment: results of a French exploratory survey. Psychooncology. 2011;20(8):841–50.

53. Jain S, Santa-Maria CA, Gradishar WJ. The role of ovarian suppression in premenopausal women with hormone receptor-positive early-stage breast cancer. Oncology. 2015;29(7):473–8.

54. Baumgart J, Nilsson K, Stavreus-Evers A, Kask K, Villman K, Lindman H, et al. Urogenital disorders in women with adjuvant endocrine therapy after early breast cancer. Am J Obstet Gynecol. 2011;204(1):26. e1–7.

55. Rosenberg SM, Partridge AH. Premature menopause in young breast cancer: effects on quality of life and treatment interventions. J Thorac Dis. 2013;5(Suppl 1):S55–61.

56. Anchan RM, Ginsburg ES. Fertility concerns and preservation in younger women with breast cancer. Crit Rev Oncol Hematol. 2010;74(3):175–92.

57. Shuster LT, Rhodes DJ, Gostout BS, Grossardt BR, Rocca WA. Premature menopause or early menopause: long-term health consequences. Maturitas. 2010;65(2):161–6.

58. Burstein HJ, Lacchetti C, Anderson H, Buchholz TA, Davidson NE, Gelmon KE, et al. Adjuvant endocrine therapy for women with hormone receptor-positive breast Cancer: American Society of Clinical Oncology clinical practice guideline update. J OncolPract. 2015;12:390–3.

59. Paluch-Shimon S, Pagani O, Partridge AH, Abulkhair O, Cardoso MJ, Dent RA, et al. ESO-ESMO 3rd international consensus guidelines for breast cancer in young women (BCY3). Breast. 2017;35:203–17.

60. Ribi K, Luo W, Bernhard J, Francis PA, Burstein HJ, Ciruelos E, et al. Adjuvant Tamoxifen plus ovarian function suppression versus Tamoxifen alone in premenopausal women with early breast Cancer: patient-reported outcomes in the sup-pression of ovarian function trial. J Clin Oncol. 2016;34:1601–10.

61. Lewis RW, Fugl-Meyer KS, Corona G, Hayes RD, Laumann EO, Moreira ED Jr, et al. Definitions/epidemiology/risk factors for sexual dysfunction. J Sex Med. 2010;7(4 Pt 2):1598–607.

62. Laumann EO, Paik A, Rosen RC. Sexual dysfunction in the United States: prevalence and predictors. JAMA. 1999;281(6):537–44.

63. Goldfarb S. Endocrine therapy and its effect on sexual function. Am Soc Clin Oncol Educ Book. 2015;2015:e575–81.

64. Layeequr Rahman R, Baker T, Crawford S, Kauffman R. SOFT trial can be very hard on young women. Breast. 2015;24(6):767–8.

65. Francis PA, Pagani O, Fleming GF, Walley BA, Colleoni M, Lang I, et al. Tailoring adjuvant endocrine therapy for premenopausal breast cancer. N Engl J Med. 2018;379(2):122–37.

66. Francis PA, Regan MM, Fleming GF, Lang I, Ciruelos E, Bellet M, et al. Adjuvant ovarian suppression in premenopausal breast cancer. N Engl J Med. 2015;372(5):436–46.

67. Frechette D, Paquet L, Verma S, Clemons M, Wheatley-Price P, Gertler SZ, et al. The impact of endocrine therapy on sexual dysfunction in postmenopausal women with early stage breast cancer: encouraging results from a prospective study. Breast Cancer Res Treat. 2013;141(1):111–7.

68. Finch A, Metcalfe KA, Chiang JK, Elit L, McLaughlin J, Springate C, et al. The impact of prophylactic salpingo-oophorectomy on menopausal symptoms and sexual function in women who carry a BRCA mutation. Gynecol Oncol. 2011;121(1):163–8.

69. Tucker PE, Bulsara MK, Salfinger SG, Tan JJ-S, Green H, Cohen PA. Prevalence of sexual dysfunction after risk-reducing salpingo-oophorectomy. Gynecol Oncol. 2015;140(1):95–100.

70. Pezaro C, James P, McKinley J, Shanahan M, Young MA, Mitchell G. The consequences of risk reducing salpingo-oophorectomy: the case for a coordinated approach to long-term follow up post surgical menopause. Familial Cancer. 2012;11(3):403–10.

71. Dizon DS. Quality of life after breast cancer: survivorship and sexuality. Breast J. 2009;15(5):500–4.

72. Emilee G, Ussher JM, Perz J. Sexuality after breast cancer: a review. Maturitas. 2010;66(4):397–407.

73. Elmir R, Jackson D, Beale B, Schmied V. Against all odds: Australian women's experiences of recovery from breast cancer. J Clin Nurs. 2010;19(17–18):2531–8.

74. Reese JB, Shelby RA, Keefe FJ, Porter LS, Abernethy AP. Sexual concerns in cancer patients: a comparison of GI and breast cancer patients. Support Care Cancer. 2010;18(9):1179–89.

75. Fobair P, Spiegel D. Concerns about sexuality after breast cancer. Cancer J. 2009;15(1):19–26.

76. Fang SY, Lin YC, Chen TC, Lin CY. Impact of marital coping on the relationship between body image and sexuality among breast cancer survivors. Support Care Cancer. 2015;23(9):2551–9.

77. Shaw LK, Sherman KA, Fitness J, Elder E. Factors associated with romantic relationship formation difficulties in women with breast cancer. Psychooncology. 2018;27(4):1270–6.
78. Kurowecki D, Fergus KD. Wearing my heart on my chest: dating, new relationships, and the reconfiguration of self-esteem after breast cancer. Psychooncology. 2014;23(1):52–64.
79. Christie KM, Meyerowitz BE, Maly RC. Depression and sexual adjustment following breast cancer in low-income Hispanic and non-Hispanic White women. Psychooncology. 2010;19(10):1069–77.
80. Giedzinska AS, Meyerowitz BE, Ganz PA, Rowland JH. Health-related quality of life in a multiethnic sample of breast cancer survivors. Ann Behav Med. 2004;28(1):39–51.
81. Siegel RL, Miller KD, Jemal A. Cancer statistics, 2016. CA Cancer J Clin. 2016;66(1):7–30.
82. Ashing-Giwa KT, Padilla G, Tejero J, Kraemer J, Wright K, Coscarelli A, et al. Understanding the breast cancer experience of women: a qualitative study of African American, Asian American, Latina and Caucasian cancer survivors. Psychooncology. 2004;13(6):408–28.
83. Taylor KL, Lamdan RM, Siegel JE, Shelby R, Hrywna M, Moran-Klimi K. Treatment regimen, sexual attractiveness concerns and psychological adjustment among African American breast cancer patients. Psychooncology. 2002;11(6):505–17.
84. Wilmoth MC, Sanders LD. Accept me for myself: African American women's issues after breast cancer. Oncol Nurs Forum. 2001;28(5):875–9.
85. Lewis PE, Sheng M, Rhodes MM, Jackson KE, Schover LR. Psychosocial concerns of young African American breast cancer survivors. J Psychosoc Oncol. 2012;30(2):168–84.
86. Hoffman-Goetz L. Cancer experiences of African-American women as portrayed in popular mass magazines. Psychooncology. 1999;8(1):36–45.
87. Masi CM, Gehlert S. Perceptions of breast cancer treatment among African-American women and men: implications for interventions. J Gen Intern Med. 2009;24(3):408–14.
88. Germino BB, Mishel MH, Alexander GR, Jenerette C, Blyler D, Baker C, et al. Engaging African American breast cancer survivors in an intervention trial: culture, responsiveness and community. J Cancer Surviv. 2011;5(1):82–91.
89. Schover LR, Rhodes MM, Baum G, Adams JH, Jenkins R, Lewis P, et al. Sisters peer counseling in reproductive issues after treatment (SPIRIT): a peer counseling program to improve reproductive health among African American breast cancer survivors. Cancer. 2011;117(21):4983–92.
90. Viladrich A, Yeh MC, Bruning N, Weiss R. "Do real women have curves?" paradoxical body images among Latinas in New York City. J Immigr Minor Health. 2009;11(1):20–8.
91. Gil RM, Vazquez CI. The Maria paradox: how Latinas can merge old world traditions with new world self-esteem. New York: Open Road Media; 2014.
92. Pompper D, Koenig J. Cross-cultural-generational perceptions of ideal body image: Hispanic women and magazine standards. J Mass Commun Quarterly. 2004;81(1):89–107.
93. Buki LP, Reich M, Lehardy EN. "Our organs have a purpose": body image acceptance in Latina breast cancer survivors. Psychooncology. 2016;25(11):1337–42.
94. Ashing-Giwa KT, Padilla GV, Bohorquez DE, Tejero JS, Garcia M. Understanding the breast cancer experience of Latina women. J Psychosoc Oncol. 2006;24(3):19–52.
95. Martinez-Ramos GP, Biggs MJG, Lozano Y. Quality of life of Latina breast cancer survivors: from silence to empowerment. Adv Soc Work. 2013;14:82–101.
96. Lopez-Class M, Perret-Gentil M, Kreling B, Caicedo L, Mandelblatt J, Graves KD. Quality of life among immigrant Latina breast cancer survivors: realities of culture and enhancing cancer care. J Cancer Educ. 2011;26(4):724–33.
97. Boehmer U, Glickman M, Winter M, Clark MA. Breast cancer survivors of different sexual orientations: which factors explain survivors' quality of life and adjustment? Ann Oncol. 2013;24(6):1622–30.
98. Brown MT, McElroy JA. Unmet support needs of sexual and gender minority breast cancer survivors. Support Care Cancer. 2018;26(4):1189–96.
99. Fobair P, O'Hanlan K, Koopman C, Classen C, Dimiceli S, Drooker N, et al. Comparison of lesbian and heterosexual women's response to newly diagnosed breast cancer. Psychooncology. 2001;10(1):40–51.
100. Rubin LR, Tanenbaum M. "Does that make me a woman?": breast Cancer, mastectomy, and breast reconstruction decisions among sexual minority women. Psychol Women Q. 2011;35(3):401–14.
101. Park ER, Norris RL, Bober SL. Sexual health communication during cancer care: barriers and recommendations. Cancer J. 2009;15(1):74–7.
102. Goldfarb SB, Abramsohn E, Andersen BL, Baron SR, Carter J, Dickler M, et al. A national network to advance the field of cancer and female sexuality. J Sex Med. 2013;10(2):319–25.
103. Bober S, Reese JB, Barbera L, Bradford A, Carpenter KM, Goldfarb S, et al. How to ask and what to do: a guide for clinical inquiry and intervention regarding female sexual health after cancer. Curr Opin Support Palliat Care. 2016;10:44–54.
104. Carter J, Goldfrank D, Schover LR. Simple strategies for vaginal health promotion in cancer survivors. J Sex Med. 2011;8(2):549–59.
105. Coady D, Kennedy V. Sexual health in women affected by cancer: focus on sexual pain. Obstet Gynecol. 2016;128(4):775–91.

Matteo Lambertini and Fedro A. Peccatori

15.1 Introduction

Young women with newly diagnosed breast cancer require personalized approaches in order to manage their specific age-associated needs not only in terms of optimal anticancer treatments but also related to other important quality-of-life implications [1]. Among them, fertility- and pregnancy-related issues are considered one of the priority areas of concerns for young breast cancer patients [1]. Major advances in the management of early breast cancers have substantially increased the survival of young women. However, anticancer therapies can expose premenopausal women to additional long-term side effects such as premature ovarian insufficiency (POI) and subsequent impaired fertility [2]. As shown in a large prospective study, at the time of breast cancer diagnosis, approximately half of the young women with newly diagnosed breast cancer are concerned about the possible development of treatment-induced POI and infertility [3]. These concerns can cause important psycho-social distress and impact on the decision and the adherence toward the proposed anticancer therapies [3].

Major international guidelines highlight the importance of counseling all cancer patients diagnosed during their reproductive years about the possible risk of treatment-induced POI and infertility and then informing interested patients about the different available options for fertility preservation [4, 5]. Nowadays, oncofertility counseling should be considered standard of care in all newly diagnosed young cancer patients [6, 7]. To help oncologists addressing these issues and to improve adherence to guidelines, several services and resources are now available [8–12]. However, despite the development of specific programs to support clinicians in discussing concerns related to fertility and pregnancy with young patients [13], there are still several barriers on this regard and not all patients are adequately informed, thus limiting the access to fertility preservation procedures and reducing the chance of future pregnancies [14, 15]. Hence, even though other personal issues might interfere with the desire of motherhood, the percentage of patients who achieve a pregnancy after the end of treatment remains low, especially among breast cancer survivors [16].

The aim of the present chapter is to highlight the risk of treatment-induced POI and infertility in young women with breast cancer, to review the available data on the different fertil-

M. Lambertini
Department of Medical Oncology, Clinica di
Oncologia Medica, Policlinico San Martino-IST,
University of Genova, Genoa, Italy

F. A. Peccatori (✉)
Fertility and Procreation Unit, Division of
Gynecologic Oncology, European Institute of
Oncology, Milan, Italy
e-mail: fedro.peccatori@ieo.it

ity preservation options in these patients, and to discuss the safety issues of pregnancy in breast cancer survivors.

15.2 Anticancer Treatments and Gonadal Function

The development of treatment-induced POI and infertility are possible additional consequences of anticancer therapies in patients treated during their reproductive years [2]. Of note, the majority of the studies that investigated the risk of developing this side effect used amenorrhea and resumption of menstrual function as surrogate indicators of POI and preserved ovarian function, respectively [17]. However, resumption of menses does not imply intact ovarian function and fertility potential, and women with prior exposure to chemotherapy may have diminished ovarian reserve despite the return of cyclical menstruation [18]. Using amenorrhea to assess the impact of chemotherapy on ovarian function, the most commonly administered regimens in breast cancer including cyclophosphamide, anthracyclines, and taxanes are associated with a rate of treatment-induced POI around 40–60% [2, 19].

Nevertheless, this risk can vary according to type and dose of chemotherapy regimens, age of the patients at the time of treatment, and need for adjuvant endocrine therapy which are the main factors impacting on the likelihood of developing treatment-induced POI in young breast cancer patients [2]. The effect of these three factors has been clearly shown in the amenorrhea sub-study conducted within the National Surgical Adjuvant Breast and Bowel Project (NSABP) B-30 trial that compared three different adjuvant chemotherapy regimens (sequential doxorubicin [A] and cyclophosphamide [C] followed by docetaxel [T; AC → T], AT, and TAC) [20]. Amenorrhea rates differed significantly according to patients' age at the time of treatment, ranging from 61% in those younger than 40 years to 100% in women older than 50 years. Amenorrhea rates were also significantly different between treatment arms, ranging from 37.9% for AT to 57.7% for TAC to 69.8%

for AC → T. Finally, the addition of tamoxifen increased the risk of treatment-induced amenorrhea [20].

Although the mechanisms that are responsible for chemotherapy-induced ovarian damage have not been fully elucidated, the direct induction of oocytes and follicle apoptosis and the vascular damage to the ovary seem to be the two major determinants of the toxic effect of anticancer agents [21, 22].

15.3 Fertility Preservation Strategies

Embryo and oocyte cryopreservation, ovarian tissue cryopreservation, and temporary ovarian suppression with gonadotropin-releasing hormone analogs (GnRHa) during chemotherapy are the available fertility preservation strategies in breast cancer patients. During oncofertility counseling, the specific pro and contra of each procedure should be clearly discussed, including access to services, reimbursability, and out-of-pocket costs (Table 15.1).

15.3.1 Embryo and Oocyte Cryopreservation

According to major international guidelines, embryo and oocyte cryopreservation are standard strategies for fertility preservation in all female cancer patients [1, 4, 5, 23]. In infertile women without cancer, these options demonstrated the most reliable results in terms of subsequent pregnancies. Their success is strongly dependent by the age of the patients at the time of the procedure with live birth rates ranging from 22.7% in women younger than 34 years to less than 10% for those older than 40 years [24].

Importantly, in cancer patients requiring gonadotoxic treatments, embryo and oocyte cryopreservation cannot preserve gonadal function during chemotherapy; they must therefore be concluded before starting cytotoxic therapy and are contraindicated in women with recent

Table 15.1 Main characteristics of the available fertility preservation strategies in breast cancer patients

Type of strategy	Pro	Contra	Main results
Embryo and oocyte cryopreservation	– Effective technique in infertile non oncologic women – Minor surgical procedure required – Good availability	– Limited data on efficacy and safety in cancer patients – No protection against treatment-induced POI – Controlled ovarian stimulation required – Possible delay in the start of anticancer treatments – Need for a facility specialized in fertility preservation	– Pregnancy rate of 51.5% (series of 33 breast cancer patients) – No apparent negative consequences on patients' survival (HR for recurrence 0.77; 95% CI, 0.28–2.13; $p = 0.61$)
Ovarian tissue cryopreservation	– Preservation of both fertility and ovarian function – Controlled ovarian stimulation not required – Minimal/no delay in the start of anticancer treatments	– Limited data on efficacy and safety in cancer patients – Need for two surgical procedures – Need for a facility specialized in fertility preservation and with the adequate expertise in this technique – Risk of reintroducing malignant cells with transplantation	– Estimated live birth rate of 25% – Expected ovarian function recovery within 3–6 months (with possible sustained longevity) – More than 80 babies born worldwide
Temporary ovarian suppression with GnRHa	– Consistent data on preservation of ovarian function – Controlled ovarian stimulation not required – No delay in the start of anticancer treatments – No surgical procedure required – Wide availability	– Limited data on fertility preservation – Not to be used as the only strategy in patients interested in fertility preservation – No data on long-term preservation of ovarian function (age at menopause)	– Significant reduction in POI risk (OR, 0.36; 95% CI, 0.23–0.57; $p < 0.001$) – Higher number of patients achieving a subsequent pregnancy (33 vs. 19 women; OR, 1.83; 95% CI, 1.02–3.28; $p = 0.041$)

Abbreviations: *POI* premature ovarian insufficiency, *GnRHa* gonadotropin-releasing hormone analogs, *HR* hazard ratio, *CI* confidence intervals, *OR* odds ratio

exposure to such treatments due to the possible occurrence of morphologic/genetic abnormalities in the retrieved oocytes [25].

Embryo and oocyte cryopreservation require the need of performing a controlled ovarian stimulation (COS) lasting between 10 and 16 days with subsequent potential delay in treatment initiation and exposure to supraphysiological estradiol levels [26]. To avoid a possible detrimental impact on cancer cell proliferation, specific protocols for COS have been developed for breast cancer patients with the concomitant administration of letrozole [27, 28] or tamoxifen [29–31].

The letrozole-associated COS protocol was developed by Oktay and colleagues [27, 28]. Despite the conflicting results reported on the performance of letrozole-associated COS [32, 33], the largest cohort that investigated the success of this technique in 33 breast cancer patients showed a similar live birth rate (45%) as the one expected in the general infertile population of a similar age [31]. The largest study that investigated the safety of embryo and oocyte cryopreservation in young women with breast cancer included a prospective cohort of 120 patients who underwent letrozole-associated COS for fertility preservation and 217 matched patients who did not undergo any fertility-preserving procedure [34]. After a mean follow-up of approximately 5 years, no survival difference between the two groups was observed with a hazard ratio (HR) for recurrence after embryo cryopreservation of 0.77 (95% confidence intervals [CI], 0.28–2.13; $p = 0.61$) [34].

Tamoxifen-associated COS can be an alternative to letrozole-associated COS in breast cancer patients [26]. Results with the use of tamoxifen-associated COS appear to be similar than those after COS without tamoxifen [30]. Nevertheless, some safety issues should be considered with this COS, mainly related to the delay (approximately 2 months) in achieving steady state for tamoxifen and its bioactive metabolite endoxifen [35].

Conventionally, COS is initiated at the beginning of the follicular phase to optimize oocyte harvest. This has been challenged by recently developed protocols that allow a "random start" of COS, including late follicular and luteal phase start, without impairment in clinical results [36]. This strategy allows a prompt initiation of chemotherapy immediately after COS and the possibility to perform a double stimulation in specific circumstances, thus increasing the number of harvested oocytes [37].

When COS is not feasible due to time constraints or safety concerns on risk of breast cancer recurrence, immature oocytes collected at any phase of the menstrual cycle followed by in vitro maturation (IVM) may be considered [38, 39]. Although IVM seems to be less efficient than standard in vitro fertilization (IVF) procedures, IVM might be an interesting alternative option for fertility preservation in selected cases [40].

15.3.2 Ovarian Tissue Cryopreservation

Ovarian tissue cryopreservation is an effective, yet still experimental, fertility preservation strategy in patients receiving anticancer therapies [1, 4, 5, 23]. Ovarian tissue either from the whole ovary or more commonly from ovarian biopsies is collected by laparoscopy, and small fragments are then cryopreserved for a possible future autotransplantation after the end of anticancer treatments to restore ovarian function and fertility. Immature oocytes can be also collected ex vivo and cryopreserved after IVM when ovarian tissue cryopreservation is performed before the start of gonadotoxic treatment.

The main advantages over embryo and oocyte cryopreservation are the possibility to preserve not only fertility but also ovarian function and the fact that a COS before the procedure is not needed. Thus, this procedure can be discussed when neoadjuvant chemotherapy is planned and a prompt

initiation of treatment is mandatory. However, ovarian tissue cryopreservation requires two surgical procedures and, although not demonstrated yet for breast cancer patients, there is a potential risk of reintroducing malignant cells when the tissue is transplanted [41]. Despite being considered still experimental, ovarian tissue cryopreservation can be proposed to selected breast cancer patients as those scheduled for treatments with a high gonadotoxic risk who cannot delay anticancer therapies or those with prior exposure to chemotherapy, or in women with contraindications to COS [42]. While the harvesting of the tissue can be performed locally, subsequent sample freezing and storage should preferably be performed in few referral centers with the appropriate expertise to optimize freezing methods and cancer cell detection techniques [42].

In terms of success of the procedure, a recovery of ovarian function is expected in almost all cases within 3–6 months, with possible sustained longevity of function of the transplanted tissue [43, 44]. Although it is basically impossible to be calculated due to the lack of exact data on the number of patients transplanted after the end of treatment, the pregnancy rate (i.e., ratio between the number of women who conceived and the number of transplanted women) with the use of this strategy seems to be approximately 25% [45] but appears to be increasing over the years [46]. More than 80 babies were born worldwide after ovarian tissue transplantation [47, 48]. Of note, the success of the technique is strongly dependent on the age and ovarian reserve of the patients at the time of the procedure; hence, it should not be proposed to women older than 35 years or with reduced baseline ovarian reserve [42].

15.3.3 Temporary Ovarian Suppression with GnRHa

Pharmacological protection of the ovaries during chemotherapy with the administration of GnRHa is an attractive option to preserve gonadal function and fertility due to both its wide availability and the fact that no controlled ovarian stimulation before the procedure nor a delay in the initiation of anticancer treatments is needed [49].

Over the past years, despite the availability of many randomized trials and meta-analyses on the topic, there has been an active debate on the effective role and clinical application of this strategy [50–53]. However, recent data reporting long-term results on ovarian function recovery and pregnancies after treatment have supported the efficacy of temporary ovarian suppression with GnRHa during chemotherapy in breast cancer patients [54].

Specifically, the three largest randomized trials on this topic (PROMISE-GIM6, POEMS-SWOG S0230, and Anglo Celtic Group OPTION trials) have shown similar and consistent results on the efficacy of this strategy in reducing the risk of developing treatment-induced POI [55–57]. A meta-analysis of 12 randomized trials including 1231 breast cancer patients confirmed that concurrent administration of GnRHa and chemotherapy was associated with both a reduction of treatment-induced POI risk (odds ratio [OR], 0.36; 95% CI, 0.23–0.57; $p < 0.001$) and an increased chance of having a pregnancy after the end of treatment (OR, 1.83; 95% CI, 1.02–3.28; $p = 0.041$) [58]. Following the publication of these results, some guidelines have incorporated the use of temporary ovarian suppression with GnRHa during chemotherapy as a standard strategy to preserve ovarian function and potential fertility in breast cancer patients [1, 59, 60].

Of note, this strategy should not be considered an alternative to cryopreservation options in patients interested in fertility preservation [1, 59, 60]. Temporary ovarian suppression with GnRHa during chemotherapy can be used following cryopreservation procedures or in patients with no access to these strategies as well as in patients interested in ovarian function preservation only, as the delay of premature menopause has a great impact on patients' well-being, particularly for those that do not require prolonged ovarian suppression [59].

15.4 Pregnancy After Breast Cancer

Approximately half of young women with newly diagnosed breast cancer desire to have a subsequent pregnancy after treatment [61]. However, as reported in the literature, the percentage of breast cancer survivors achieving at least one full-term pregnancy after treatment remains very low ranging between 5% and 15% [55, 62]. Female cancer survivors have lower pregnancy rates than age-matched individuals from the general population (HR, 0.61; 95% CI, 0.58–0.64) [16]. Of note, among cancer survivors, young women with breast cancer are those with the lowest pregnancy rate with a 67% reduction in the chance of achieving a pregnancy after treatment as compared to the general population (HR, 0.33; 95% CI, 0.27–0.39) [16]. This observation reflects both the iatrogenic damage to patients' ovarian reserve following the use of anticancer gonadotoxic treatments and the potential concerns of both patients and providers related to the possible negative impact of pregnancy on the evolution of breast cancer being a hormonally driven tumor.

Recent surveys have shown that a significant proportion of oncologists believe that pregnancy after breast cancer may negatively impair on patients' prognosis [14, 15], and 49% of them supported the statement that a rise in estrogen levels during pregnancy can potentially stimulate the growth of hidden tumor cells [14]. However, the available data so far on the topic suggest that pregnancy in breast cancer survivors does not have a negative impact on patients' survival, irrespectively of the hormone receptor status of the tumor. A recent updated metanalysis including 19 studies for a total of 1829 pregnant patients and 21,907 nonpregnant controls showed that pregnancy following breast cancer diagnosis has no negative prognostic impact [63]. On the contrary, patients with a pregnancy after breast cancer have a significantly reduced risk of death (HR, 0.63; 95% CI, 0.51–0.79) [63]. Although these results could be partially confounded by selection biases and lack of specific information in women with hormone receptor-positive disease, a large multicenter retrospective cohort study adjusting for these confounding factors confirmed the safety of pregnancy in breast cancer survivors, even in patients with endocrine-sensitive tumors [64]. In this study, including 333 pregnant patients and 874 matched nonpregnant controls, no difference in disease-free survival

(DFS) between the two groups was observed in the whole study population (HR, 0.84; 95% CI, 0.66–1.06; $p = 0.14$), but also in the subgroups of women with estrogen receptor-positive (HR, 0.91; 95% CI, 0.67–1.24; $p = 0.55$) and estrogen receptor-negative (HR, 0.75; 95% CI, 0.51–1.08; $p = 0.12$) tumors. The pregnant group showed better OS (HR, 0.72; 95% CI, 0.54–0.97; $p = 0.03$), with no interaction according to estrogen receptor status ($p = 0.11$) [64]. Updated long-term results from this study, at more than 10 years of follow-up, confirmed the safety of pregnancy in breast cancer survivors irrespective of hormone receptor status [65].

According to these findings, current recommendations support the statement that, after adequate treatment and follow-up, pregnancy in cancer survivors including patients with endocrine-sensitive breast cancer should not be discouraged [2, 42].

Finally, another issue in this field that remains not clearly elucidated is the ideal interval between the end of anticancer treatments and the time for trying to have a pregnancy. According to experts' recommendation, the timing should be "personalized" taking into account patients' age and ovarian reserve, individual risk of relapse, previous treatments, and time of their completion [5]. Moreover, in patients with hormone receptor-positive disease, the need for adjuvant endocrine therapy up to 5–10 years can further hinder the chances of future pregnancies [55]. An international prospective study conducted by the International Breast Cancer Study Group (IBCSG) in collaboration with the Breast International Group (BIG) and the North American Breast Cancer Groups (NABCG) is currently ongoing to assess the safety of a temporary interruption of endocrine therapy to allow pregnancy in these patients (POSITIVE–IBCSG 48-14 NCT02308085 study) [66].

Of note, egg donation, surrogacy, and adoption represent other potential options for breast cancer patients whenever available and allowed by national laws and regulations [67].

15.5 Conclusions

Fertility preservation and concerns related to the possibility of having a subsequent pregnancy in young women with breast cancer have received a growing attention over the past years and should be discussed with all patients diagnosed during their reproductive age.

Patients concerned about the risk of treatment-induced infertility should be referred as soon as possible to fertility clinics to have access to embryo and oocyte cryopreservation (or to ovarian tissue cryopreservation in selected cases) followed by the administration of GnRHa during chemotherapy (Fig.15.1). In patients concerned about the risk of treatment-induced POI but not interested in fertility preservation procedures, temporary ovarian suppression with GnRHa during chemotherapy should be offered (Fig.15.1).

Young breast cancer survivors wishing to have a pregnancy after having received the adequate anticancer treatment should be counseled that this can be considered safe and should not be discouraged anymore. For patients with hormone receptor-positive breast cancer who are candidates to 5–10 years of adjuvant endocrine therapy, the results of the POSITIVE study are awaited to counsel them about the safety of a temporary interruption of endocrine therapy to allow pregnancy.

Despite a growing amount of data have become available on both the safety and efficacy of fertility preservation strategies as well as the feasibility of having a pregnancy after treatment, further studies are needed to improve the oncofertility counseling of young breast cancer patients on these issues. Several prospective efforts are currently ongoing in this setting including the HOHO study in the United States and Europe [3], the Italian PREFER study [68, 69], the PYNK program in Canada [70], and the Mexican Joven y Fuerte program [71], among others. Furthermore, reproduction studies to address the specific issues faced by women with hereditary breast tumors should be considered a research priority consider-

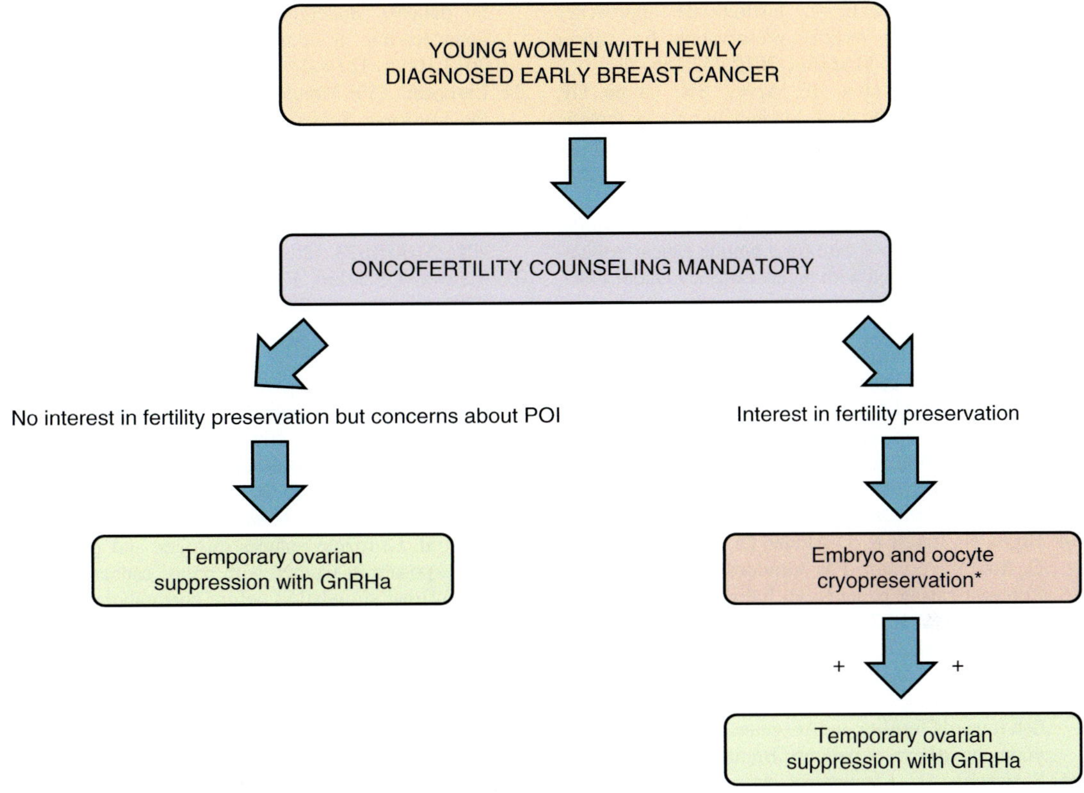

Fig. 15.1 Oncofertility counseling in newly diagnosed breast cancer patients. Abbreviations: *POI* premature ovarian insufficiency, *GnRHa* gonadotropin-releasing hormone analogs

ing that the majority of breast cancer patients are nowadays candidates to receive a genetic test at the time of diagnosis [72, 73].

References

1. Paluch-Shimon S, Pagani O, Partridge AH, Abulkhair O, Cardoso M-J, Dent RA, et al. ESO-ESMO 3rd international consensus guidelines for breast cancer in young women (BCY3). Breast. 2017;35:203–17.
2. Lambertini M, Goldrat O, Clatot F, Demeestere I, Awada A. Controversies about fertility and pregnancy issues in young breast cancer patients: current state of the art. Curr Opin Oncol. 2017;29(4):243–52.
3. Ruddy KJ, Gelber SI, Tamimi RM, Ginsburg ES, Schapira L, Come SE, et al. Prospective study of fertility concerns and preservation strategies in young women with breast cancer. J Clin Oncol. 2014;32(11):1151–6.
4. Loren AW, Mangu PB, Beck LN, Brennan L, Magdalinski AJ, Partridge AH, et al. Fertility preservation for patients with cancer: American Society of Clinical Oncology clinical practice guideline update. J Clin Oncol. 2013;31(19):2500–10.
5. Peccatori FA, Azim HA Jr, Orecchia R, Hoekstra HJ, Pavlidis N, Kesic V, et al. Cancer, pregnancy and fertility: ESMO clinical practice guidelines for diagnosis, treatment and follow-up. Ann Oncol. 2013;24(Suppl 6):vi160–70.
6. Lambertini M, Anserini P, Levaggi A, Poggio F, Del Mastro L. Fertility counseling of young breast cancer patients. J Thorac Dis. 2013;5(Suppl 1):S68–80.
7. Woodruff TK, Smith K, Gradishar W. Oncologists' role in patient fertility care: a call to action. JAMA Oncol. 2016;2(2):171–2.
8. Quinn GP, Vadaparampil ST, Gwede CK, Reinecke JD, Mason TM, Silva C. Developing a referral system for fertility preservation among patients with newly diagnosed cancer. J Natl Compr Cancer Netw. 2011;9(11):1219–25.

9. Kelvin JF, Reinecke J. Institutional approaches to implementing fertility preservation for cancer patients. Adv Exp Med Biol. 2012;732:165–73.

10. Reinecke JD, Kelvin JF, Arvey SR, Quinn GP, Levine J, Beck LN, et al. Implementing a systematic approach to meeting patients' cancer and fertility needs: a review of the fertile Hope centers of excellence program. J Oncol Pract. 2012;8(5):303–8.

11. Partridge AH, Ruddy KJ, Kennedy J, Winer EP. Model program to improve care for a unique cancer population: young women with breast cancer. J Oncol Pract. 2012;8(5):e105–10.

12. Clayman ML, Harper MM, Quinn GP, Reinecke J, Shah S. Oncofertility resources at NCI-designated comprehensive cancer centers. J Natl Compr Cancer Netw. 2013;11(12):1504–9.

13. Kelvin JF, Thom B, Benedict C, Carter J, Corcoran S, Dickler MN, et al. Cancer and fertility program improves patient satisfaction with information received. J Clin Oncol. 2016;34(15):1780–6.

14. Biglia N, Torrisi R, D'Alonzo M, Codacci Pisanelli G, Rota S, Peccatori FA. Attitudes on fertility issues in breast cancer patients: an Italian survey. Gynecol Endocrinol. 2015;31(6):458–64.

15. Lambertini M, Di Maio M, Pagani O, Curigliano G, Poggio F, Del Mastro L, et al. The BCY3/BCC 2017 survey on physicians' knowledge, attitudes and practice towards fertility and pregnancy-related issues in young breast cancer patients. Breast. 2018;42:41–9.

16. Stensheim H, Cvancarova M, Møller B, Fosså SD. Pregnancy after adolescent and adult cancer: a population-based matched cohort study. Int J Cancer. 2011;129(5):1225–36.

17. Lee SJ, Schover LR, Partridge AH, Patrizio P, Wallace WH, Hagerty K, et al. American Society of Clinical Oncology recommendations on fertility preservation in cancer patients. J Clin Oncol. 2006;24(18):2917–31.

18. Reh A, Oktem O, Oktay K. Impact of breast cancer chemotherapy on ovarian reserve: a prospective observational analysis by menstrual history and ovarian reserve markers. Fertil Steril. 2008;90(5):1635–9.

19. Lambertini M, Ceppi M, Cognetti F, Cavazzini G, De Laurentiis M, De Placido S, et al. Dose-dense adjuvant chemotherapy in premenopausal breast cancer patients: a pooled analysis of the MIG1 and GIM2 phase III studies. Eur J Cancer. 2017;71:34–42.

20. Ganz PA, Land SR, Geyer CE Jr, Cecchini RS, Costantino JP, Pajon ER, et al. Menstrual history and quality-of-life outcomes in women with node-positive breast cancer treated with adjuvant therapy on the NSABP B-30 trial. J Clin Oncol. 2011;29(9):1110–6.

21. Bedoschi G, Navarro PA, Oktay K. Chemotherapy-induced damage to ovary: mechanisms and clinical impact. Future Oncol. 2016;12(20):2333–44.

22. Codacci-Pisanelli G, Del Pup L, Del Grande M, Peccatori FA. Mechanisms of chemotherapy-induced ovarian damage in breast cancer patients. Crit Rev Oncol Hematol. 2017;113:90–6.

23. Practice Committee of the American Society for Reproductive Medicine. Fertility preservation in patients undergoing gonadotoxic therapy or gonadectomy: a committee opinion. Fertil Steril. 2013;100(5):1214–23.

24. European IVF-Monitoring Consortium (EIM) for the European Society of Human Reproduction and Embryology (ESHRE), Calhaz-Jorge C, de Geyter C, Kupka MS, de Mouzon J, Erb K, et al. Assisted reproductive technology in Europe, 2012: results generated from European registers by ESHRE. Hum Reprod. 2016;31(8):1638–52.

25. Meirow D, Schiff E. Appraisal of chemotherapy effects on reproductive outcome according to animal studies and clinical data. J Natl Cancer Inst Monogr. 2005;2005(34):21–5.

26. Lambertini M, Pescio MC, Viglietti G, Goldrat O, Del Mastro L, Anserini P, Demeestere I. Methods of controlled ovarian stimulation for embryo/oocyte cryopreservation in breast cancer patients. Expert Rev Qual Life Cancer Care. 2017;2(1):47–59.

27. Oktay K, Hourvitz A, Sahin G, Oktem O, Safro B, Cil A, et al. Letrozole reduces estrogen and gonadotropin exposure in women with breast cancer undergoing ovarian stimulation before chemotherapy. J Clin Endocrinol Metab. 2006;91(10):3885–90.

28. Azim AA, Costantini-Ferrando M, Oktay K. Safety of fertility preservation by ovarian stimulation with letrozole and gonadotropins in patients with breast cancer: a prospective controlled study. J Clin Oncol. 2008;26(16):2630–5.

29. Oktay K, Buyuk E, Davis O, Yermakova I, Veeck L, Rosenwaks Z. Fertility preservation in breast cancer patients: IVF and embryo cryopreservation after ovarian stimulation with tamoxifen. Hum Reprod. 2003;18(1):90–5.

30. Meirow D, Raanani H, Maman E, Paluch-Shimon S, Shapira M, Cohen Y, et al. Tamoxifen co-administration during controlled ovarian hyperstimulation for in vitro fertilization in breast cancer patients increases the safety of fertility-preservation treatment strategies. Fertil Steril. 2014;102(2):488–495.e3.

31. Oktay K, Turan V, Bedoschi G, Pacheco FS, Moy F. Fertility preservation success subsequent to concurrent aromatase inhibitor treatment and ovarian stimulation in women with breast Cancer. J Clin Oncol. 2015;33(22):2424–9.

32. Revelli A, Porcu E, Levi Setti PE, Delle Piane L, Merlo DF, Anserini P. Is letrozole needed for controlled ovarian stimulation in patients with estrogen receptor-positive breast cancer? Gynecol Endocrinol. 2013;29(11):993–6.

33. Pereira N, Hancock K, Cordeiro CN, Lekovich JP, Schattman GL, Rosenwaks Z. Comparison of ovarian stimulation response in patients with breast cancer undergoing ovarian stimulation with letrozole and gonadotropins to patients undergoing ovarian stimulation with gonadotropins alone for elective cryopreservation of oocytes†. Gynecol Endocrinol. 2016;32(10):823–6.

34. Kim J, Turan V, Oktay K. Long-term safety of Letrozole and gonadotropin stimulation for fertil-

ity preservation in women with breast Cancer. J Clin Endocrinol Metab. 2016;101(4):1364–71.

35. Balkenende EME, Dahhan T, Linn SC, Jager NGL, Beijnen JH, Goddijn M. A prospective case series of women with estrogen receptor-positive breast cancer: levels of tamoxifen metabolites in controlled ovarian stimulation with high-dose tamoxifen. Hum Reprod. 2013;28(4):953–9.

36. Cakmak H, Katz A, Cedars MI, Rosen MP. Effective method for emergency fertility preservation: random-start controlled ovarian stimulation. Fertil Steril. 2013;100(6):1673–80.

37. Kuang Y, Chen Q, Hong Q, Lyu Q, Ai A, Fu Y, et al. Double stimulations during the follicular and luteal phases of poor responders in IVF/ICSI programmes (Shanghai protocol). Reprod Biomed Online. 2014;29(6):684–91.

38. Shalom-Paz E, Almog B, Shehata F, Huang J, Holzer H, Chian R-C, et al. Fertility preservation for breast-cancer patients using IVM followed by oocyte or embryo vitrification. Reprod Biomed Online. 2010;21(4):566–71.

39. Chian R-C, Uzelac PS, Nargund G. In vitro maturation of human immature oocytes for fertility preservation. Fertil Steril. 2013;99(5):1173–81.

40. Walls ML, Hunter T, Ryan JP, Keelan JA, Nathan E, Hart RJ. In vitro maturation as an alternative to standard in vitro fertilization for patients diagnosed with polycystic ovaries: a comparative analysis of fresh, frozen and cumulative cycle outcomes. Hum Reprod. 2015;30(1):88–96.

41. Rosendahl M, Greve T, Andersen CY. The safety of transplanting cryopreserved ovarian tissue in cancer patients: a review of the literature. J Assist Reprod Genet. 2013;30(1):11–24.

42. Lambertini M, Del Mastro L, Pescio MC, Andersen CY, Azim HA, Peccatori FA, et al. Cancer and fertility preservation: international recommendations from an expert meeting. BMC Med. 2016;14(1):1.

43. Kim SS, Lee WS, Chung MK, Lee HC, Lee HH, Hill D. Long-term ovarian function and fertility after heterotopic autotransplantation of cryobanked human ovarian tissue: 8-year experience in cancer patients. Fertil Steril. 2009;91(6):2349–54.

44. Andersen CY, Silber SJ, Bergholdt SH, Berghold SH, Jorgensen JS, Ernst E. Long-term duration of function of ovarian tissue transplants: case reports. Reprod Biomed Online. 2012;25(2):128–32.

45. Donnez J, Dolmans M-M, Pellicer A, Diaz-Garcia C, Ernst E, Macklon KT, et al. Fertility preservation for age-related fertility decline. Lancet. 2015;385(9967):506–7.

46. Andersen CY. Success and challenges in fertility preservation after ovarian tissue grafting. Lancet. 2015;385(9981):1947–8.

47. Van der Ven H, Liebenthron J, Beckmann M, Toth B, Korell M, Krüssel J, et al. Ninety-five orthotopic transplantations in 74 women of ovarian tissue after cytotoxic treatment in a fertility preservation network: tissue activity, pregnancy and delivery rates. Hum Reprod. 2016;31(9):2031–41.

48. Jensen AK, Macklon KT, Fedder J, Ernst E, Humaidan P, Andersen CY. 86 successful births and 9 ongoing pregnancies worldwide in women transplanted with frozen-thawed ovarian tissue: focus on birth and perinatal outcome in 40 of these children. J Assist Reprod Genet. 2017;34(3):325–36.

49. Lambertini M, Ginsburg ES, Partridge AH. Update on fertility preservation in young women undergoing breast cancer and ovarian cancer therapy. Curr Opin Obstet Gynecol. 2015;27(1):98–107.

50. Turner NH, Partridge A, Sanna G, Di Leo A, Biganzoli L. Utility of gonadotropin-releasing hormone agonists for fertility preservation in young breast cancer patients: the benefit remains uncertain. Ann Oncol. 2013;24(9):2224–35.

51. Del Mastro L, Lambertini M. Temporary ovarian suppression with gonadotropin-releasing hormone agonist during chemotherapy for fertility preservation: toward the end of the debate? Oncologist. 2015;20(11):1233–5.

52. Lambertini M, Peccatori FA, Moore HCF, Del Mastro L. Reply to the letter to the editor "can ovarian suppression with gonadotropin releasing hormone analogs (GnRHa) preserve fertility in cancer patients?" by Rodriguez-Wallberg et al. Ann Oncol. 2016;27(3):548–9.

53. Lambertini M, Falcone T, Unger JM, Phillips K-A, Del Mastro L, Moore HCF. Debated role of ovarian protection with gonadotropin-releasing hormone agonists during chemotherapy for preservation of ovarian function and fertility in women with Cancer. J Clin Oncol. 2017;35(7):804–5.

54. Lambertini M, Poggio F, Vaglica M, Blondeaux E, Del Mastro L. News on the medical treatment of young women with early-stage HER2-negative breast cancer. Expert Opin Pharmacother. 2016;17(12):1643–55.

55. Lambertini M, Boni L, Michelotti A, Gamucci T, Scotto T, Gori S, et al. Ovarian suppression with Triptorelin during adjuvant breast Cancer chemotherapy and long-term ovarian function, pregnancies, and disease-free survival: a randomized clinical trial. JAMA. 2015;314(24):2632–40.

56. Leonard RCF, Adamson DJA, Bertelli G, Mansi J, Yellowlees A, Dunlop J, et al. GnRH agonist for protection against ovarian toxicity during chemotherapy for early breast cancer: the Anglo Celtic group OPTION trial. Ann Oncol. 2017;28(8):1811–6.

57. Moore HCF, Unger JM, Phillips K-A, Boyle F, Hitre E, Moseley A, et al. Final analysis of the prevention of early menopause study (POEMS)/SWOG intergroup S0230. J Natl Cancer Inst. 2019;111(2):210–3. Epub ahead of print

58. Lambertini M, Ceppi M, Poggio F, Peccatori FA, Azim HA, Ugolini D, et al. Ovarian suppression using luteinizing hormone-releasing hormone agonists during chemotherapy to preserve ovarian function and fertility of breast cancer patients: a meta-analysis of randomized studies. Ann Oncol. 2015;26(12):2408–19.

59. Lambertini M, Cinquini M, Moschetti I, Peccatori FA, Anserini P, Valenzano Menada M, et al. Temporary

ovarian suppression during chemotherapy to preserve ovarian function and fertility in breast cancer patients: a GRADE approach for evidence evaluation and recommendations by the Italian Association of Medical Oncology. Eur J Cancer. 2017;71:25–33.

60. Oktay K, Harvey BE, Partridge AH, Quinn GP, Reinecke J, Taylor HS, et al. Fertility preservation in patients with Cancer: ASCO clinical practice guideline update. J Clin Oncol Off J Am Soc Clin Oncol. 2018;36(19):1994–2001.

61. Letourneau JM, Smith JF, Ebbel EE, Craig A, Katz PP, Cedars MI, et al. Racial, socioeconomic, and demographic disparities in access to fertility preservation in young women diagnosed with cancer. Cancer. 2012;118(18):4579–88.

62. Moore HCF, Unger JM, Phillips K-A, Boyle F, Hitre E, Porter D, et al. Goserelin for ovarian protection during breast-cancer adjuvant chemotherapy. N Engl J Med. 2015;372(10):923–32.

63. Hartman EK, Eslick GD. The prognosis of women diagnosed with breast cancer before, during and after pregnancy: a meta-analysis. Breast Cancer Res Treat. 2016;160(2):347–60.

64. Azim HA Jr, Kroman N, Paesmans M, Gelber S, Rotmensz N, Ameye L, et al. Prognostic impact of pregnancy after breast cancer according to estrogen receptor status: a multicenter retrospective study. J Clin Oncol. 2013;31(1):73–9.

65. Lambertini M, Kroman N, Ameye L, Cordoba O, Pinto A, Benedetti G, et al. Long-term safety of pregnancy following breast cancer according to estrogen receptor status. J Natl Cancer Inst. 2018;110(4):426–9.

66. Pagani O, Ruggeri M, Manunta S, Saunders C, Peccatori F, Cardoso F, et al. Pregnancy after breast cancer: are young patients willing to participate in clinical studies? Breast. 2015;24(3):201–7.

67. Luke B, Brown MB, Missmer SA, Spector LG, Leach RE, Williams M, et al. Assisted reproductive technology use and outcomes among women with a history of cancer. Hum Reprod. 2016;31(1):183–9.

68. Lambertini M, Anserini P, Fontana V, Poggio F, Iacono G, Abate A, et al. The PREgnancy and FERtility (PREFER) study: an Italian multicenter prospective cohort study on fertility preservation and pregnancy issues in young breast cancer patients. BMC Cancer. 2017;17(1):346.

69. Lambertini M, Fontana V, Massarotti C, Poggio F, Dellepiane C, Iacono G, et al. Prospective study to optimize care and improve knowledge on ovarian function and/or fertility preservation in young breast cancer patients: results of the pilot phase of the PREgnancy and FERtility (PREFER) study. Breast. 2018;41:51–6.

70. Cohen L, Hamer J, Helwig C, Fergus K, Kiss A, Mandel R, et al. Formal evaluation of PYNK: breast cancer program for young women-the patient perspective. Curr Oncol. 2016;23(2):e102–8.

71. Villarreal-Garza C, Platas A, Martinez-Cannon BA, Bargalló-Rocha E, Aguilar-González CN, Ortega-Leonard V, et al. Information needs and internet use of breast cancer survivors in Mexico. Breast J. 2017;23(3):373–5.

72. Lambertini M, Goldrat O, Toss A, Azim HA, Peccatori FA, Ignatiadis M, et al. Fertility and pregnancy issues in BRCA-mutated breast cancer patients. Cancer Treat Rev. 2017;59:61–70.

73. Peccatori FA, Mangili G, Bergamini A, Filippi F, Martinelli F, Ferrari F, et al. Fertility preservation in women harboring deleterious BRCA mutations: ready for prime time? Hum Reprod. 2018;33(2):181–7.

Lifestyle Changes and Prevention: Unique Issues for Young Women

Nathalie Levasseur, Rinat Yerushalmi, and Karen A. Gelmon

16.1 Introduction

While prevention has classically been studied according to etiological elements, it has become clear that a number of unique issues present challenges to preventing breast cancer in young women, which extend beyond the traditional concepts. A growing body of research for prevention and therapeutic interventions has been mainly focused on older women and often does not emphasize the increased risk of younger individuals given the lack of applicable risk stratification models. Primary prevention poses a number of challenges, including reaching a younger target population, as prevention strategies are often not geared toward young women. Accessibility to primary care is also variable globally and has become a relevant issue. Furthermore, there are a number of competing general health initiatives for a younger age group which may often take precedence during preventative care appointments. Likewise, secondary prevention in young women encompasses other critical considerations that are different than those applied to an unselected breast cancer population who are generally older and mostly postmenopausal. These points raise an important question: should distinct biological, pharmacological, surgical, and lifestyle prevention strategies be applied to young women?

One of the most noteworthy aspects of breast cancer in young women is undoubtedly the importance of biological and genetic factors. This has been the focus of many conventional prevention strategies, such as genetic testing and screening guidelines including early adoption of screening imaging for those identified to be at higher risk. However, with the evolution of cancer genetics research, pharmacological and surgical strategies for prevention are constantly being refined to integrate novel findings and translate these to clinical practice. Unfortunately, few studies enroll women under 40, limiting the applicability of the results to a younger age group. Specific biological factors such as breast density, parity, and breast feeding, to name a few, are also more relevant for this age group and are associated with specific considerations. Lastly, a number of environmental and lifestyle factors such as smoking, alcohol, radiation, diet, exercise, and shift work have been associated with an increased relative risk of cancer, especially during developmental years, and should be taken into consideration when discussing effective prevention strategies. Noteworthy developments

N. Levasseur · K. A. Gelmon (✉)
BC Cancer Agency, Vancouver Cancer Centre,
Vancouver, BC, Canada
e-mail: Nathalie.Levasseur@bccancer.bc.ca;
kgelmon@bccancer.bc.ca

R. Yerushalmi
Davidoff Cancer Center, Rabin Medical Center,
Petah Tikva, Israel
e-mail: rinaty@clait.org.il

© Springer Nature Switzerland AG 2020
O. Gentilini et al. (eds.), *Breast Cancer in Young Women*,
https://doi.org/10.1007/978-3-030-24762-1_16

have been made in the identification of lifestyle factors and environmental factors which correlate with a higher risk of developing breast cancer. Ultimately, the early adoption of prevention strategies for breast cancer is crucial, but recognizing and understanding the specific challenges in young women is the first step toward achieving effective change. Furthermore, finding ways to inspire societal change and achieve sustainable change within individuals remains an area of unmet need. This chapter consequently focuses on the unique issues for prevention and lifestyle changes for young women.

16.2 Risk Prediction Models

Over the last few decades, a number of models have been developed to statistically estimate the probability of developing breast cancer based on various risk factors, over a predefined period of time. The results, in turn, should allow for modifications in breast cancer screening and counseling on risk-reducing options such as pharmacoprevention, surgical prevention, or lifestyle change for individuals identified to be at higher risk than the general population. However, it is well recognized that these models are associated with a wide range of calibration performance and discriminatory accuracy [1, 2]. The Gail model, one of the most well-validated risk assessment tools, helps to determine the 5-year and lifetime risk of breast cancer in women without a history of invasive or in situ breast cancers using data from the Breast Detection Demonstration Project (BCDDP) [3–5]. This model includes age at menarche, age of first live birth, number of prior benign breast biopsies, and number of first-degree relatives with breast cancer. It was then recalibrated to data from the National Cancer Institute (NCI) Surveillance, Epidemiology, and End Results (SEER) database. However, models such as the Gail model have not been validated in patients with known mutations such as BRCA1, BRCA2, and other hereditary syndromes associated with breast cancer or in patients with a family history beyond first-degree relatives. Furthermore, the risk for patients with atypical

ductal hyperplasia and family history may be underestimated by this model. Most importantly, this model, like many others, was not designed to estimate risk in women aged less than 35 as the data used from the BCDDP and SEER data recruited women between 35 and 74 years of age with a median age of 50 years old.

Building on the Gail model, alternative models such as the Chen model integrated breast density into their algorithm, in addition to age of first live birth, number of affected first-degree relatives (mothers or sisters), number of previous benign breast biopsies, and weight. This was based on a significant association with breast cancer risk from an independently conducted multivariable model [6]. Results suggested a higher attributable risk of breast cancer associated with these features in women under 50, but also predicted higher risks than the Gail model for women with a higher percentage of dense breast area, although this poses issues for the screening of young women given the limited sensitivity and specificity of diagnostic imaging. This model was also developed based on 1744 Caucasian women, limiting its applicability to individuals of other ethnic backgrounds. Addressing some of these issues, the Barlow model was designed using prospective data from one million women undergoing screening mammography, with separate logistic regression risk models for premenopausal and postmenopausal women [7]. In premenopausal women, age, breast density, family history of breast cancer, and a prior breast procedure were found to have a strong association with breast cancer risk, although none of these factors are targets for new preventative strategies, and it remains unclear if a reduction in breast density translates into a decreased risk of breast cancer.

Moreover, genetics are clearly more relevant in young women, which has led to the development of models such as BOADICEA (Breast and Ovarian Analysis of Disease Incidence and Carrier Estimation Algorithm), to estimate the likelihood of detecting a mutation in a cancer susceptibility gene for an individual [8–10]. The most recent version of the model was based on 2785 families and was the first polygenic breast cancer risk model. However, this model, similar to others like it, including the BRCAPRO, IBIS, and extended Claus models (eCLAUS), is also associated with a wide range of diagnostic accuracy [11–14].

Ultimately, the use of predictive models in women younger than 40 has not been well established, and the accuracy of models to predict the likelihood of a young patient harboring a deleterious mutation is limited. Decisions regarding screening and preventative measures therefore remain quite complex and should take all patient characteristics into account to make personalized recommendations.

16.3 Biological Prevention Strategies

16.3.1 Prevention Guided by Genetics

Biological factors such as germline and somatic mutations are of great interest for the development of effective prevention strategies against breast cancer in young women. While testing has traditionally only included BRCA gene testing for high risk individuals, based on their individual or familial history, contemporary testing now comprises multigene panel testing, including genes functionally related to BRCA 1 and/or BRCA 2 such as CHEK2 and PALB2, as well as testing for other known hereditary cancer syndromes such as p53 (Li-Fraumeni syndrome), PTEN (Cowden syndrome), STK11 (Peutz-Jeghers syndrome), and CDH1 [15, 16]. However, as research into cancer genetics evolves, it is increasingly recognized that many cancers associated with genetic mutations do not always correlate with an individual's family history [17–19]. Notably, recent studies have identified BRCA1 or BRCA2 mutations in up to 14% of patients unselected for family history with triple-negative breast cancers, with a higher incidence in very young women [20]. Furthermore, up to 10% of high-risk patients without BRCA1 or BRCA2 mutations have been found to harbor mutations in a number of other genes conferring a predisposi-

tion to breast cancer, with the use of new hereditary cancer multigene panel testing [21].

However, current expert opinion from North American guidelines continues to reserve genetic counseling for individuals with a family history of BRCA mutation, a relative with two or more primary breast cancers, two or more relatives with breast cancer on the same side of the family with at least one diagnosed before the age of 50, a relative with ovarian cancer, a close family member with breast cancer before the age of 45, a family history of male breast cancer, or individuals with Ashkenazi Jewish ancestry [22]. Similarly, guidelines in Europe are also somewhat restrictive and suggest testing individuals with three or more relatives with breast and ovarian including at least one below the age of 50, two relatives with breast cancer below the age of 40, a male relative with breast cancer, or individuals of Ashkenazi Jewish heritage with breast cancer before the age 60 [16, 23]. Certain countries use testing criteria based on a 10–20% probability of finding a mutation based on predictive models such as the ones discussed previously, including the BOADICEA and BRCAPRO models [16].

In the context of the difficulties associated with the identification of truly high-risk individuals, it becomes increasingly difficult to recommend pharmacological and surgical methods of prevention which apply to a distinct but heterogeneous cohort of young women. There have also been concerns regarding the limitations of multigene panel testing, which include multiple genes with variable levels of penetrance, an unknown level of risk, and many variants of unknown significance, complicating the interpretation of test results in clinical practice [21, 22]. Finally, there is currently no standard panel for multigene testing globally, given the lack of supportive evidence that preventative measures can be effective if the mutation is identified earlier. As well, increased testing of the tumor genomics may lead to new recommendations for germline testing based on tumor findings.

With regard to breast examination and screening imaging in patients fulfilling high-risk criteria, namely BRCA gene mutation carriers, current recommendations suggest annual screening with breast magnetic resonance imaging (MRI) starting at age 25, screening mammograms beginning at age 30, biannual clinical breast examinations by an experienced clinician starting at age 25 or 10 years before the youngest breast cancer diagnosis in the family, and optional monthly self-breast examinations which can be beneficial in combination with other screening methods [24–27].

16.3.2 Ethnic Variations in Breast Cancer Biology

Other well-recognized biological factors correlated with the incidence of breast cancer are related to ethnic background. While it has been speculated that breast cancer outcomes are directly related to disparities in social and economic factors limiting access to cancer care among various ethnic groups, there is also data suggesting a difference in the biology of breast cancer related to ethnic background [28]. With regard to the incidence, it remains clear that this is highest in women of Caucasian background or European descent with rates of 128 per 100,000 women per year as compared to 123 per 100,000 for African-American women [29, 30]. However, breast cancers in women of African background are more frequently associated with unfavorable characteristics, such as a higher-grade and negative hormone receptor status at the time of presentation, regardless of age, which may contribute to the increased mortality seen in this particular group [31–34]. African-American women are also more likely to be diagnosed prior to the age of 50 as compared to their Caucasian counterparts, and this difference is most pronounced in women younger than 35 with a 1.4 to 2 times higher likelihood compared to Caucasian women [35].

Furthermore, data from the SEER database reports that although incidence rates are highest in Caucasian women, mortality rates are highest in African-American women at 30.6 per 100,000 versus 21.7 per 100,000 [36–38]. Recent corroborative studies from the United Kingdom and Australia also report more advanced stages at presentation and a lower likelihood of having a screen-detected cancer in this same ethnic group [39]. Similarly, a population case-control study revealed a higher prevalence of basal-like breast cancer subtype and lower luminal A subtype in premenopausal African women as compared to postmenopausal African women and non-African women [40, 41]. Some have postulated that this may be related to increased parity and lower rates of breastfeeding in women of African background, although these results remain hypothesis generating [42]. Regardless, breastfeeding may prove to be an important prevention strategy for African-American women. While the exact mechanisms by which outcomes are worse, it is important to realize that differences in biology exist and the development of prevention strategies should therefore be designed to identify higher-risk individuals, who typically present with high-grade, basal-type tumors with higher stages of disease, which behave more aggressively.

16.3.3 Breast Density and Malignant Potential

In addition to the well-recognized risk of breast cancer associated with deleterious germline mutations and ethnic background, there are a number of other important biological features thought to be associated with the risk of breast cancer. One of the factors with the strongest association with breast cancer is breast density, which has been found to be a strong predictor of breast cancer incidence, proportional to the increase in breast density [43]. While the exact mechanisms remain speculative, the risk may be attributed to reduced visibility of small tumors on screening mammograms, although an independent relationship to the malignant potential of dense breast tissue has also been postulated [43]. Furthermore, higher local recurrence rates have been associated with a higher breast density [44–46]. However, despite conferring a higher risk of recurrence, data on breast density as a predictor for overall survival remains conflicting, with some studies suggesting the detection of larger screen-detected tumors, but no effect on overall survival in both a British and American cohort [47, 48], whereas a larger study of a Swedish cohort comprising over 15,000 women aged 45 to 59 showed a significant association with breast cancer mortality [RR = 1.91 (1.26–2.91)] [49]. These differences may be attributed to methodological differences, given that the British and American studies used the Breast Imaging Reporting and Data System (BI-RADS) density classification whereas the Swedish study used a different but translatable system, the Tabar classification system. These studies therefore support shorter screening intervals to detect breast cancer recurrence or new primaries, although none were designed for younger women, once again limiting their applicability to a younger patient cohort. Interestingly, in a case-control study of 1112 pairs, 25% of all breast cancers and 50% of cancers detected less than 12 months after a negative screening test in women younger than the median age of 56 were attributed to density exceeding 50% [50]. Younger age and higher breast density were also independently associated with higher rates of interval breast cancers in screening programs [51].

Moreover, the use of alternative imaging techniques in women with dense breast tissue may be considered, including new methods to improve the accuracy of existing diagnostic methods including mammography, with recent studies showing a prediction accuracy greater than 80% as compared to traditional methods, which achieved an accuracy between 55 and 65% [52]. Ultrasound may also be considered as an adjunct to mammography as an alternative in centers where MRIs are unavailable. However, the use of supplemental screening modalities should be tailored based on individual risk assessment [53].

Notwithstanding this information, it remains unclear if a temporal change in breast density is correlated with a reduced risk of breast cancer. While it is well known that a number of non-modifiable risk factors are associated with breast density, including genetics, age, and menopausal status, it is also recognized that other lifestyle factors such as the number of live births, use of hormonal therapy, diet, alcohol intake, weight, and exercise are also associated with breast density [54–61]. These are therefore interesting areas of research as they could influence breast density, and it could be hypothesized that changes in these parameters could lead to therapeutic gains.

16.3.4 Reproductive Factors and Breast Cancer Risk

Additional biological considerations linked to the development of breast cancer are directly related to hormonal and reproductive factors, including age at menarche, age at menopause, age at the time of first live birth, total number of pregnancies, and exposure to endogenous and exogenous hormones.

With regard to age of menarche and age of menopause, it is thought that the cumulative exposure to estrogen is associated with an increased risk of breast cancer. Although it was traditionally thought that the total exposure was most important, recent studies have suggested that early life exposure associated with early menarche carries the greatest risk, suggesting that timing may be more critical than cumulative exposure to estrogen [62, 63]. Notably, breast cancer risk has been reported to increase by 5% for each year younger at the time of menarche [64] and to decrease significantly if menarche occurred beyond age 13 [63].

Additionally, associations between parity and the risk of breast cancer have been an evolving topic over the last 20 years. Specifically, low or late parity is thought to be associated with a higher cumulative risk of breast cancer, consisting predominantly of hormone receptor-positive breast cancers [65]. However, it remains controversial as to whether parity directly influences the subtype of breast cancer, with some studies suggesting an association between breast cancer subtype and age of first live birth/number of full-term pregnancies [66], whereas other studies did not show this [67]. In a Swedish case-control study of over 12,000 women, it was found that increasing parity was associated with a risk reduction of 10% in breast cancer with each additional birth, with a proportional increase in risk dependant on age at first birth [68]. Indeed, it is thought that having a child before the age of 24 decreases the risk of breast cancer by about half by the time women reach the age of menopause [69], but that childbearing after age 35 may actually confer a higher risk [67]. Similarly, in a retrospective cohort study of women carrying a BRCA1 or BRCA2 gene mutation, a statistically significant decrease in the risk of breast cancer was observed among women who had full-term pregnancies and multiple births whereas delayed childbirth was associated with an increased risk of breast cancer [70]. Interestingly, although parity conferred some protection to BRCA gene mutation carriers, no link was observed with breastfeeding, contradicting other published works.

16.3.5 Breast Feeding and Its Preventative Role

While a number of historical studies have suggested a risk reduction in women who have breastfed, the protective effect of breastfeeding has been widely debated. Namely, older multicenter population-based case-control studies of over 14,000 women suggested that even after adjustment for parity, age at first delivery, and risk factors, breastfeeding was associated with a reduction in the risk of breast cancer among premenopausal women [71]. The prospective Nurses' Health Study also suggested that breastfeeding for 4 months or longer reduced the risk of basal-like breast cancer by 40% as compared to women who had never breastfed. This has also been corroborated by a recent meta-analysis [72]. Similar studies conducted in women harboring a BRCA gene mutation were equally found to have a reduced risk of breast cancer with breastfeeding [73]. Other interesting observations relating to breastfeeding include a possible higher risk of invasive triple-negative breast cancer in women who did not breastfeed, independent of other risk factors [42, 74, 75], and that longer periods of breastfeeding were associated with lower odds of developing triple-negative breast cancer [66, 67].

16.3.6 Exogenous Hormone Exposure and Prevention

It is also well recognized that exposure to hormone-replacement therapy and exogenous estrogens is associated with a higher risk of breast cancer. Importantly, it is also thought that mammary glands in younger individuals are more susceptible than that of older individuals, although the exact mechanisms remain speculative [62]. The role of the oral contraceptive pill has also been questioned, and its use has also been linked with a higher incidence of breast cancer [76, 77] and possibly a higher incidence of triple-negative breast cancers [78]. This is particularly true for young women aged less than 35 and appears to be correlated with both high and low concentrations of estradiol, although the risk was greatest with pills containing a higher level of progestins [79]. Other studies in women aged 35 or greater did not reveal this same risk [80]. Nevertheless, two large case-control studies did not reveal an effect on mortality [81], while other studies suggested that the risk returns to baseline after 4–10 years of discontinuation [77, 79].

In summary, there are a number of biological factors directly related to the risk of breast cancer in young women, and many younger women present with more aggressive tumor biology, namely with more triple-negative, triple-positive, and HER2-positive tumors [34]. Genetic factors remain important to identify high-risk patients and guide screening and preventative pharmacological and surgical methods. However, other factors such as breast density, parity, and breastfeeding are potentially actionable variables which could be further utilized in future risk-reducing strategies for younger women.

16.4 Pharmacological Prevention Strategies

Pharmacoprevention remains one of the most widely discussed strategies in women considered to be at higher risk for breast cancer, allowing for a reduction in estrogen receptor-positive invasive and in situ breast cancers with the use of selective estrogen receptor modulators (SERMs) such as tamoxifen or raloxifene [82–86]. However, meta-analysis data suggests no difference in breast cancer-specific survival or overall survival, although none of the trials were powered for these endpoints [87]. Another important consideration is that the use of SERMs was associated with a greater risk of thromboembolic disease and endometrial cancer, although these events were infrequent and generally did not affect quality of life significantly. Eligibility criteria varied among trials, but enrolled almost exclusively women aged 35 years of age or greater [84]. Given the paucity of data in women aged younger than 40, current guidelines recommend the use of pharmacoprevention exclusively in women aged greater than 35 [88] with a particular benefit for those aged 35–50 with a 5-year projected breast cancer risk $\geq 1.66\%$, according to the National Cancer Institute Breast Cancer Risk Assessment Tool based on the Gail model, or for women with LCIS. This limits the applicability of data to women younger than 35 who may still be considered at higher risk of developing breast cancer. Furthermore, no evidence exists for raloxifene in premenopausal women and therefore should not be considered in this patient population. In addition, observational studies conducted among women with a confirmed BRCA mutation suggested an equal but small reduction in hormone receptor-positive breast cancers.

It is now also recognized that aromatase inhibitors have a limited ability to reduce circulating estrogen in premenopausal women and may actually be detrimental, therefore limiting their role in the premenopausal population [89]. The additional benefit of ovarian suppression in this setting has also not been well established and is not considered a standard practice, as compared to the adjuvant setting for young women with a history of high-risk invasive disease, based on results of the SOFT and TEXT trials [90, 91].

16.5 Surgical Prevention Strategies

Taking the limitations of genetic screening into account, preventative surgical strategies, such as prophylactic bilateral mastectomies and bilateral salpingo-oophorectomy, remain a pillar of risk reduction strategies in women found to harbor a deleterious BRCA1 or BRCA2 mutation for the prevention of breast cancer. However, this data is mostly based on prospective cohort studies regarding the prophylactic role of surgery for risk reduction. Indeed, some studies suggest up to a 90% relative risk reduction in the development of subsequent breast cancer with the use of prophylactic bilateral mastectomies (PBM) [92–95]. More recently, a prospective multicenter cohort study of 2482 women with BRCA 1 and BRCA2 mutations detected between 1974 and 2008 and conducted in North America and Europe also revealed a significant risk reduction of breast cancer with mastectomy and a survival benefit with salpingo-oophorectomy. The potential long-term impacts on body image, sexuality, and other aspects of quality of life should be extensively discussed prior to embarking on this route. Alternative options for risk-reducing surgery have also been explored, including skin-sparing and nipple-sparing procedures [96]. Regardless of which method is selected, it is recommended that breast reconstruction options be discussed with the patient in advance, with access to immediate reconstruction, if desired [16, 97].

Furthermore, prophylactic bilateral salpingo-oophorectomy (BSO) has also been shown to be effective for risk reduction of breast cancer in premenopausal BRCA carriers, with a risk reduction of nearly 50% if completed prior to menopause [98]. It is also strongly recommended due to the lack of effective ovarian cancer screening modalities. Laparoscopic approaches should be favored and discussed, after age 35 or when childbearing is complete. Meta-analyses also suggest a reduction in all-cause mortality favoring the individuals who have undergone a BSO [99]. However, careful consideration of the impact of facing premature menopausal for young women should be addressed, including regular bone density measurements, assessment of cardiovascular risk factors, and the possible need of hormone replacement therapy [26]. Data suggesting that the fallopian tubes are the origin of ovarian cancers advocates that salpingectomy alone may be considered in very young women, with a plan for oophorectomy closer to the time of natural menopause, sparing the woman a precocious menopause [100].

Nevertheless, although the preventative role of these surgical interventions has been demonstrated for patients harboring a BRCA mutation, their preventative role in women with other predisposing mutations has yet to be established. Therefore, surgical prevention may be considered in carriers of a BRCA mutation although this same strategy should not be applied to women with a moderate to high risk without a mutation given the lack of robust evidence.

16.6 Environmental Factors and Prevention Strategies in Young Women

16.6.1 Socioeconomic Status, Ethnicity, and Cancer Care

While preventative strategies have long focused on the biological and clinical aspects, it has become increasingly recognized that there is significant interplay between environmental factors and breast cancer risk, especially in younger individuals. One of the most noteworthy aspects of this topic is undoubtedly the significant role of socioeconomic status and ethnic background on disparities in cancer care. Indeed, it has been shown that 5-year relative survival from breast cancer is linked to socioeconomic status, with a relative improvement in survival for women residing in more prosperous areas, indicating that the benefits of medical advances have not benefited diverse populations equally [29, 30]. Notably, cancer death rates for individuals with the least education were more than double that of the individuals with the most education, as detailed in a SEER report from 2011 [101]. The adherence to primary prevention and screening programs is also associated with a much lower uptake in individuals belonging to lower socioeconomic status [102], and this remains true on a global level [103].

Review of the incidence rates, mortality, and breast cancer-specific mortality reveals the highest incidence rates of breast cancer among Caucasian women and the lowest incidence rate among individuals of Asian or Pacific Island background. However, it is widely recognized that health disparities persist and that women belonging to minority groups generally fare worse compared to their Caucasian counterparts [104, 105]. Notably, individuals belonging to minority groups tend to present with more advanced stage of disease at diagnosis and are less often involved in clinical trials [74, 106]. Moreover, an inverse correlation with survival exists among women of African and Hispanic background, with much lower reported rates of 5-year breast cancer-specific survival [29, 30]. Although these differences may be partially attributed to differences in tumor biology, it has also been shown that young women of African-American and Hispanic background are also more likely to experience delays in diagnosis and treatment of breast cancer [107–109]. The health inequity among women belonging to minority groups seems to be particularly important in young women given the difficulty in spreading awareness of the importance of breast health and cancer screening [110]. While it may be encouraging that advances in access to oncological care through large cancer centers have translated into a reduction of this disproportionate difference, access remains problematic in smaller communities, especially among young women belonging to minority groups [109].

16.6.2 Risk of Radiation

Another important factor at the forefront of preventative strategies is radiation. It is now increasingly acknowledged that radiation confers a significantly higher risk of breast cancer, particularly in young individuals with developing breasts up until the age of 30, with the highest risk associated with puberty [111, 112]. There are a number of studies showing that pediatric cancer survivors are at particularly high risk for developing breast cancer later on in life, especially for those who have received mantle radiation in the context of lymphoma [113–116]. However, this effect is not limited to therapeutic radiation, but also to diagnostic radiation and overall radiation exposure in an occupational or environmental setting which has also been directly linked to breast cancer incidence [117–119]. In a retrospective study of nearly 2000 female carriers of BRCA1 and BRCA2 mutations, it was found that there is a significant association between exposure to diagnostic radiation prior to the age of 30 and breast cancer risk (HR 1.90 [1.20–3.00]) with a dose-response pattern [120]. Similarly, a study of carriers of a BRCA mutation with early initiation of mammographic screening had an increase in radiation-induced breast cancer mortality [121], supporting to current guidelines to delay mammography screening after age 30 [16, 22]. Furthermore, a better culture around occupational safety and limits to radiation exposure in addition to limitation of diagnostic imaging may serve as preventative strategies to mitigate risk.

16.6.3 Alcohol Intake and the Risk of Cancer

Another important but frequently forgotten target for risk reduction is alcohol consumption, which has been found to be an independent risk factor for breast cancer [122]. Epidemiological studies have linked alcohol consumption to the risk of breast cancer, with an increase in the order of 4% with one drink per day, increasing up to 40–50% with heavy alcohol consumption [123]. This is thought to be related to increased levels of estrogen which in turn increases carcinogenesis through a number of mechanisms [124]. It is also thought that alcohol directly affects breast density and may be correlated with an increased risk of breast cancer because of this association [125, 126]. Based on data from 53 epidemiological studies comprising nearly 60,000 women with breast cancer compared to a non-cancer cohort, it was noted that the relative risk of breast cancer was 30% greater in women with an average alcohol consumption and up to 46% greater in those with a higher than average intake when compared

to those that did not consume alcohol [127]. The relative risk also increased by 7% for each additional daily alcoholic beverage intake. Similarly, the prospective Nurses' Health Study found that even usual alcohol intake, defined as 3–6 drinks per week, was associated with an increased risk of breast cancer, with an independent association for those aged 18–40 years of age [128]. Interestingly, there was also a strong association with hormone receptor-positive status. Perhaps what is most interesting is that alcohol intake and associated risk may also be associated to age, with a higher risk if consumed before first pregnancy [129–131]. Data from the Nurses' Health Study also revealed that alcohol intake between the time of menarche and age of first birth is directly related to an increase in proliferative benign lesions, but also of invasive breast cancer among premenopausal women [128]. Furthermore, younger women are more likely to partake in binge drinking, making this an important topic of discussion during preventative care visits, noting that timing to reach young women is especially important.

16.6.4 Smoking and the Risk of Cancer

In an attempt to identify other preventative strategies, research has been done on the risk of smoking and the incidence of breast cancer, both in the active form and in the passive form by means of second-hand smoke exposure. Interestingly, studies suggest that the risk associated with smoking increased by sevenfold when it took place within 5 years of menarche in parous women, but also in nulliparous women who smoked more than 20 cigarettes daily with a cumulative pack-year smoking history of 20 or greater [132]. The correlation between smoking initiation prior to menarche or at least 11 years before first birth and breast cancer risk is also supported by meta-analysis data in the United States [133] and in Europe, with a study of more than 300,000 Norwegian woman revealing that women who began smoking more than 10 years before the birth of their first child was at 60% increased risk of breast cancer compared to never smokers [134]. It was also suggested that this risk may be even higher for women with a genetic predisposition to breast cancer. With regard to passive smoking, five case-control studies concluded that there was a significant increase in risk of breast cancer when compared to those who had not been exposed [135] and that those with the most extensive exposure to passive smoking had a greater than 30% increased risk of breast cancer when the exposure was greater than 10 years during childhood or adulthood at work or greater than 20 years of exposure at home during adulthood [136].

16.7 Lifestyle Modifications and Their Impact

The final and possibly the most important component of preventative strategies is lifestyle change and its potential impact on breast cancer risk. While biological factors may not necessary yield actionable areas of change, lifestyle factors can be modified at a low cost to public health care with minimal resources.

16.7.1 Obesity and BMI in Breast Cancer

One of the first factors worth mentioning is weight and BMI as a predictor of cancer risk [137]. Obesity is an underrecognized contributor to cancer incidence and accounts for up to 20% of cancer-related mortality [138–142]. Hypotheses surrounding this are related to increased aromatization by adipose tissue leading to increased estrogen, insulin resistance, proinflammatory cytokines, oxidative stress, and the activation of insulin-like growth factor pathways in obese women [143, 144]. However, most of this data applies to postmenopausal women and remains controversial with regard to premenopausal women. A population-based cohort study conducted in the United Kingdom in over 5 million participants concluded that obesity was only associated with a higher risk of postmenopausal breast cancers, whereas an inverse association

was observed for premenopausal breast cancers [145]. While it has been speculated that this is due to reduced progesterone levels in obese premenopausal women, this difference remains misunderstood [146].

Similarly, a meta-analysis of seven prospective cohort studies in Europe suggested a higher risk of postmenopausal breast cancers in obese women [147]. Further evidence suggests that postmenopausal breast cancer risk is directly associated with adiposity and negatively affects breast cancer recurrence and survival in women via inflammation of mammary adipose tissue, which can occur early during hypertrophy. Conversely, truncal fat might be more predictive in premenopausal women [148]. The California Teachers Study cohort also suggested that obesity at adolescence did not increase the risk of breast cancer as compared to adiposity changes later in adulthood [149]. In contrast, other studies suggest that being overweight or obese is an independent prognostic factor for women with triple-negative breast cancer, conferring a greater risk of death when compared to women of normal weight [150]. Given the available information, it remains difficult to make recommendations regarding weight changes for premenopausal women given the lack of clear evidence that this alters outcomes, although a clear link exists with postmenopausal breast cancers.

16.7.2 The Role of Diet and Prevention

Although no clear link to premenopausal breast cancer could be established with weight, a number of studies on dietary habits have been linked to the risk of breast cancer. Notably, total dietary fiber intake during early adulthood was associated with a 20% lower risk of breast cancer in the Nurses' Health Study II [151]. Interestingly, earlier results from the Nurses' Health Study II suggested that carbohydrate intake and glycemic load varied based on baseline BMI and could either mitigate the risk in individuals with low BMI or increase the risk in individuals with high BMI [152].

The role of fruit and vegetable intake on breast cancer risk has also been a topic of interest with mixed results. This was explored by a meta-analysis of 26 studies, suggesting a 25% decrease in relative risk of breast cancer with high vegetable intake and to a lesser degree with fruit intake [153], although the European Prospective Investigation into Cancer and Nutrition study of 285,000 women did not suggest an association [154]. However, some studies have suggested that a higher vegetable intake was related to less hormone receptor-negative tumors, although this was not seen for hormone receptor-positive tumors [155, 156].

Moreover, the effect of meat intake was also explored based on data from the Nurses' Health Study II, suggesting that a greater consumption of red meat during adolescence was associated with a 42% increase in premenopausal breast cancer risk [157]. A particularly noteworthy finding is that replacement of one serving of red meat per day during adolescence with poultry, fish, legumes, and nuts was associated with a 15% lower risk of breast cancer [157]. Comparison of the highest vegetable eaters to the lowest also revealed a significant decrease in the risk of premenopausal breast cancer in the range of 35%.

While there are a number of other preventative strategies which have been explored, a few worth mentioning include the relationship with soy intake and a decrease in premenopausal breast cancer, although the effect was different in Asia as compared to Western countries which may be related to the balance of soy with other nutrients [158]. A case-cohort analysis has also shown better outcomes including overall survival with higher levels of 25-hydroxyvitamin D [159], which could also serve as a prevention strategy.

16.7.3 Exercise and Risk Mitigation

A large component of lifestyle change is physical activity, and a number of studies over the last two decades have attempted to identify the role of exercise in cancer prevention. Review of epidemiological evidence from 73 studies conducted globally reveals a 25% average risk reduction across studies among physically active women as compared to their inactive counterparts [160]. Associations were greatest with activities of moderate to vigorous intensity (>4.5 METs, equivalent to mowing the lawn) and those which were performed regularly [161]. Review of 29 other case-control studies has also suggested an inverse association between exercise and breast cancer risk, although the effect was much less pronounced in premenopausal women around 15–20% [162]. There was, however, evidence of a dose-response relationship in the higher-quality studies included in this review, with a decrease of up to 6% for every additional hour of physical activity per week, assuming this would be sustained [162]. While all this data seems generally in favor of exercise for breast cancer prevention, a number of inconsistencies make the application to clinical practice difficult. This is partially due to the fact that it is unclear if the late adoption of an active lifestyle can be initiated early enough to translate into meaningful change, but also due to the significant variability of physical activity across studies; the effect also varies according to subgroups and different tumor biology. Nonetheless, exercise has so many other health benefits that its adoption as a prevention strategy for other medical conditions, including breast cancer, should not be discounted.

16.7.4 Sleep, Shift Work, and Its Effect on Cancer Risk

Finally, short sleep duration, sleep quality, and changes to circadian rhythm have been shown to have adverse metabolic implications which have been linked to worse cancer outcomes, putting young women at high risk [163]. Furthermore, 6 of 8 epidemiological studies noted a modestly increase risk of breast cancer among individuals who worked night shifts as compared to those who worked day shifts, with one study estimating up to 36% increase in breast cancer risk following 30 years of shift work [164]. This is thought to be related to disruption of the circadian rhythm, light at night, suppression of melatonin, and sleep deprivation [165–167]. The International Agency for Research on Cancer (IARC) has since then stated that "shift work involving circadian disruption is probably carcinogenic to humans" [164]. This may be attributed to hypoxia, inflammatory response, immune response, and endocrine and neurological factors although no clear explanation has been definitely supported. A large prospective Japanese study of nearly 24,000 women also reported that shorter sleep duration was associated with a higher risk of breast cancer compared to those who slept 7 h per night [168]. Thus, while shift work is unavoidable in certain industries, the ramifications are much larger than previously believed, and adoption of good sleep hygiene should be recommended as part of cancer prevention.

16.8 Summary

While there are a number of attractive lifestyle interventions which can be utilized as protective strategies, the prevention of breast cancer in young women remains different and complex. Biological factors are clearly more relevant, and breast cancers in a younger age group are more likely to be due to hereditary causes, more likely to be found at a later stage and more aggressive in nature. Furthermore, breast density and reproductive factors are of considerable importance in the development of breast cancer in younger women. Environmental exposure in earlier stages of life appears to be associated with greater risk, notably with regard to radiation, alcohol, and smoking. The study of lifestyle interventions as preventative strategies, as they relate to diet, exercise, and sleep disturbances, also warrants further evaluation.

Instigating change is difficult at the individual level, and a number of strategies have been utilized, such as the 5 A's model, which consists of asking what is the current behavior, advising on appropriate changes, assessing the barriers or opportunities for change, assisting with behavior modification, and arranging follow-up to ensure the new behavior is maintained [169–171]. However, it is vital that the punitive aspect of prevention be avoided. From a societal standpoint,

the importance of prevention among young women must be emphasized, and further research on the impact of prevention strategies is needed. Furthermore, the disproportionate shift in breast cancer-related mortality in young minority groups should be addressed, with an emphasis on engaging young women in prevention programs. The dissemination of information regarding biological factors, environmental factors, and lifestyle factors is crucial to the adoption of better behaviors, and the recognition of risk factors may ultimately lead to innovative risk-modifying opportunities.

Given the uncertainty and variable diagnostic accuracy of prediction models, individualized risk assessments must be performed, which also poses a challenge to the implementation of targeted prevention programs. Current initiatives include the Bring your Brave Campaign, led by the Centers for Disease Control and Prevention (CDC), designed to reach young women with information relating to breast cancer. Other programs have also been developed, such as the Know BRCA, to provide women with easily accessible resources which may help them with health-related decisions. Ultimately, although research has generally been focused on all ages, there is a large unmet need for preventative research tailored to young women.

References

1. Arrospide A, Forne C, Rue M, Tora N, Mar J, Bare M. An assessment of existing models for individualized breast cancer risk estimation in a screening program in Spain. BMC Cancer. 2013;13:587. https://doi.org/10.1186/1471-2407-13-587.
2. Anothaisintawee T, Teerawattananon Y, Wiratkapun C, Kasamesup V, Thakkinstian A. Risk prediction models of breast cancer: a systematic review of model performances. Breast Cancer Res Treat. 2012;133(1):1–10.
3. Decarli A, Calza S, Masala G, Specchia C, Palli D, Gail MH. Gail model for prediction of absolute risk of invasive breast cancer: independent evaluation in the Florence-European Prospective Investigation Into Cancer and Nutrition cohort. J Natl Cancer Inst. 2006;98(23):1686–93.
4. Gail MH, Brinton LA, Byar DP, Corle DK, Green SB, Schairer C, et al. Projecting individualized

probabilities of developing breast cancer for white females who are being examined annually. J Natl Cancer Inst. 1989;81(24):1879–86.

5. Costantino JP, Gail MH, Pee D, Anderson S, Redmond CK, Benichou J, et al. Validation studies for models projecting the risk of invasive and total breast cancer incidence. J Natl Cancer Inst. 1999;91(18):1541–8.

6. Chen J, Pee D, Ayyagari R, Graubard B, Schairer C, Byrne C, et al. Projecting absolute invasive breast cancer risk in white women with a model that includes mammographic density. J Natl Cancer Inst. 2006;98(17):1215–26.

7. Barlow WE, White E, Ballard-Barbash R, Vacek PM, Titus-Ernstoff L, Carney PA, et al. Prospective breast cancer risk prediction model for women undergoing screening mammography. J Natl Cancer Inst. 2006;98(17):1204–14.

8. Antoniou AC, Cunningham AP, Peto J, Evans DG, Lalloo F, Narod SA, et al. The BOADICEA model of genetic susceptibility to breast and ovarian cancers: updates and extensions. Br J Cancer. 2008;98(8):1457–66.

9. Lee AJ, Cunningham AP, Kuchenbaecker KB, Mavaddat N, Easton DF, Antoniou AC, et al. BOADICEA breast cancer risk prediction model: updates to cancer incidences, tumour pathology and web interface. Br J Cancer. 2014;110(2):535–45.

10. Antoniou AC, Pharoah PP, Smith P, Easton DF. The BOADICEA model of genetic susceptibility to breast and ovarian cancer. Br J Cancer. 2004;91(8):1580–90.

11. Fischer C, Kuchenbacker K, Engel C, Zachariae S, Rhiem K, Meindl A, et al. Evaluating the performance of the breast cancer genetic risk models BOADICEA, IBIS, BRCAPRO and Claus for predicting BRCA1/2 mutation carrier probabilities: a study based on 7352 families from the German Hereditary Breast and Ovarian Cancer Consortium. J Med Genet. 2013;50(6):360–7.

12. Berry DA, Iversen ES Jr, Gudbjartsson DF, Hiller EH, Garber JE, Peshkin BN, et al. BRCAPRO validation, sensitivity of genetic testing of BRCA1/BRCA2, and prevalence of other breast cancer susceptibility genes. J Clin Oncol. 2002;20(11):2701–12.

13. Tyrer J, Duffy SW, Cuzick J. A breast cancer prediction model incorporating familial and personal risk factors. Stat Med. 2004;23(7):1111–30.

14. Claus EB, Risch N, Thompson WD. Autosomal dominant inheritance of early-onset breast cancer. Implications for risk prediction. Cancer. 1994;73(3):643–51.

15. Turnbull C, Rahman N. Genetic predisposition to breast cancer: past, present, and future. Annu Rev Genomics Hum Genet. 2008;9:321–45.

16. Paluch-Shimon S, Cardoso F, Sessa C, Balmana J, Cardoso MJ, Gilbert F, et al. Prevention and screening in BRCA mutation carriers and other breast/ovarian hereditary cancer syndromes: ESMO Clinical Practice Guidelines for cancer prevention and screening. Ann Oncol. 2016;27(Suppl 5):v103–10.

17. Gonzalez-Angulo AM, Timms KM, Liu S, Chen H, Litton JK, Potter J, et al. Incidence and outcome of BRCA mutations in unselected patients with triple receptor-negative breast cancer. Clin Cancer Res. 2011;17(5):1082–9.

18. Hartman AR, Kaldate RR, Sailer LM, Painter L, Grier CE, Endsley RR, et al. Prevalence of BRCA mutations in an unselected population of triple-negative breast cancer. Cancer. 2012; 118(11):2787–95.

19. Grindedal EM, Heramb C, Karsrud I, Ariansen SL, Maehle L, Undlien DE, et al. Current guidelines for BRCA testing of breast cancer patients are insufficient to detect all mutation carriers. BMC Cancer. 2017;17(1):438. https://doi.org/10.1186/s12885-017-3422-2.

20. Couch FJ, Hart SN, Sharma P, Toland AE, Wang X, Miron P, et al. Inherited mutations in 17 breast cancer susceptibility genes among a large triple-negative breast cancer cohort unselected for family history of breast cancer. J Clin Oncol. 2015;33(4):304–11.

21. LaDuca H, Stuenkel AJ, Dolinsky JS, Keiles S, Tandy S, Pesaran T, et al. Utilization of multigene panels in hereditary cancer predisposition testing: analysis of more than 2,000 patients. Genet Med. 2014;16(11):830–7.

22. The NCCN Clinical Practice Guidelines in Oncology. Genetic/Familial High-Risk Assessment: Breast and Ovarian V2.2019. National Comprehensive Cancer Network.

23. National Collaborating Centre for Cancer (UK). 2013.

24. Warner E, Plewes DB, Hill KA, Causer PA, Zubovits JT, Jong RA, et al. Surveillance of BRCA1 and BRCA2 mutation carriers with magnetic resonance imaging, ultrasound, mammography, and clinical breast examination. JAMA. 2004;292(11):1317–25.

25. Kriege M, Brekelmans CT, Boetes C, Besnard PE, Zonderland HM, Obdeijn IM, et al. Efficacy of MRI and mammography for breast-cancer screening in women with a familial or genetic predisposition. N Engl J Med. 2004;351(5):427–37.

26. Horsman D, Wilson BJ, Avard D, Meschino WS, Kim Sing C, Plante M, et al. Clinical management recommendations for surveillance and risk-reduction strategies for hereditary breast and ovarian cancer among individuals carrying a deleterious BRCA1 or BRCA2 mutation. J Obstet Gynaecol Can. 2007;29(1):45–60.

27. Chiarelli AM, Prummel MV, Muradali D, Majpruz V, Horgan M, Carroll JC, et al. Effectiveness of screening with annual magnetic resonance imaging and mammography: results of the initial screen from the ontario high risk breast screening program. J Clin Oncol. 2014;32(21):2224–30.

28. Daly B, Olopade OI. A perfect storm: how tumor biology, genomics, and health care delivery patterns

collide to create a racial survival disparity in breast cancer and proposed interventions for change. CA Cancer J Clin. 2015;65(3):221–38.

29. DeSantis CE, Lin CC, Mariotto AB, Siegel RL, Stein KD, Kramer JL, et al. Cancer treatment and survivorship statistics, 2014. CA Cancer J Clin. 2014;64(4):252–71.

30. DeSantis C, Siegel R, Bandi P, Jemal A. Breast cancer statistics, 2011. CA Cancer J Clin. 2011;61(6):409–18.

31. Chlebowski RT, Chen Z, Anderson GL, Rohan T, Aragaki A, Lane D, et al. Ethnicity and breast cancer: factors influencing differences in incidence and outcome. J Natl Cancer Inst. 2005;97(6):439–48.

32. Cunningham JE, Montero AJ, Garrett-Mayer E, Berkel HJ, Ely B. Racial differences in the incidence of breast cancer subtypes defined by combined histologic grade and hormone receptor status. Cancer Causes Control. 2010;21(3):399–409.

33. Kurian AW, Fish K, Shema SJ, Clarke CA. Lifetime risks of specific breast cancer subtypes among women in four racial/ethnic groups. Breast Cancer Res. 2010;12(6):R99.

34. Howlader N, Altekruse SF, Li CI, Chen VW, Clarke CA, Ries LA, et al. US incidence of breast cancer subtypes defined by joint hormone receptor and HER2 status. J Natl Cancer Inst. 2014;106(5):dju055. https://doi.org/10.1093/jnci/dju055.

35. Clarke CA, West DW, Edwards BK, Figgs LW, Kerner J, Schwartz AG. Existing data on breast cancer in African-American women: what we know and what we need to know. Cancer. 2003;97(1 Suppl):211–21.

36. Surveillance, Epidemiology, and End Results program. National Cancer Institute. Surveillance, Epidemiology, and End Results (SEER) stat fact sheets: breast cancer.

37. Hunt BR, Whitman S, Hurlbert MS. Increasing Black:White disparities in breast cancer mortality in the 50 largest cities in the United States. Cancer Epidemiol. 2014;38(2):118–23.

38. Iqbal J, Ginsburg O, Rochon PA, Sun P, Narod SA. Differences in breast cancer stage at diagnosis and cancer-specific survival by race and ethnicity in the United States. JAMA. 2015;313(2):165–73.

39. Brennan M. Breast cancer in ethnic minority groups in developed nations: case studies of the United Kingdom and Australia. Maturitas. 2017; 99:16–9.

40. Carey LA, Perou CM, Livasy CA, Dressler LG, Cowan D, Conway K, et al. Race, breast cancer subtypes, and survival in the Carolina Breast Cancer Study. JAMA. 2006;295(21):2492–502.

41. O'Brien KM, Cole SR, Tse CK, Perou CM, Carey LA, Foulkes WD, et al. Intrinsic breast tumor subtypes, race, and long-term survival in the Carolina Breast Cancer Study. Clin Cancer Res. 2010;16(24):6100–10.

42. Palmer JR, Viscidi E, Troester MA, Hong CC, Schedin P, Bethea TN, et al. Parity, lactation, and breast cancer subtypes in African American women: results from the AMBER Consortium. J Natl Cancer Inst. 2014;106(10):dju237. https://doi.org/10.1093/jnci/dju237.

43. McCormack VA, dos Santos Silva I. Breast density and parenchymal patterns as markers of breast cancer risk: a meta-analysis. Cancer Epidemiol Biomarkers Prev. 2006 Jun;15(6):1159–69.

44. Cil T, Fishell E, Hanna W, Sun P, Rawlinson E, Narod SA, et al. Mammographic density and the risk of breast cancer recurrence after breast-conserving surgery. Cancer. 2009;115(24):5780–7.

45. Eriksson L, Czene K, Rosenberg L, Humphreys K, Hall P. Possible influence of mammographic density on local and locoregional recurrence of breast cancer. Breast Cancer Res. 2013;15(4):R56.

46. Park CC, Rembert J, Chew K, Moore D, Kerlikowske K. High mammographic breast density is independent predictor of local but not distant recurrence after lumpectomy and radiotherapy for invasive breast cancer. Int J Radiat Oncol Biol Phys. 2009;73(1):75–9.

47. Porter GJ, Evans AJ, Cornford EJ, Burrell HC, James JJ, Lee AH, et al. Influence of mammographic parenchymal pattern in screening-detected and interval invasive breast cancers on pathologic features, mammographic features, and patient survival. AJR Am J Roentgenol. 2007;188(3):676–83.

48. Gierach GL, Ichikawa L, Kerlikowske K, Brinton LA, Farhat GN, Vacek PM, et al. Relationship between mammographic density and breast cancer death in the Breast Cancer Surveillance Consortium. J Natl Cancer Inst. 2012;104(16):1218–27.

49. Chiu SY, Duffy S, Yen AM, Tabar L, Smith RA, Chen HH. Effect of baseline breast density on breast cancer incidence, stage, mortality, and screening parameters: 25-year follow-up of a Swedish mammographic screening. Cancer Epidemiol Biomarkers Prev. 2010;19(5):1219–28.

50. Boyd NF, Guo H, Martin LJ, Sun L, Stone J, Fishell E, et al. Mammographic density and the risk and detection of breast cancer. N Engl J Med. 2007;356(3):227–36.

51. Boyd NF, Huszti E, Melnichouk O, Martin LJ, Hislop G, Chiarelli A, et al. Mammographic features associated with interval breast cancers in screening programs. Breast Cancer Res. 2014;16(4):417. https://doi.org/10.1186/s13058-014-0417-7.

52. Yan S, Wang Y, Aghaei F, Qiu Y, Zheng B. Applying a new bilateral mammographic density segmentation method to improve accuracy of breast cancer risk prediction. Int J Comput Assist Radiol Surg. 2017;12(10):1819–28.

53. Melnikow J, Fenton JJ, Whitlock EP, Miglioretti DL, Weyrich MS, Thompson JH, et al. Supplemental screening for breast cancer in women with dense breasts: a systematic review for the U.S. preventive services task force. Ann Intern Med. 2016;164(4):268–78.

54. Greendale GA, Reboussin BA, Slone S, Wasilauskas C, Pike MC, Ursin G. Postmenopausal hormone therapy and change in mammographic density. J Natl Cancer Inst. 2003;95(1):30–7.
55. Lee E, Ingles SA, Van Den Berg D, Wang W, Lavallee C, Huang MH, et al. Progestogen levels, progesterone receptor gene polymorphisms, and mammographic density changes: results from the Postmenopausal Estrogen/Progestin Interventions Mammographic Density Study. Menopause. 2012;19(3):302–10.
56. Singletary KW, Gapstur SM. Alcohol and breast cancer: review of epidemiologic and experimental evidence and potential mechanisms. JAMA. 2001;286(17):2143–51.
57. Harvey JA, Bovbjerg VE. Quantitative assessment of mammographic breast density: relationship with breast cancer risk. Radiology. 2004;230(1):29–41.
58. Heine JJ, Malhotra P. Mammographic tissue, breast cancer risk, serial image analysis, and digital mammography. Part 1. Tissue and related risk factors. Acad Radiol. 2002;9(3):298–316.
59. Heine JJ, Malhotra P. Mammographic tissue, breast cancer risk, serial image analysis, and digital mammography. Part 2. Serial breast tissue change and related temporal influences. Acad Radiol. 2002;9(3):317–35.
60. Sellers TA, Vachon CM, Pankratz VS, Janney CA, Fredericksen Z, Brandt KR, et al. Association of childhood and adolescent anthropometric factors, physical activity, and diet with adult mammographic breast density. Am J Epidemiol. 2007;166(4):456–64.
61. Vachon CM, Kushi LH, Cerhan JR, Kuni CC, Sellers TA. Association of diet and mammographic breast density in the Minnesota breast cancer family cohort. Cancer Epidemiol Biomarkers Prev. 2000;9(2):151–60.
62. Dall GV, Britt KL. Estrogen effects on the mammary gland in early and late life and breast cancer risk. Front Oncol. 2017;7:110.
63. Collaborative Group on Hormonal Factors in Breast Cancer. Menarche, menopause, and breast cancer risk: individual participant meta-analysis, including 118 964 women with breast cancer from 117 epidemiological studies. Lancet Oncol. 2012;13(11):1141–51.
64. Sisti JS, Bernstein JL, Lynch CF, Reiner AS, Mellemkjaer L, Brooks JD, et al. Reproductive factors, tumor estrogen receptor status and contralateral breast cancer risk: results from the WECARE study. Springerplus. 2015;30(4):825. https://doi.org/10.1186/s40064-015-1642-y. eCollection 2015
65. Anderson KN, Schwab RB, Martinez ME. Reproductive risk factors and breast cancer subtypes: a review of the literature. Breast Cancer Res Treat. 2014;144(1):1–10.
66. Chen L, Li CI, Tang MT, Porter P, Hill DA, Wiggins CL, et al. Reproductive factors and risk of luminal, HER2-overexpressing, and triple-negative breast cancer among multiethnic women. Cancer Epidemiol Biomarkers Prev. 2016;25(9):1297–304.
67. Gaudet MM, Press MF, Haile RW, Lynch CF, Glaser SL, Schildkraut J, et al. Risk factors by molecular subtypes of breast cancer across a population-based study of women 56 years or younger. Breast Cancer Res Treat. 2011;130(2):587–97.
68. Lambe M, Hsieh CC, Chan HW, Ekbom A, Trichopoulos D, Adami HO. Parity, age at first and last birth, and risk of breast cancer: a population-based study in Sweden. Breast Cancer Res Treat. 1996;38(3):305–11.
69. Rao CV. Protective effects of human chorionic gonadotropin against breast cancer: how can we use this information to prevent/treat the disease? Reprod Sci. 2017;24(8):1102–10.
70. Andrieu N, Goldgar DE, Easton DF, Rookus M, Brohet R, Antoniou AC, et al. Pregnancies, breast-feeding, and breast cancer risk in the International BRCA1/2 Carrier Cohort Study (IBCCS). J Natl Cancer Inst. 2006;98(8):535–44.
71. Newcomb PA, Storer BE, Longnecker MP, Mittendorf R, Greenberg ER, Clapp RW, et al. Lactation and a reduced risk of premenopausal breast cancer. N Engl J Med. 1994;330(2):81–7.
72. Lambertini M, Santoro L, Del Mastro L, Nguyen B, Livraghi L, Ugolini D, et al. Reproductive behaviors and risk of developing breast cancer according to tumor subtype: A systematic review and meta-analysis of epidemiological studies. Cancer Treat Rev. 2016;49:65–76.
73. Jernstrom H, Lubinski J, Lynch HT, Ghadirian P, Neuhausen S, Isaacs C, et al. Breast-feeding and the risk of breast cancer in BRCA1 and BRCA2 mutation carriers. J Natl Cancer Inst. 2004;96(14):1094–8.
74. Downing NS, Shah ND, Neiman JH, Aminawung JA, Krumholz HM, Ross JS. Participation of the elderly, women, and minorities in pivotal trials supporting 2011–2013 U.S. Food and Drug Administration approvals. Trials. 2016;17:199. https://doi.org/10.1186/s13063-016-1322-4.
75. Shinde SS, Forman MR, Kuerer HM, Yan K, Peintinger F, Hunt KK, et al. Higher parity and shorter breastfeeding duration: association with triple-negative phenotype of breast cancer. Cancer. 2010;116(21):4933–43.
76. Soroush A, Farshchian N, Komasi S, Izadi N, Amirifard N, Shahmohammadi A. The role of oral contraceptive pills on increased risk of breast cancer in Iranian populations: a Meta-analysis. J Cancer Prev. 2016;21(4):294–301.
77. Charlton BM, Rich-Edwards JW, Colditz GA, Missmer SA, Rosner BA, Hankinson SE, et al. Oral contraceptive use and mortality after 36 years of follow-up in the Nurses' Health Study: prospective cohort study. BMJ. 2014;349:g6356.
78. Li L, Zhong Y, Zhang H, Yu H, Huang Y, Li Z, et al. Association between oral contraceptive use as a risk factor and triple-negative breast cancer: a sys-

tematic review and meta-analysis. Mol Clin Oncol. 2017;7(1):76–80.

79. Althuis MD, Brogan DR, Coates RJ, Daling JR, Gammon MD, Malone KE, et al. Hormonal content and potency of oral contraceptives and breast cancer risk among young women. Br J Cancer. 2003;88(1):50–7.

80. Marchbanks PA, McDonald JA, Wilson HG, Folger SG, Mandel MG, Daling JR, et al. Oral contraceptives and the risk of breast cancer. N Engl J Med. 2002;346(26):2025–32.

81. Lu Y, Ma H, Malone KE, Norman SA, Sullivan-Halley J, Strom BL, et al. Oral contraceptive use and survival in women with invasive breast cancer. Cancer Epidemiol Biomarkers Prev. 2011;20(7):1391–7.

82. Cuzick J, Powles T, Veronesi U, Forbes J, Edwards R, Ashley S, et al. Overview of the main outcomes in breast-cancer prevention trials. Lancet. 2003;361(9354):296–300.

83. Fisher B, Costantino JP, Wickerham DL, Cecchini RS, Cronin WM, Robidoux A, et al. Tamoxifen for the prevention of breast cancer: current status of the National Surgical Adjuvant Breast and Bowel Project P-1 study. J Natl Cancer Inst. 2005;97(22):1652–62.

84. Cuzick J, Forbes J, Edwards R, Baum M, Cawthorn S, Coates A, et al. First results from the International Breast Cancer Intervention Study (IBIS-I): a randomised prevention trial. Lancet. 2002;360(9336):817–24.

85. Powles TJ, Ashley S, Tidy A, Smith IE, Dowsett M. Twenty-year follow-up of the Royal Marsden randomized, double-blinded tamoxifen breast cancer prevention trial. J Natl Cancer Inst. 2007;99(4):283–90.

86. Veronesi U, Maisonneuve P, Rotmensz N, Bonanni B, Boyle P, Viale G, et al. Tamoxifen for the prevention of breast cancer: late results of the Italian Randomized Tamoxifen Prevention Trial among women with hysterectomy. J Natl Cancer Inst. 2007;99(9):727–37.

87. Nelson HD, Smith ME, Griffin JC, Fu R. Use of medications to reduce risk for primary breast cancer: a systematic review for the U.S. Preventive Services Task Force. Ann Intern Med. 2013;158(8):604–14.

88. Visvanathan K, Lippman SM, Hurley P, Temin S, American Society of Clinical Oncology Clinical Practice Guideline. American Society of Clinical Oncology clinical practice guideline update on the use of pharmacologic interventions including tamoxifen, raloxifene, and aromatase inhibition for breast cancer risk reduction. Gynecol Oncol. 2009;115(1):132–4.

89. Winer EP. Optimizing endocrine therapy for breast cancer. J Clin Oncol. 2005;23(8):1609–10.

90. Pagani O, Regan MM, Walley BA, Fleming GF, Colleoni M, Lang I, et al. Adjuvant exemestane with ovarian suppression in premenopausal breast cancer. N Engl J Med. 2014;371(2):107–18.

91. Saha P, Regan MM, Pagani O, Francis PA, Walley BA, Ribi K, et al. Treatment efficacy, adherence, and quality of life among women younger than 35 years in the international breast cancer study group TEXT and SOFT adjuvant endocrine therapy trials. J Clin Oncol. 2017;35(27):3113–22. https://doi.org/10.1200/JCO.2016.72.0946.

92. Hartmann LC, Sellers TA, Schaid DJ, Frank TS, Soderberg CL, Sitta DL, et al. Efficacy of bilateral prophylactic mastectomy in BRCA1 and BRCA2 gene mutation carriers. J Natl Cancer Inst. 2001;93(21):1633–7.

93. Rebbeck TR, Friebel T, Lynch HT, Neuhausen SL, van 't Veer L, Garber JE, et al. Bilateral prophylactic mastectomy reduces breast cancer risk in BRCA1 and BRCA2 mutation carriers: the PROSE Study Group. J Clin Oncol. 2004;22(6):1055–62.

94. Heemskerk-Gerritsen BA, Brekelmans CT, Menke-Pluymers MB, van Geel AN, Tilanus-Linthorst MM, Bartels CC, et al. Prophylactic mastectomy in BRCA1/2 mutation carriers and women at risk of hereditary breast cancer: long-term experiences at the Rotterdam Family Cancer Clinic. Ann Surg Oncol. 2007;14(12):3335–44.

95. Evans DG, Baildam AD, Anderson E, Brain A, Shenton A, Vasen HF, et al. Risk reducing mastectomy: outcomes in 10 European centres. J Med Genet. 2009;46(4):254–8.

96. Chung AP, Sacchini V. Nipple-sparing mastectomy: where are we now? Surg Oncol. 2008;17(4):261–6.

97. Morrow M, Mehrara B. Prophylactic mastectomy and the timing of breast reconstruction. Br J Surg. 2009;96(1):1–2.

98. Rebbeck TR, Kauff ND, Domchek SM. Meta-analysis of risk reduction estimates associated with risk-reducing salpingo-oophorectomy in BRCA1 or BRCA2 mutation carriers. J Natl Cancer Inst. 2009;101(2):80–7.

99. Marchetti C, De Felice F, Palaia I, Perniola G, Musella A, Musio D, et al. Risk-reducing salpingo-oophorectomy: a meta-analysis on impact on ovarian cancer risk and all cause mortality in BRCA 1 and BRCA 2 mutation carriers. BMC Womens Health. 2014;14:150. https://doi.org/10.1186/s12905-014-0150-5.

100. Erickson BK, Conner MG, Landen CN Jr. The role of the fallopian tube in the origin of ovarian cancer. Am J Obstet Gynecol. 2013;209(5):409–14.

101. Siegel R, Ward E, Brawley O, Jemal A. Cancer statistics, 2011: the impact of eliminating socioeconomic and racial disparities on premature cancer deaths. CA Cancer J Clin. 2011;61(4):212–36.

102. Hirth JM, Laz TH, Rahman M, Berenson AB. Racial/Ethnic differences affecting adherence to cancer screening guidelines among women. J Womens Health (Larchmt). 2016;25(4):371–80.

103. Belkic K, Cohen M, Wilczek B, Andersson S, Berman AH, Marquez M, et al. Imaging surveillance programs for women at high breast cancer risk in Europe: are women from ethnic minority

groups adequately included? (Review). Int J Oncol. 2015;47(3):817–39.

104. Bigby J, Holmes MD. Disparities across the breast cancer continuum. Cancer Causes Control. 2005;16(1):35–44.

105. Reeder-Hayes KE, Wheeler SB, Mayer DK. Health disparities across the breast cancer continuum. Semin Oncol Nurs. 2015;31(2):170–7.

106. Yedjou CG, Tchounwou PB, Payton M, Miele L, Fonseca DD, Lowe L, et al. Assessing the racial and ethnic disparities in breast cancer mortality in the United States. Int J Environ Res Public Health. 2017;14(5):E486. https://doi.org/10.3390/ijerph14050486.

107. Gorin SS, Heck JE, Cheng B, Smith SJ. Delays in breast cancer diagnosis and treatment by racial/ethnic group. Arch Intern Med. 2006;166(20):2244–52.

108. Gwyn K, Bondy ML, Cohen DS, Lund MJ, Liff JM, Flagg EW, et al. Racial differences in diagnosis, treatment, and clinical delays in a population-based study of patients with newly diagnosed breast carcinoma. Cancer. 2004;100(8):1595–604.

109. Parsons HM, Lathrop KI, Schmidt S, Mazo-Canola M, Trevino-Jones J, Speck H, et al. Breast cancer treatment delays in a majority minority community: is there a difference? J Oncol Pract. 2015;11(2):e144–53.

110. Kidd AD, Colbert AM, Jatoi I. Mammography: review of the controversy, health disparities, and impact on young African American women. Clin J Oncol Nurs. 2015;19(3):E52–8.

111. Guibout C, Adjadj E, Rubino C, Shamsaldin A, Grimaud E, Hawkins M, et al. Malignant breast tumors after radiotherapy for a first cancer during childhood. J Clin Oncol. 2005;23(1):197–204.

112. Kenney LB, Yasui Y, Inskip PD, Hammond S, Neglia JP, Mertens AC, et al. Breast cancer after childhood cancer: a report from the Childhood Cancer Survivor Study. Ann Intern Med. 2004;141(8):590–7.

113. Bluhm EC, Ronckers C, Hayashi RJ, Neglia JP, Mertens AC, Stovall M, et al. Cause-specific mortality and second cancer incidence after non-Hodgkin lymphoma: a report from the Childhood Cancer Survivor Study. Blood. 2008;111(8):4014–21.

114. Hancock SL, Tucker MA, Hoppe RT. Breast cancer after treatment of Hodgkin's disease. J Natl Cancer Inst. 1993;85(1):25–31.

115. Swerdlow AJ, Barber JA, Hudson GV, Cunningham D, Gupta RK, Hancock BW, et al. Risk of second malignancy after Hodgkin's disease in a collaborative British cohort: the relation to age at treatment. J Clin Oncol. 2000;18(3):498–509.

116. Bhatia S, Yasui Y, Robison LL, Birch JM, Bogue MK, Diller L, et al. High risk of subsequent neoplasms continues with extended follow-up of childhood Hodgkin's disease: report from the Late Effects Study Group. J Clin Oncol. 2003; 21(23):4386–94.

117. Marcus PM, Newman B, Millikan RC, Moorman PG, Baird DD, Qaqish B. The associations of adolescent cigarette smoking, alcoholic beverage consumption, environmental tobacco smoke, and ionizing radiation with subsequent breast cancer risk (United States). Cancer Causes Control. 2000;11(3):271–8.

118. Preston DL, Kitahara CM, Freedman DM, Sigurdson AJ, Simon SL, Little MP, et al. Breast cancer risk and protracted low-to-moderate dose occupational radiation exposure in the US Radiologic Technologists Cohort, 1983–2008. Br J Cancer. 2016;115(9):1105–12.

119. Rajaraman P, Doody MM, Yu CL, Preston DL, Miller JS, Sigurdson AJ, et al. Cancer risks in U.S. radiologic technologists working with fluoroscopically guided interventional procedures, 1994–2008. AJR Am J Roentgenol. 2016;206(5):1101–8. quiz 1109

120. Pijpe A, Andrieu N, Easton DF, Kesminiene A, Cardis E, Nogues C, et al. Exposure to diagnostic radiation and risk of breast cancer among carriers of BRCA1/2 mutations: retrospective cohort study (GENE-RAD-RISK). BMJ. 2012;345:e5660.

121. Berrington de Gonzalez A, Berg CD, Visvanathan K, Robson M. Estimated risk of radiation-induced breast cancer from mammographic screening for young BRCA mutation carriers. J Natl Cancer Inst. 2009;101(3):205–9.

122. McDonald JA, Goyal A, Terry MB. Alcohol intake and breast cancer risk: weighing the overall evidence. Curr Breast Cancer Rep. 2013;5:3. https://doi.org/10.1007/s12609-013-0114-z.

123. Seitz HK, Pelucchi C, Bagnardi V, La Vecchia C. Epidemiology and pathophysiology of alcohol and breast cancer: update 2012. Alcohol Alcohol. 2012;47(3):204–12.

124. Oyesanmi O, Snyder D, Sullivan N, Reston J, Treadwell J, Schoelles KM. Alcohol consumption and cancer risk: understanding possible causal mechanisms for breast and colorectal cancers. Evid Rep Technol Assess (Full Rep). 2010;197:1–151.

125. Boyd NF, Martin LJ, Yaffe MJ, Minkin S. Mammographic density and breast cancer risk: current understanding and future prospects. Breast Cancer Res. 2011;13(6):223.

126. Conroy SM, Koga K, Woolcott CG, Dahl T, Byrne C, Nagata C, et al. Higher alcohol intake may modify the association between mammographic density and breast cancer: an analysis of three case-control studies. Cancer Epidemiol. 2012;36(5):458–60.

127. Hamajima N, Hirose K, Tajima K, Rohan T, Calle EE, Heath CW Jr, et al. Alcohol, tobacco and breast cancer--collaborative reanalysis of individual data from 53 epidemiological studies, including 58,515 women with breast cancer and 95,067 women without the disease. Br J Cancer. 2002;87(11):1234–45.

128. Chen WY, Rosner B, Hankinson SE, Colditz GA, Willett WC. Moderate alcohol consumption during adult life, drinking patterns, and breast cancer risk. JAMA. 2011;306(17):1884–90.

129. Jayasekara H, MacInnis RJ, Hodge AM, Room R, Milne RL, Hopper JL, et al. Is breast cancer risk associated with alcohol intake before first full-term pregnancy? Cancer Causes Control. 2016;27(9):1167–74.

130. Colditz GA, Bohlke K, Berkey CS. Breast cancer risk accumulation starts early: prevention must also. Breast Cancer Res Treat. 2014;145(3):567–79.

131. Liu Y, Colditz GA, Rosner B, Berkey CS, Collins LC, Schnitt SJ, et al. Alcohol intake between menarche and first pregnancy: a prospective study of breast cancer risk. J Natl Cancer Inst. 2013;105(20):1571–8.

132. Band PR, Le ND, Fang R, Deschamps M. Carcinogenic and endocrine disrupting effects of cigarette smoke and risk of breast cancer. Lancet. 2002;360(9339):1044–9.

133. Gaudet MM, Gapstur SM, Sun J, Diver WR, Hannan LM, Thun MJ. Active smoking and breast cancer risk: original cohort data and meta-analysis. J Natl Cancer Inst. 2013;105(8):515–25.

134. Bjerkaas E, Parajuli R, Weiderpass E, Engeland A, Maskarinec G, Selmer R, et al. Smoking duration before first childbirth: an emerging risk factor for breast cancer? Results from 302,865 Norwegian women. Cancer Causes Control. 2013;24(7):1347–56.

135. Johnson KC. Accumulating evidence on passive and active smoking and breast cancer risk. Int J Cancer. 2005;117(4):619–28.

136. Luo J, Margolis KL, Wactawski-Wende J, Horn K, Messina C, Stefanick ML, et al. Association of active and passive smoking with risk of breast cancer among postmenopausal women: a prospective cohort study. BMJ. 2011;342:d1016.

137. Calle EE, Rodriguez C, Walker-Thurmond K, Thun MJ. Overweight, obesity, and mortality from cancer in a prospectively studied cohort of U.S. adults. N Engl J Med. 2003;348(17):1625–38.

138. Ligibel JA, Alfano CM, Courneya KS, Demark-Wahnefried W, Burger RA, Chlebowski RT, et al. American Society of Clinical Oncology position statement on obesity and cancer. J Clin Oncol. 2014;32(31):3568–74.

139. Renehan AG, Zwahlen M, Egger M. Adiposity and cancer risk: new mechanistic insights from epidemiology. Nat Rev Cancer. 2015;15(8):484–98.

140. Arnold M, Pandeya N, Byrnes G, Renehan AG, Stevens GA, Ezzati M, et al. Global burden of cancer attributable to high body-mass index in 2012: a population-based study. Lancet Oncol. 2015;16(1):36–46.

141. National Cancer Institute. NC: Fact sheet: Obesity and cancer risk.

142. Protani M, Coory M, Martin JH. Effect of obesity on survival of women with breast cancer: systematic review and meta-analysis. Breast Cancer Res Treat. 2010;123(3):627–35.

143. Engin A. Obesity-associated breast cancer: analysis of risk factors. Adv Exp Med Biol. 2017;960:571–606.

144. Schmidt S, Monk JM, Robinson LE, Mourtzakis M. The integrative role of leptin, oestrogen and the insulin family in obesity-associated breast cancer: potential effects of exercise. Obes Rev. 2015;16(6):473–87.

145. Bhaskaran K, Douglas I, Forbes H, dos-Santos-Silva I, Leon DA, Smeeth L. Body-mass index and risk of 22 specific cancers: a population-based cohort study of 5.24 million UK adults. Lancet. 2014;384(9945):755–65.

146. Dowsett M, Folkerd E. Reduced progesterone levels explain the reduced risk of breast cancer in obese premenopausal women: a new hypothesis. Breast Cancer Res Treat. 2015;149(1):1–4.

147. Freisling H, Arnold M, Soerjomataram I, O'Doherty MG, Ordonez-Mena JM, Bamia C, et al. Comparison of general obesity and measures of body fat distribution in older adults in relation to cancer risk: meta-analysis of individual participant data of seven prospective cohorts in Europe. Br J Cancer. 2017;116(11):1486–97.

148. Vaysse C, Lomo J, Garred O, Fjeldheim F, Lofteroed T, Schlichting E, et al. Inflammation of mammary adipose tissue occurs in overweight and obese patients exhibiting early-stage breast cancer. NPJ Breast Cancer. 2017;3:19. https://doi.org/10.1038/s41523-017-0015-9. eCollection 2017

149. Horn-Ross PL, Canchola AJ, Bernstein L, Neuhausen SL, Nelson DO, Reynolds P. Lifetime body size and estrogen-receptor-positive breast cancer risk in the California Teachers Study cohort. Breast Cancer Res. 2016;18(1):132. https://doi.org/10.1186/s13058-016-0790-5.

150. Al Jarroudi O, Abda N, Seddik Y, Brahmi SA, Overweight AS. Is it a prognostic factor in women with triple-negative breast cancer? Asian Pac J Cancer Prev. 2017;18(6):1519–23.

151. Farvid MS, Eliassen AH, Cho E, Liao X, Chen WY, Willett WC. Dietary fiber intake in young adults and breast cancer risk. Pediatrics. 2016;137(3):e20151226. Epub 2016 Feb 1

152. Cho E, Spiegelman D, Hunter DJ, Chen WY, Colditz GA, Willett WC. Premenopausal dietary carbohydrate, glycemic index, glycemic load, and fiber in relation to risk of breast cancer. Cancer Epidemiol Biomarkers Prev. 2003;12(11 Pt 1):1153–8.

153. Gandini S, Merzenich H, Robertson C, Boyle P. Meta-analysis of studies on breast cancer risk and diet: the role of fruit and vegetable consumption and the intake of associated micronutrients. Eur J Cancer. 2000;36(5):636–46.

154. Bradbury KE, Appleby PN, Key TJ. Fruit, vegetable, and fiber intake in relation to cancer risk: findings from the European Prospective Investigation into Cancer and Nutrition (EPIC). Am J Clin Nutr. 2014;100(Suppl 1):394S–8S.

155. Emaus MJ, Peeters PH, Bakker MF, Overvad K, Tjonneland A, Olsen A, et al. Vegetable and fruit consumption and the risk of hormone receptor-

defined breast cancer in the EPIC cohort. Am J Clin Nutr. 2016;103(1):168–77.

156. Jung S, Spiegelman D, Baglietto L, Bernstein L, Boggs DA, van den Brandt PA, et al. Fruit and vegetable intake and risk of breast cancer by hormone receptor status. J Natl Cancer Inst. 2013;105(3):219–36.

157. Farvid MS, Cho E, Chen WY, Eliassen AH, Willett WC. Adolescent meat intake and breast cancer risk. Int J Cancer. 2015;136(8):1909–20.

158. Chen M, Rao Y, Zheng Y, Wei S, Li Y, Guo T, et al. Association between soy isoflavone intake and breast cancer risk for pre- and post-menopausal women: a meta-analysis of epidemiological studies. PLoS One. 2014;9(2):e89288.

159. Yao S, Kwan ML, Ergas IJ, Roh JM, Cheng TD, Hong CC, et al. Association of serum level of Vitamin D at diagnosis with breast cancer survival: a case-cohort analysis in the pathways study. JAMA Oncol. 2017;3(3):351–7.

160. Friedenreich CM, Neilson HK, Lynch BM. State of the epidemiological evidence on physical activity and cancer prevention. Eur J Cancer. 2010;46(14):2593–604.

161. Lee IM. Physical activity and cancer prevention-data from epidemiologic studies. Med Sci Sports Exerc. 2003;35(11):1823–7.

162. Monninkhof EM, Elias SG, Vlems FA, van der Tweel I, Schuit AJ, Voskuil DW, et al. Physical activity and breast cancer: a systematic review. Epidemiology. 2007;18(1):137–57.

163. Schmid SM, Hallschmid M, Schultes B. The metabolic burden of sleep loss. Lancet Diabetes Endocrinol. 2015;3(1):52–62.

164. Erren TC, Morfeld P, Stork J, Knauth P, von Mulmann MJ, Breitstadt R, et al. Shift work, chronodisruption and cancer?--The IARC 2007 challenge for research and prevention and 10 theses from the Cologne Colloquium 2008. Scand J Work Environ Health. 2009;35(1):74–9.

165. Haus EL, Smolensky MH. Shift work and cancer risk: potential mechanistic roles of circadian disruption, light at night, and sleep deprivation. Sleep Med Rev. 2013;17(4):273–84.

166. Stevens RG, Brainard GC, Blask DE, Lockley SW, Motta ME. Breast cancer and circadian disruption from electric lighting in the modern world. CA Cancer J Clin. 2014;64(3):207–18.

167. Blask DE. Melatonin, sleep disturbance and cancer risk. Sleep Med Rev. 2009;13(4):257–64.

168. Kakizaki M, Kuriyama S, Sone T, Ohmori-Matsuda K, Hozawa A, Nakaya N, et al. Sleep duration and the risk of breast cancer: the Ohsaki Cohort Study. Br J Cancer. 2008;99(9):1502–5.

169. Grandes G, Sanchez A, Cortada JM, Balague L, Calderon C, Arrazola A, et al. Is integration of healthy lifestyle promotion into primary care feasible? Discussion and consensus sessions between clinicians and researchers. BMC Health Serv Res. 2008;8:213. https://doi.org/10.1186/1472-6963-8-213.

170. Jamal A, Dube SR, Malarcher AM, Shaw L, Engstrom MC. Centers for Disease Control and Prevention (CDC). Tobacco use screening and counseling during physician office visits among adults-National Ambulatory Medical Care Survey and National Health Interview Survey, United States, 2005–2009. MMWR Suppl. 2012;61(2):38–45.

171. Sherson EA, Yakes Jimenez E, Katalanos N. A review of the use of the 5 A's model for weight loss counselling: differences between physician practice and patient demand. Fam Pract. 2014;31(4):389–98.

Supportive Care and Psycho-oncology Issues During and Beyond Diagnosis and Treatment

Luzia Travado and Julia H. Rowland

So this is what it feels like to be told you have cancer. Shock, numbness, fear, unreality—this cannot actually be happening to me. (…) Suddenly I was out of control of my life; cancer had invaded my body and horror was fast invading my mind. [1]

(Scott H., Me: Why Me?—One Patient's Story, 1994, p. xiii).

17.1 Impact of Cancer and Its Consequences

17.1.1 Overview

The discovery of a breast lump by the woman herself or secondary to an otherwise routine breast screening examination is a highly anxiety producing experience. The anxiety is driven by the fear of receiving a diagnosis of cancer, which is still considered by many as a "death sentence" [2, 3], and represents a significant threat to a woman's physical and psychological integrity. A cancer diagnosis often forces people to confront their own mortality, precipitating a search for ways to negotiate uncertainty about the disease and the future. As illustrated in the above personal narrative, uncertainty, anxiety, a state of confusion and shock, denial, and feelings of

L. Travado (✉)
Psycho-Oncology, Neuropsychiatry Unit,
Champalimaud Clinical Center, Champalimaud
Foundation, Lisbon, Portugal

J. H. Rowland
Smith Center for Healing and the Arts,
Washington, DC, USA

Department of Psychiatry, Georgetown University
School of Medicine, Washington, DC, USA

anger or rage are characteristic of individuals who are confronted with an acute crisis such as a diagnosis of cancer. A variety of factors enter into a woman's adaptation to her diagnosis including the nature of her illness (stage, treatment options, likely side effects and late risks), what she brings to the experience in terms of personal and psychosocial resources, the social context within which her illness and treatment occur, and, importantly, the supportive care she receives along the way. Age at time of diagnosis exerts a unique influence on adaptation.

17.1.2 Breast Cancer in the Younger Woman

While women of all ages may worry about threat to life and future health, as well as the potential for disfigurement, disability, and discomfort associated with treatment, these fears are often heightened in younger women (those under age 40 as defined by the BCY Consensus Guidelines [4]) for whom the diagnosis of cancer is experienced as being "off-time" in their expected life course. Median age at diagnosis of breast cancer in the USA is 62; as of January 1, 2018, an estimated 63% of breast cancer survivors are aged 65

© Springer Nature Switzerland AG 2020
O. Gentilini et al. (eds.), *Breast Cancer in Young Women*,
https://doi.org/10.1007/978-3-030-24762-1_17

or older [5]. By comparison, breast cancer in a younger woman is less common.

The diagnosis and management of cancer in a young woman sets her on a potential collision course with normal personal and family development stages [4]. Young women are usually leading very active lives; many are striving to attain or are at the peak of their professional careers; many will be married or in committed relationships, or if single wishing to date or seek life partnerships; many will have children at home, or wish to have a child; all are fully engaged in their life projects and social life. Beyond the disruption of multiple active roles, there is the perception of having more to lose, an anticipated threat to nascent career and family aspirations, and, at the extreme, a potentially foreshortened future.

Although younger women represent a minority of breast cancer cases, they tend to be overrepresented among those experiencing the poorest psychosocial adjustment during and following treatment. Worse quality of life and depressive symptoms have been shown to be more frequent and severe in breast cancer survivors age 50 or younger when compared to the general age-matched population and older women (age > 50) with cancer [6]. Concerns most frequently reported in this age group pertain to body image, sexual functioning, fertility, relationships, fear of cancer recurrence, and caring for children; failure of healthcare providers to initiate conversations to educate women about treatment side effects early on and/or safely discuss sensitive issues; and the lack of widespread availability of professional psychosocial programs that are tailored to the unique needs of this age group [7]. Unchecked and unattended, these concerns are intrusive at the emotional and cognitive level and may interfere with social function and concentration.

17.2 Adaptation to Breast Cancer: A Phase Approach

Adaptation to cancer, a major stressor for anyone, varies widely from individual to individual and is influenced by a variety of factors. Among these are disease stage and where the person is in the disease trajectory [8].

17.2.1 Diagnosis of Cancer: A Crisis Event

Why me? What did I do wrong? Did I cause the cancer? Did someone wish this on me – who was it? Is this punishment? Am I going to die? These are some of the common questions a woman may ask. Fear, anxiety, depression, denial, psychic numbness, confusion, confronting one's mortality, terror, anger, and loss of trust in God, in self, in one's body, and in others are common feelings and reactions that women may exhibit [9].

A diagnosis of cancer introduces many alterations in a person's life that require adjustment, effective problem-solving, and active coping. Integrating the reality of the diagnosis into one's personal life, tolerating emotional turmoil and stress, accepting help and some dependency, adjusting to the milieu of the healthcare system, planning regular daily routines to undergo treatment, making decisions about treatment options, communicating about the illness/diagnosis and its implications to family and friends (specifically for younger patients, their children, and/or parents), and searching for meaning in the adverse episode they are living are some of the coping tasks identified in the early phase of dealing with diagnosis. All of these must be juggled while the woman simultaneously focuses on trying to get the best care possible or available with the least disruption to life [9].

In looking back, the early phase of care is reported by many women to be the most stressful of their breast cancer experience, that is, living with the uncertainty and trying to come to grips with a new reality while also making the "right" decisions about what to do next. As information about the recommended course of care emerges, and a plan of treatment is determined and therapy actually begins, anxiety generally tends to diminish.

17.2.2 Treatment: A Varied Journey

Although breast cancer treatment saves lives and has increased survival enormously in the past decades bringing new hope for cancer patients, it nevertheless entails, in most cases, complex, multimodal regimens that produce significant side effects with both short- and long-term consequences for the individual. Cancer and its treatment have the capacity to affect virtually all areas of the woman's life: physical, psychological, social, and spiritual, each of which may interfere with the woman's well-being and quality of life (see Table 17.1) [10, 11].

At the physical level, the type of available treatments may involve disfigurement (e.g., amputations, alopecia) or unpleasant symptoms (e.g., pain, nausea and vomiting, fatigue), as well as interfere with the body and its functions (including premature menopause, infertility).

Table 17.1 Adverse psychosocial and behavioral responses to cancer and its treatment[a,b]

Surgery	Altered body image (response to amputation, reconstruction, scarring), disfigurement/mutilation, loss of self-esteem
Radiation	Disfigurement (burns, fibrous breasts/tissue, tattooing)
Chemotherapy	Adherence issues, altered body image (alopecia/hair loss, skin changes, weight gain/loss), cognitive changes (problems with concentration and attention), sexual dysfunction (premature menopause, hot flashes, loss of libido/desire, infertility)
Hormonal therapy	Adherence issues, cognitive changes (problems with concentration and attention), sexual dysfunction (premature menopause, hot flashes, loss of libido/desire, infertility), weight gain
Cancer in general	Altered interpersonal relationships, anger, anxiety, cancer-related posttraumatic stress, blame (of others and/or self), depression, existential plight (Why me? Why now? What now?), fear of recurrence/second malignancy, financial worries, guilt, isolation, problems coping with number and/or intensity of physical side effects (e.g., nausea and vomiting, pain, fatigue, sleep disruption), sense of foreshortened future, social disruption (family, work), spiritual threat, stigmatization

[a]Responses are listed alphabetically, not in order of prevalence or importance which can vary across populations and for each woman respectively
[b]Adverse reactions to the newer biological and immunotherapies are still emerging and are not listed here. Given that many of these are taken over long periods of time, consideration should be given to the challenges of adherence

Combined, these can have significant consequences for patients' body image, sense of well-being, and performance in daily life activities [10, 11]. Innovative surgical procedures, including breast conservation (lumpectomy or partial breast surgery) and post-mastectomy reconstruction, have improved aesthetic outcomes for women, sparing them the deforming consequences of the more aggressive procedures performed in the past (e.g., radical mastectomy); they have also contributed to improved psychosocial outcomes [12–14]. New antiemetics (to control severe nausea and vomiting) and other supportive drugs are now commonly used to reduce the side effects of chemotherapy. The use of novel cold caps can even help prevent or reduce alopecia in women facing chemotherapy [15].

Therapy may also affect patients' neurocognitive function, resulting in decreased attention, poor concentration, and memory impairment [16]; generate fatigue [17]; and cause other effects such as problems with sleep [18], appetite [19], and sexual function [20].The most common physical symptoms reported by breast cancer patients are pain, fatigue, arm impairment, and postmenopausal complaints [13]. The stage of the disease at diagnosis and its characteristics, whether it is an initial stage or more advanced cancer, also have different implications in terms of the physical and psychological burden of symptoms (e.g., pain, depression, and delirium), with the advanced stages being associated with a heavier burden of illness (see following section on recurrence and advanced disease) [20]. For young women, hormone therapy, with its side effects of induced menopause, reduced libido, and vaginal dryness, can have a major impact on the woman's comfort with intimacy and sexuality with a partner.

From the psychological point of view, myriad reactions can contribute to distress. These include perceived loss of health, uncertainty about the future, threat of possible death, concern about physical symptoms and functional limitations, emotional lability (e.g., roller coaster feelings of fear, anxiety, worry, sadness, despair, change in body image), loss of control and autonomy, the need to rely on others, and the change in perspective about self and the future. These reactions may be more or less intense and lead to increased suffering for patients and their families, further contributing to the psychological distress associated with cancer [10, 21].

The family, social, and interpersonal dimensions are also affected by the disease and its treatments. When cancer strikes, the individual's social and family roles and routine tasks are disrupted, dismissed, or delegated to others to give priority to the demands of treatment. Feelings of loneliness or isolation, problems in returning to work, and marginalization or stigmatization are common issues reported by patients. The impact of cancer must also be considered at the spiritual and existential level. Religion and faith, the person's set of spiritual values, the meaning given to life and existence, and the perception of time and the future are often revisited in people affected by cancer or other chronic diseases in general. In particular, faith and spirituality frequently serve as central and valued components of many people's lives. These may play an important role in the cancer patient's adaptation, such that individuals with strong religious beliefs or sense of spirituality may be protected from psychological morbidity, specifically depression [22].

In addition to these diverse individual dimensions affected by the disease, another area of impact for the patient is her relationship with the healthcare system and the healthcare professionals involved in her care[23]. The type of communication and trust promoted by the healthcare staff is of utmost importance and significantly affects patients' adaptation to the disease and its treatments [23]. Further, other dimensions of cancer care delivery can create unique challenges to adaptation. These include distance from or barriers to care based on the location and accessibility of the hospital or clinic for the patient and her family, loss of privacy, the impersonal nature of treatments and procedures, and exposure to new and confusing terminology.

17.2.3 Recurrent or Metastatic Disease: Confronting Mortality

Knowledge that the cancer has returned or is found to be at an advanced stage can be devastating. If the recurrence is local and has the potential for cure, adaptation can occur over time [24]. However, even when disease is localized, levels of psychiatric morbidity can be high. When compared with disease-free survivors, women who experience a recurrence report worse physical functioning and perceived health, greater impairment in emotional well-being, more problems in family as well as healthcare provider relationships, and less hope [24].

When the disease is metastatic or stage IV at diagnosis or, despite treatment, progresses to a more advanced stage, the woman is confronted with a new set of challenges. Among these are the need for the woman to come to terms with the fact that her illness will never be cured (she will never be disease-free); rather, her cancer will become a chronic condition that must be actively managed. While there may be periods of relative relief, times of high symptoms and disease burden are also expected. Women may struggle with the lost hope for cure and accompanying need to face and prepare for end-of-life decisions and actions. In a survey conducted among women with metastatic breast cancer ($n = 618$), the most frequently reported symptoms were fatigue (98%), insomnia (84%), pain (79%), hot flashes (79%), cognitive problems (78%), hair loss (77%), sexual problems (73%), depression (66%), anxiety (59%), neuropathy (65%), loss of appetite (60%), and nausea (55%). The broad range and prevalence of symptoms experienced account for the diversity of physical as well as psychosocial needs of women in this phase [25]. In general, women with more advanced disease report higher rates of depression than those with earlier stage illness [26, 27]. Because pain is such a common—and often feared—experience in people living with advanced cancer, attention to its management as part of psychosocial care is critical.

17.2.4 Posttreatment: Embracing Survivorship

Addressing the psychosocial needs of young women treated for breast cancer does not end when treatment ends. Indeed, the unique psychosocial challenges related to the transition to recovery and life after breast cancer often catch many women, their loved ones—and even healthcare providers—by surprise. As some survivors describe the reentry phase, "It is not over when it is over!"

Women who may have adapted well during treatment can find anxiety increasing as the end of therapy approaches. A number of factors attendant to the termination of treatment serve to fan women's anxiety. These include fear that the cancer will come back once treatment stops, loss of a supportive and caring clinical environment, lack of a clear plan for future care and worry about who will provide this care as well as who to call if there is a problem, the cumulative effects of treatment (such that women often find they feel worse, not better at the end of treatment), and pressure by family and friends to return to "normal" function. Finding her "new normal" takes time, as does the recovery process. Giving women permission to take the time necessary to heal and to process the experience she has undergone is helpful in aiding recovery.

Younger breast cancer survivors report lower quality of life after treatment when compared to older women, and the largest functional deficits when compared to age-matched peers without a cancer history [28]. They talk about having to endure long-term (5–10 years) effects such as earlier menopause (with its hot flashes, lower sexual desire, vaginal dryness, reduced frequency of sexual activity), reduced breast sensitivity, infertility, menstrual changes, lymphedema, pain, sleep problems, weight gain, scars (body-image issues), and problems with physical and recreational activities due to physical limitations. They also report experiencing a disrupted sense of normalcy in their physical developmental trajectory, their womanhood, their youth and health, and their family plans and a negative impact in particular on couple well-being [28].

Despite cancer's challenges, those who have worked long term with breast cancer survivors often note their remarkable resilience; some have even studied posttraumatic growth as a benefit to surviving life-threatening illness [29]. Nevertheless, cure comes with a human cost. Research shows that breast cancer survivors are at higher risk of late morbidity which in turn can

affect their participation in the workforce [30]. Population-based data suggest that over time, carrying a cancer history puts survivors at greater risk for experiencing problems in their physical (24.5%) and mental (10.1%) health compared with 10.2% and 5.9% of adults without cancer, respectively [31]. A large, international retrospective study of suicide among long-term breast cancer survivors saw elevated risk compared to population norms for women even 25 or more years after diagnosis [32]. These findings have propelled the clinical community to recommend extending routine screening for distress and/or anxiety and depression beyond the active treatment phase [33, 34].

17.3 Risk Factors for Distress

While not always systematically assessed, the risk factors for problems in adapting to cancer are well known and described (see Table 17.2) [35–38]. These can be viewed as falling into three main categories: medical (the clinical characteristics of the situation), personal (what a woman brings to her experience, both coping assets and liabilities), and social (the context in which disease is treated and associated resources). To these are added factors that are particular to breast cancer (e.g., genetic or family history, concern about breast disfigurement). With few exceptions (age, stage at diagnosis, prior history of cancer and/or trauma), most are amenable to supportive intervention. For example, women experiencing isolation can be linked to support groups and/or seen in consultation by mental health staff; those concerned with the economic burden of cancer can be referred to financial services or agencies that help with cost of care. Even the adverse effect of low income/education can be modified by use of educational materials tailored for appropriate reading levels and referral to social services to help with transportation, child-care needs, and barriers to access to care. Some of these risk factors are embedded in current quick-screen tools such as the Distress Thermometer checklist discussed later in this chapter. Finding a way to evaluate women for each of these risk factors and considering approaches to address them in plans

Table 17.2 Risk factors for poor adaptation

1. Medical
(a) More advanced disease/worse prognosis
(b) More intense or aggressive treatment
(c) Other/multiple comorbid conditions
(d) Greater symptom burden (e.g., pain, fatigue, lymphedema)
(e) Fewer rehabilitative options
(f) Poor doctor/patient relationship
2. Personal
(a) Prior psychiatric history
(b) Past trauma history (especially physical or sexual abuse)
(c) Rigid or limited coping capacity
(d) Helpless/hopeless outlook
(e) Low income/education
(f) Multiple competing demands (e.g., work, child or other family care, economic concerns)
(g) Poor marital/interpersonal relationships
(h) Younger age (<40) or older age (>80)
(i) Having children younger than 21
3. Social
(a) Lack of social support (and/or religious affiliation) (including lack of a partner: single, divorced, widowed)
(b) Limited access to service resources
(c) Multiple stressful life events
(d) Cultural biases
(e) Social stigma or illness taboo
4. Breast cancer specific
(a) Prior breast cancer experience
• Recurrence or second breast cancer
• Loss of family or friends to breast cancer
(b) High investment in body image, in particular breasts

Source: Adapted from Weisman D. Early diagnosis of vulnerability in cancer patients Am J Med Sci 1976;271:187

for care at the outset can help reduce risk of poor adaptation later.

17.4 Prevalence of Distress, Anxiety, and Depression in Women with Breast Cancer

In the face of a cancer diagnosis and the demands of treatment, many patients develop symptoms indicative of psychological distress. Psychological suffering of cancer patients was coined as *distress* by the National Comprehensive Cancer Network (NCCN) in order to destigmatize as well as differentiate these reactions from standard mental health conditions or nomenclature, categorizations that often do not apply in the cancer setting. Cancer-related distress was defined as:

> …a multifactorial unpleasant emotional experience of a psychological (i.e., cognitive, behavioral, emotional), social and/or spiritual nature that may interfere with the ability to cope effectively with cancer, its physical symptoms, and its treatment. Distress extends along a continuum, ranging from common feelings of vulnerability, sadness and fears to problems that can become disabling, such as depression, anxiety, panic, social isolation and spiritual crisis (NCCN, 2018) [39].

Reflected in this definition is the premise that it is considered normal for patients to develop emotional reactions when confronted with cancer, such as fear, worry, or sadness. In a subset of individuals, these states may escalate into conditions with clinical significance, such as anxiety, depression, or maladjustment. These latter states are pathological and therefore termed as "psychological morbidity" versus distress. Over time, most patients adjust to the cancer experience and, as noted earlier, may even find a sense of personal growth, giving life new and more positive meanings (i.e., posttraumatic growth) [29, 40]. Nevertheless, it is still the case that for the majority of patients the initial experience of the disease and its treatments have dramatic consequences for their psychosocial equilibrium and quality of life [41].

The prevalence of distress in cancer patients has been studied in many countries worldwide. In a landmark study conducted by Zabora and colleagues in which they assessed 4496 cancer patients, the average prevalence rate of psychological distress was 35.1% and ranged from 43.4% in patients with lung cancer to 29.6% in women with gynecologic cancer, to 32.8% for patients with early stage breast cancer [42]. Other international studies report similar findings suggesting that about 4 in 10 cancer patients experience significant distress [43, 44], a prevalence figure similar to that found in younger early-stage breast cancer [45]. For metastatic breast cancer patients, prevalence of distress can be as high as 60% [46]. In their experience, Ruddy and colleagues found later stage of disease and financial difficulties increased risk for distress, whereas factors such as level of education, type of surgery, receipt of chemotherapy, employment status, marital status, having children, family history of cancer, and alcohol consumption were not found to be predictors of anxiety, depression, or overall distress [45].

Depression and anxiety have been identified as the most significant source of psychological morbidity associated with cancer [21], along with adjustment disorder [47]. In their study using the Diagnostic and Statistical Manual of Mental Disorders (DSM) or the International Classification of Diseases (ICD) criteria, Mitchell and colleagues found the prevalence of depression to be 16.5% (13.1–20.3%), adjustment disorder to be 15.4% (10.1–21.6%), and anxiety disorders to be 9.8% (6.8–13.2%) [47]. While these data pertained to single diagnosis, a combination of emotional problems was found to be frequent, with all types of depression occurring in 20.7% of patients (12.9–29.8%), depression plus adjustment disorder in 31.6% (25.0–38.7%), and any mood disorder in 38.2% (28.4–48.6%) [47]. Of note, marked distress associated with disruption of social or occupational function may show up as an adjustment disorder [48].

Not surprisingly, depression and anxiety are also the most frequent cause of psychological morbidity following the diagnosis and treatment of breast cancer [49–51]. Actual prevalence varies by study but may range from 20 to 50% for women with early-stage breast cancer in the first year after diagnosis [36, 52, 53]. In a study we conducted with Portuguese breast cancer patients who were posttreatment for their disease [54], we found the presence of anxiety in 39.1% of the women and depression in 29.1%; as many as ¼ of the women (16.1–24.5%) reported psychological morbidity. Others have confirmed this pattern [55]. Importantly, a number of studies examining quality-of-life outcomes following breast cancer report a negative association with depression and anxiety [54, 56, 57].

Depression is the psychological response to the losses the cancer patient faces in her illness trajectory and is characterized by the presence of symptoms of depressed mood and anhedonia, appetite and sleep disturbance, psychomotor agitation or retardation, decreased energy, feelings of worthlessness or guilt, difficulty concentrating, and/or suicidal ideation [58]. Depression can range on a continuum of intensity from mild subthreshold symptoms to moderate and severe symptoms, which may account for major depression [59].

Anxiety is the psychological response to the threat of life, uncertainty, and suffering the cancer patient faces in her illness trajectory and is characterized by the presence of symptoms such as fear, difficulty concentrating, irritability, sleep disturbance, excessive worry and fright, palpitations, shortness of breath, restlessness, sweats, and gastrointestinal discomfort, among others [60]. Anxiety may range from mild to severe and may have peaks at critical points or phases during the course of the disease similar to patterns reported for other life-threatening illnesses [61]. Critical anxiety-generating phases are the time of diagnosis, before and during major treatments in the acute phase (e.g., surgery, chemotherapy, radiotherapy), before and during clinical tests (e.g., biopsy, PET scan), in the chronic phase when facing symptoms that suggest a recurrence or when a relapse is diagnosed, before and after receiving clinical results, and when entering terminal phase [62]. Anxiety has been found to be more frequent in the pretreatment phases while depression is more common in the posttreatment ones [63]. The prevalence of anxiety varies according to the phase in which the patient is in the cancer trajectory. In a large cohort study of adult outpatients, 34% had significant anxiety symptoms [64].

Psychological morbidity has significant negative consequences for the patient, affecting her quality of life [65], and clinical outcomes. It has been reported in several studies that it decreases treatment compliance [66, 67], reduces the effectiveness of chemotherapy [68], shortens survival time [69, 70], increases symptom burden and functional impairment [71], results in longer hospital stays [72], and increases risk of suicide [73]. The breadth of reported negative effects of psychological morbidity on patients' clinical outcomes makes clear that in treating the cancer, the patient's psychosocial variables can play an independent role and can either facilitate or complicate health-related outcomes.

17.5 Psychological Interventions

How women adjust to their cancer is closely related to the way they evaluate their illness. According to the *transactional stress model* of Richard Lazarus [74, 75], the emotional reaction and the psychological adjustment of a person to a stressful event is determined by her appraisal of the threat and the resources perceived as being available to help her cope. This opens up the field for psychological interventions, particularly cognitive-behavioral therapy (CBT) interventions [76].

A broad array of interventions has proved successful in reducing the psychological symptoms of women with breast cancer in the various phases of the disease continuum; these have also shown efficacy in reducing symptom burden, improving overall quality of life, and facilitating psychosocial adjustment. These are well reviewed elsewhere [77–80]. A detailed review of the use of different interventions across the course of care is beyond the scope of this chapter. Interventions vary widely by type (e.g., individual vs. group), orientation (e.g., behavioral vs. cognitive vs. supportive), mode of delivery (in person vs. remote), duration (time limited vs. open-ended), and timing (before, during, and/or after treatment), as well as target audience served (early vs. advanced stage, younger than 40 vs. older, partnered vs. single, or mixed). All share a fundamental purpose, namely, to provide each woman with the skills or resources necessary to cope with her illness and improve the quality of her life and health. It is clear that work remains to be done to help us more systematically determine who needs what, delivered by whom, and when in the course of care [81]. However, a few broad generalizations can be made about use of these programs in the care and support of women treated for breast cancer and their families.

First, women who receive an intervention designed to improve well-being, and coping, or reduce distress do better than women who do not. Importantly, they are not at risk for doing worse. Women receiving some form of individual or group therapy experienced less anxiety and depression, reported increased sense of control, improved body image and better sexual function, had greater satisfaction with care, and exhibited improved medication adherence [82, 83]. In a meta-analysis, new interventions such as mindfulness-based stress reduction (MBSR) have also shown significant benefits in reducing stress, anxiety, and depression [84].

Second, in the small number of studies that compared or controlled for mode of delivery, no difference was found for outcomes between women receiving individual versus group interventions. This is reassuring as individually tailored programs (arguably the ideal for maximizing effect) are not always feasible. Some argue that group participation offers the advantage of providing a uniquely supportive and normalizing experience. Current experimentation with online, web-based, telephone, and digital (applications or apps) modalities for intervention delivery has the potential to overcome barriers of isolation, distance or access to programs, desire for privacy or anonymity, and also tailored personalization not readily attainable in less nimble, older individual and group interventions.

Third, the use of psychosocial and behavioral interventions in cancer continues to rise. The use of these services reflects both patient demand and growing awareness that addressing psychosocial distress may improve physical outcomes for survivors. Current opinion is that such interventions do *not* prolong survival [85, 86], but do help women "live better," although there is provocative evidence to suggest that women in the highest risk groups for medical and psychological morbidity (see Table 17.1) may realize a survival benefit [87, 88]. These techniques and therapies are important resources for the clinician to have for use in the psychological treatment of women as part of quality cancer care. Based on the literature to date, evidence-based psychosocial interventions addressing cancer patients' psychosocial needs have proven beneficial to patients' psychological adjustment. When appropriately administered, they have the potential to significantly reduce psychological symptoms of depression and anxiety, prevent psychological morbidity, increase treatment compliance, improve quality of life and well-being, facilitate the recovery process and return to work, and, in limited instances, may even increase survival time [59, 62, 85–88]. In addition to reducing the human cost of cancer, psychosocial interventions have the potential to reduce the long-term economic cost of this disease, which may be of keen interest to overburdened healthcare systems [89]. When systematically integrated into cancer care, and to the extent that they result in adequate support for and rehabilitation of patients with respect to their unique individual, social, and economic need, psychosocial care can be expected to help reduce healthcare costs. This effect is reported in *The Scientific Evidence of Cost-Effectiveness of Psychological Interventions in Health Care*, prepared by the Portuguese College of Psychologists in 2011 [90].

17.6 Standards and Clinical Guidelines

To achieve the best clinical outcomes for patients, quality cancer care nowadays demands that patients' psychosocial needs be regularly assessed and that psychosocial oncology services and/or specialists are available to address those needs as an integral part of comprehensive cancer treatment and care [10, 91–95]. To guide the clinical practice of psychosocial oncology in cancer care, some scientific bodies and some countries have developed clinical guidelines in this area that serve not only to assist the clinician in choosing best practices but also to regulate and standardize delivery of this care (i.e., contribute to quality care standards). A number of standards and clinical practice guidelines for the provision of psychosocial cancer care have been published in the last dozen years, and a number of international recommendations have been issued that call for (a) the integration of psychosocial care into routine cancer practice, (b) implementation of regular distress screening, and (c) inclusion of

psychosocial care as a unique component of cancer policy documents [4, 10, 11, 39, 96–98].

The National Comprehensive Cancer Network (NCCN) Distress Management guideline, one of the first efforts in this area, was originally created by the US-based NCCN in 1997 and is updated annually. The guideline incorporates use of a screening tool for distress, called the Distress Thermometer, and a checklist of symptoms and problems that may contribute to distress. The measure is simple, brief, and easy to administer in the clinic, allowing for rapid identification of areas of need, and helpful in guiding patients to appropriate referral for specialized professionals per the guidelines provided by NCCN for distress management [39]. This tool has been validated in most countries throughout the world that have a cancer policy and have psychosocial oncology care available for their cancer patients [63, 99, 100] and is presently being used in a number of settings to screen for patients' distress and psychosocial needs.

Other countries have advanced efforts to provide cancer care for the whole patient by developing their own clinical guidelines [101], embracing the assertion that "Today, it is not possible to deliver good-quality cancer care without using existing approaches, tools, and resources to address patients' psychosocial health needs. All patients with cancer and their families should expect and receive cancer care that ensures the provision of appropriate psychosocial health services." [10]

Despite broad recognition of the importance of psychosocial well-being to quality cancer care, and notwithstanding the existence of published recommendations and clinical guidelines to address this domain of care, the psychosocial needs of patients with cancer continue to be frequently dismissed or underestimated. Psycho-oncology services are not yet offered on a regular basis as part of the treatment of cancer patients [102, 103], creating a major gap in cancer care and the rehabilitation of cancer patients.

A recent report conducted by the European Commission Initiative on Breast Cancer (ECIBC), which focused on the development of a voluntary European quality assurance (QA) scheme for breast cancer, identified an irregular landscape regarding the provision of psycho-oncological support for women treated for breast cancer in the European Breast Units [104]. The report noted that the identified gaps in care could be overcome by making provision of psycho-oncological care a requirement for the accreditation of Breast Units, a goal which the working group intends to pursue.

To overcome the many disparities in the treatment and survival of European cancer patients across countries, two guides for informing European cancer policy were recently produced co-financed by the European Commission: (1) the *European Guide for Quality National Cancer Control Programmes* (NCCPs), which features a chapter on Psychosocial Oncology Care discussing the necessary program elements for quality psycho-oncological care delivery [97], and (2) the *European Guide for Quality Improvement in Comprehensive Cancer Control*, which includes a chapter on Survivorship and Rehabilitation [98] that contains guidance on how to provide and implement quality rehabilitation and survivorship care.

Clear in all of this work is that guidelines alone do not change behavior. Rather, finding ways to systematically incorporate best psychosocial practices into standard oncology care will be needed if we are to truly change outcomes for cancer patients at large and for young breast cancer patients and survivors specifically. To do this, engaging all relevant stakeholders in the effort will be key: patients, healthcare providers, administrators, healthcare delivery systems, payors (individual and/or governmental), and policymakers.

17.7   Special Issues in Adaptation

Because of the central role they play in the adaptation of those diagnosed with cancer, two additional topics are covered here briefly: the impact of cancer on sexual function and the impact of cancer on and role of family/partners in survivors' health and function.

17.7.1   Sexual Functioning

The impact of cancer and its treatment on sexual health and function is a concern for all women but may take on particular importance for younger women for whom sexual role and capacity are often more central to self-esteem than among older breast cancer patients and for whom planned treatment may involve added threat to fertility [6]. Once rarely discussed, cancer's effect on sexual well-being has garnered research attention due both to compelling advocacy by women for greater attention to these issues and to the large number of women for whom treatment causes significant problems in this valued area of function. A range of changes in women's sexual function after breast cancer has been documented, including disruption in normative sexual processes (e.g., desire, arousal, lubrication, and orgasm), along with diminished sexual activity and pleasure. Most of these effects are secondary to chemotherapy and hormonal therapy, with surgery conferring a more limited impact (e.g., alterations in body image, interference with function due to lymphedema or persistent postoperative pain syndromes, decrease in breast sensitivity) [105].

A key barrier to addressing sexual dysfunction when it occurs is avoidance of this sensitive topic by both provider and patient. In addition to the discomfort most people feel when discussing sex, practitioners must contend with limited time and often lack of privacy to raise these issues, lack of awareness that sexual problems are being encountered, or, when present, knowledge about local resources to address them. Currently, this last barrier is diminishing as education about effective therapies for common problems, such as vaginal dryness, hot flashes, painful intercourse, and loss of desire, is becoming more broadly disseminated. Clinical guidelines for management of fertility [106–108], and more recently sexual problems broadly [109], are now available. Central to the recommendations addressed in these documents is that it is the responsibility of the clinician to raise this topic and to do so early in the course of care so that plans can be made to manage women's needs and concerns about sexual function during and after cancer.

17.7.2 Cancer and the Family/Partner

Social support and connection are linked not only to an individual's mental health but also to his/her morbidity and mortality, a finding seen in the general population [110], and also among breast cancer survivors [111, 112]. The advocacy community has long recognized the importance of informal cancer caregivers, largely family members, in their loved one's well-being, including these individuals in the definition of survivors [39].

It is well documented that cancer, along with being a significant stressor for patients, also precipitates a crisis for family, increasing members' emotional distress and affecting their physical health and well-being [113]. Caregivers, predominantly women and spouses, report significant caregiver-related burden, stress, and depression, feeling unprepared for caregiver tasks they perform, and receiving limited training for their role [114, 115]. Caregivers often balance other life responsibilities (e.g., work, caring for children or other adults) [116, 117], often have their own health issues, and frequently neglect aspects of self-care [114, 115, 118]. Studies show their psychosocial well-being may be interdependent on that of their care recipient such that when one member of the dyad does poorly so does the other [119]. By consequence, interventions that improve the well-being of one can positively influence the function of the other [119].

Because family is important for patient well-being, both in practical terms (e.g., transportation to clinic, management of daily living arrangements, overseeing medications, providing food, funds, and other resources) and psycho-emotional (e.g., providing love, reassurance, support, nurturing, meaning), engaging and supporting family in the process of care and allocating specific additional psychosocial resources for them should be part of comprehensive care. It has been reported that, in the case of the patient's death, a family that has had no psychosocial support throughout the patient's disease trajectory has an increased risk of traumatic or complicated grief [120]. Fortunately, work is progressing on interventions designed to promote couples' adaptation [121]. Attending to the concerns of both parties regarding threats to good communication and relationship maintenance may be particularly helpful [122].

17.7.3 Cancer and the Family/ Children

When young children are involved, a family's adaptation can be challenging. In one US report, it was estimated that 24% of adults with cancer are parenting children younger than 18 [123]. Children and teens whose parents are diagnosed with cancer are more likely to experience increased levels of anxiety and distress. Problems with self-esteem may also occur [124–126]. Manifestations of distress may be reflected in physical symptoms (e.g., pain, discomfort), changes in mood and school performance, as well as altered social and interpersonal relationships [127]. Children's emotional and behavioral reactions can be diverse and also fluctuate over time. Developmental differences in how children cope with a parent's illness can also be seen. Preschool children are most affected by changes in their routine, especially variations in who is caring for them; they are more likely to experience separation anxiety, depression, and attachment problems. School age and adolescents are at risk for feelings of hopelessness. They are also vulnerable to anger about the diagnosis and its associated impact on emotional isolation, or potentially guilt and feelings of being responsible for the parent's illness [127]. Teens are often expected to assume increased personal responsibilities while one parent spends more time caring for the ill parent, leading to less free time during a period when being with peers is critical for social development [125, 128]. The diagnosis of breast cancer in the mother may be particularly difficult for adolescent girls who may focus on the long-term implications of the illness and worry if a similar fate awaits them [129, 130].

It is important to note that parents often under-report or fail to recognize the intensity of their child/children's distress when compared to children's own self-report. It is also the case that each parent may perceive different challenges in parenting during this journey and use different coping strategies and resources to manage them [131].

In addition to a widening set of published and online cancer-related resources [132–134], a variety of interventions for parents, children, or both have proven beneficial to family function. Which interventions are expected to be most beneficial for whom and when remains unclear [135]. Generally, providing support early in these situations works best. However, those designing program delivery need to take into account that the time around diagnosis is often overwhelming for all members of a family and hence not always the ideal moment to introduce more complex issues to consider and tasks to assume [124]. Overall, the literature suggests that key to helping children cope with a parent's illness is open and direct communication. Taking time to think about when and how to have important conversations, what to say, and the choice of words to use is important. In addition to using age-appropriate language, children may need help in communicating with parents, other family members, and healthcare professionals. Further, assuring that there is an environment where they feel comfortable sharing positive/negative emotions and can have their experiences normalized among peers is also important [135]. For young children, keeping the family routine as close to normal as possible is recommended [136]. Monitoring school performance and talking with teachers about what is going on at home can help support school-age children's coping and also set in place a way to ensure that if problems occur, the family can intervene early as needed. Ensuring that adolescents have time for themselves also promotes healthy adaptation. If the cancer is advanced, many families have found that having the ill parent write letters to their children that they can keep as manifestations of their mother's love and concern for them can have a profoundly comforting effect. These serve as tangible legacies, help-ing children as they mature in the absence of a parent [137]. When problems persist, consideration should be given to seeking counseling with someone knowledgeable with both cancer and child development. Finding and participating in support groups of other parents, as well as identifying groups for children dealing with parental illness, can be an additional way to foster effective problem solving and reduce isolation among both parents and affected children [124, 135].

17.8 Conclusion

In summary, although differences exist concerning the exact percentage of young breast cancer patients/survivors who experience psychological morbidity (generally the result of variations in the measures used to study this effect, cancer populations screened, and timing of the assessments performed), findings point to a consistent subset of individuals whose levels of psychological distress and morbidity, and range of psychosocial needs, require specialized attention and care. The number of individuals affected, often ranging from a quarter to a third or more of samples evaluated, is important for understanding the relevance of psychosocial care in cancer and the critical need to make delivery of psychosocial services a part of high-quality cancer care. What the woman brings to her experience with respect to her strengths and vulnerabilities, the medical and treatment realities she faces, and the social environment, both personal and medical, in which she is cared for all contribute to her immediate and long-term adaptation. Further, her needs and capacity for adaptation will vary over time, depending on where she is in the trajectory of care and recovery.

Clear from this review is that to minimize cancer's adverse effects, women's psychosocial needs must be assessed at diagnosis and across the course of care, and referral to evidence-based programs of supportive care or interventions made as needed. These interventions may be particularly critical for the young breast cancer patient already at higher risk for problems coping. Attention to asking about sexual function is an important aspect of this care, as is attending to the needs of the partner or family caregivers in their efforts to support the woman living with, through and beyond a breast cancer diagnosis.

Enormous progress has been made internationally in the development and promulgation of guidelines for the incorporation of psychosocial care as part of high-quality, comprehensive cancer care. It is critical to recognize, however, that these are insufficient to ensure psychosocial needs will be met in the absence of a collective will and, importantly, the resources to do so. Looking to the future, it may be necessary for individuals in diverse practice settings to be identified as responsible for the coordination and oversight of the psychosocial component of care and to work collaboratively with key stakeholders to ensure that published standards for care are met. Also national and international regulatory bodies, such as the accreditation of Breast Units, should make it mandatory that psycho-oncology specialized professionals are available to provide psychosocial care for patients, partners, and children. Ensuring cancer care for the whole patient will optimize clinical outcomes for patients and families and be of important societal value.

References

1. Scott H. "Me: why me?"- One patient story. In: Barraclough J, editor. Cancer and emotion: a practical guide to psycho-oncology. Chichester: John Wiley and Sons; 1994. p. xiii.
2. Travado L, Reis J. What do they think about their illness? Breast cancer patients' conceptions about their illness and recovery. Psycho-Oncology. 2000;9(5):386.
3. Travado L, Reis JC. Breast cancer meanings: a cognitive-developmental study. Psychooncology. 2013;22(9):2016–23. https://doi.org/10.1002/pon.3246. Epub 2013 Feb 18.
4. Paluch-Shimon S, Pagani O, Partridge AH, Abulkhair O, Cardoso MJ, Dent RA, Gelmon K, Gentilini O, Harbeck N, Margulies A, Meirow D, Pruneri G, Senkus E, Spanic T, Sutliff M, Travado L, Peccatori F, Cardoso F. ESO-ESMO 3rd international consensus guidelines for breast cancer in young women (BCY3). Breast. 2017;35:203–17. https://doi.org/10.1016/j.breast.2017.07.017. Epub 2017 Aug 17. http://www.thebreastonline.com/article/S0960-9776(17)30548-9/pdf
5. Rowland JH, Mariotto A, Elena JW. Epidemiology of cancer survivorship: past, current and future. In: Feuerstein M, Nekhlyudov L, editors. Handbook of cancer survivorship. Philadelphia: Springer Verlag; 2018.
6. Howard-Anderson J, Ganz PA, Bower JE, et al. Quality of life, fertility concerns and behavioral health outcomes in younger breast cancer survivors: a systematic review. J Natl Cancer Inst. 2012;104:386–405.
7. Ahmad S, Fergus K, McCarthy M. Psychosocial issues experienced by young women with breast cancer: the minority group with the majority of need. Curr Opin Support Palliat Care. 2015;9(3):271–8.
8. Stanton AL, Wiley JF, Krull JL, et al. Depressive episodes, symptoms, and trajectories in women recently diagnosed with breast cancer. Breast Cancer Res Treat. 2015;154:105–15.
9. Loscalzo M, BrintzenhofeSzoc K. Brief crisis counseling. In: Holland J, editor. Psycho-oncology. New York: Oxford University Press; 1998. p. 662–75.
10. Adler NE, Page AEK. Cancer care for the whole patient: meeting psychosocial health needs. Washington, DC: The National Academies Press; 2008.
11. Grassi L, Travado L. The role of psychosocial oncology in cancer care. In: Coleman MP, Alexe D, Albreht T, McKee M, editors. Responding to the challenge of cancer in Europe. Ljubljana: Institute of Public Health of the Republic of Slovenia; 2008. p. 209–29.
12. Monteiro-Grillo I, Marques-Vidal P, Jorge M. Psychosocial effect of mastectomy versus conservative surgery in patients with early breast cancer. Clin Transl Oncol. 2005;7(11):499–503.
13. Montazeri A. Health-related quality of life in breast cancer patients: a bibliographic review of the literature from 1974 to 2007. J Exp Clin Cancer Res. 2008;27:32.
14. Al-Ghazal SK, Fallowfield L, Blamey RW. Comparison of psychological aspects and patient satisfaction following breast conserving surgery, simple mastectomy and breast reconstruction. Eur J Cancer. 2000;36:1938–43.
15. Cigler T, Isseroff D, Fiederlein B, et al. Efficacy of scalp cooling in preventing chemotherapy-induced alopecia in breast cancer patients receiving adjuvant docetaxel and cyclophosphamide chemotherapy. Clin Breast Cancer. 2015;15(5):332–4.
16. Ahles TA, Correa DD. Neuropsychological impact of cancer and cancer treatments. In: Holland J, Breitbart W, Jacobsen P, Lederberg M, Loscalzo M, McCorkle R, editors. Psycho-oncology. New York: Oxford University Press; 2010. p. 251–7.
17. Goedendorp MM, Jacobsen PB, Andrykowski MA. Fatigue screening in breast cancer patients: identifying likely cases of cancer-related fatigue. Psycho-Oncology. 2016;25(3):275–81. https://doi.org/10.1002/pon.3907.

18. Yue HJ, Dimsdale JE. Sleep and cancer. In: Holland J, Breitbart W, Jacobsen P, Lederberg M, Loscalzo M, McCorkle R, editors. Psycho-oncology. New York: Oxford University Press; 2010. p. 259–69.

19. Fleishman SB, Chadha JS. Weight and appetite loss in cancer. In: Holland J, Breitbart W, Jacobsen P, Lederberg M, Loscalzo M, McCorkle R, editors. Psycho-oncology. New York: Oxford University Press; 2010. p. 270–4.

20. Roth AJ, Carter J, Nelson CJ. Sexuality after cancer. In: Holland J, Breitbart W, Jacobsen P, Lederberg M, Loscalzo M, McCorkle R, editors. Psycho-oncology. New York: Oxford University Press; 2010. p. 245–50.

21. Grassi L, Travado L, Gil F, Sabato S, Rossi E, The SEPOS Group. Psychosocial morbidity and its correlates in cancer patients of the Mediterranean area: findings from the southern European psycho-oncology study (SEPOS). J Affect Disord. 2004;83:243–8.

22. Travado L, Grassi L, Gil F, Martins C, Ventura C, Bairradas J, The SEPOS Group. Do spirituality and faith make a difference? Report from the southern European psycho-oncology study (SEPOS). Palliat Support Care. 2010;8:405–13.

23. Epstein RM, Street RL Jr. Patient-centered communication in cancer care: promoting healing and reducing suffering. Bethesda: MD: National Cancer Institute., NIH Publication No. 07–6225; 2007.

24. Yang HC, Thornton LM, Shapiro CL, et al. Surviving recurrence: psychological and quality-of-life recovery. Cancer. 2008;112:1178–87.

25. MayerM, GroberS. Silent voices: women with metastatic breast cancer share their needs and preferences for information, support and practical services. Living Beyond Breast Cancer. 2006. http://www.advancedbc.org/content/silent-voices. Accessed 24 Jan 2018

26. Grabsch B, Clarke DM, Love A, McKenzie DP, Snyder RD, Bloch S, Smith G, Kissane DW. Psychological morbidity and quality of life in women with advanced breast cancer: a cross-sectional survey. Palliat Support Care. 2006;4:47–56.

27. Lo C, et al. Longitudinal study of depressive symptoms in patients with metastatic gastrointestinal and lung cancer. J Clin Oncol. 2010;28:3084–9.

28. Baucom DH, Porter LS, Kirby JS, Gremore TM, Keefe FJ. Psychosocial Issues confronting young women with breast cancer. Breast Dis. 2005–2006;23:103–13.

29. Bellizzi KM, Smith AW, Reeve BB, et al. Posttraumatic growth and health-related quality of life in a racially diverse cohort of breast cancer survivors. J Health Psychol. 2010;15:615–26.

30. Bradley CJ, Neumark D, Luo Z. Employment and cancer: findings from a longitudinal study of breast and prostate cancer survivors. Cancer Investig. 2007;25:47–54.

31. Weaver KE, Forsythe LP, FReeve BB, et al. Mental and physical health-related quality of life among U.S. cancer survivors: population estimates from the 2010 National Health Interview Survey. Cancer Epidemiol Biomark Prev. 2012;21:2108–17.

32. Schairer C, Brown LM, Chen BE, et al. Suicide after breast cancer: an international population-based study of 723,810 women. J Natl Cancer Inst. 2006;98(19):1416–9.

33. Andersen BL, Rowland JH, Somerfield MR. Screening, assessment, and care of anxiety and depressive symptoms in adults with cancer: an American Society of Clinical Oncology guidelines adaptation. J Oncol Pract. 2015;11(2):133–4.

34. Andersen BL, DeRubeis RJ, Berman BS, et al. Screening, assessment, and care of anxiety and depressive symptoms in adults with cancer: an American Society of Clinical Oncology guidelines adaptation. J Clin Oncol. 2014;20(32):1605–19.

35. Brandao T, Schulz MS, Matos PM. Psychological adjustment after breast cancer: a systematic review of longitudinal studies. Psychooncology. 2017;26(7):917–26.

36. Burgess C, Cornelius V, Love S, Graham J, Richards M, Ramirez A. Depression and anxiety in women with early breast cancer: five year observational cohort study. Br Med J. 2005;330(7493):702–5.

37. Janz NK, Mujahid M, Lantz PM, Fagerlin A, Salem B, Morrow M, Deapen D, Katz SJ. Population-based study of the relationship of treatment and sociodemographics on quality of life for early stage breast cancer. Qual Life Res. 2005;14(6):1467–79.

38. Miller KL, Rowland JH, Massie MJ. Psychosocial adaptation during and after breast cancer. In: Harris JR, Lippman ME, Morrow M, Osborne CK, editors. Diseases of the breast. 5th ed. Philadelphia: Wolters Kluwer; 2014. p. 1138–54.

39. National Comprehensive Cancer Network. Clinical practice guidelines in oncology™. Distress management. Version 1. 2018. http://www.nccn.org/professionals/physician_gls/default.asp

40. Stanton A. Positive consequences of the experience of cancer: perceptions of growth and meaning. In: Holland J, Breitbart W, Jacobsen P, Lederberg M, Loscalzo M, McCorkle R, editors. Psycho-oncology. New York: Oxford University Press; 2010. p. 547–50.

41. Spijker A, Trijsburg RW, Duivenvoorden DJ. Psychological sequelae of cancer diagnosis: a meta-analytical review of 58 studies after 1980. Psychosom Med. 1997;59:280–93.

42. Zabora J, BrintzenhofeSzoc K, Curbow B, Hooker C, Piantadosi S. The prevalence of psychological distress by cancer site. Psycho-Oncology. 2001;10:19–28.

43. Carlson LE, et al. High levels of untreated distress and fatigue in cancer patients. Br J Cancer. 2004b;90:2297–304.

44. Carlson LE, Waller A, Mitchell AJ. Screening for distress and unmet needs in patients with cancer: review and recommendations. J Clin Oncol. 2012;30:1160–77.

45. Ruddy K, Gelber S, Tamimi R, Mayer E, Schapira L, Come S, Meyer M, Winer E, Partridge A. Prevalence and predictors of distress in young women with newly diagnosed early stage breast cancer. Cancer Res. 2009;69(24 Suppl):abs 1067.

46. Mosher CE, DuHamel KN. An examination of distress, sleep, and fatigue in metastatic breast cancer patients. Psycho-Oncology. 2012;21(1):100–7. https://doi.org/10.1002/pon.1873.

47. Mitchell AJ, et al. Prevalence of depression, anxiety, and adjustment disorder in oncological, haematological, and palliative-care settings: a meta-analysis of 94 interview-based studies. Lancet Oncol. 2011;12(2):160–74.

48. Li M, Hales S, Rodin G. Adjustment disorders. In: Holland JC, et al., editors. Psycho-oncology. 2nd ed. New York: Oxford University Press; 2010.

49. Fann J. Major depression after breast cancer: a review of epidemiology and treatment. Gen Hosp Psychiatry. 2008;30(2):112–26.

50. Mehnert A, Koch U. Psychological comorbidity and health-related quality of life and its association with awareness, utilization, and need for psychosocial support in a cancer register-based sample of long-term breast cancer survivors. J Psychosom Res. 2008;64(4):383–91.

51. Reich M, Lesur A, Perdrizet-Chevallier C. Depression, quality of life and breast cancer: a review of the literature. Breast Cancer Res Treat. 2008;110:9–17.

52. Akechi T, Okuyama T, Imoto S, Yamawaki S, Uchitomi Y. Biomedical and psychosocial determinants of psychiatric morbidity among postoperative ambulatory breast cancer patients. Breast Cancer Res Treat. 2001;65:195–202.

53. Hopwood P, Sumo G, Mills J, Haviland J, Bliss JM. The course of anxiety and depression over 5 years of follow-up and risk factors in women with early breast cancer: results from UK Standardization of Radiotherapy Trials (START). Breast. 2010;19(2):84–91.

54. Travado L, Ventura C, Martins C. Breast cancer patients' psychosocial profile: a study with a Portuguese population. Psycho-Oncology. 2006;15(S2):1023.

55. Jassim GA, Whitford DL, Grey IM. Psychological interventions for women with non-metastatic breast cancer. Cochrane Database Syst Rev. 2015;5:CD008729. https://doi.org/10.1002/14651858.CD008729.

56. Longman AJ, Braden CJ, Mishel MH. Side-effects burden, psychological adjustment, and life quality in women with breast cancer: pattern of association over time. Oncol Nurs Forum. 1999;26(5):909–15.

57. Okamura M, Yamawaki S, Akechi T, Tanigychi K, Uchitomi Y. Psychiatric disorders following first breast cancer recurrence: prevalence, associated factors and relationship to quality of life. Jpn J Clin Oncol. 2005;35(6):302–9.

58. Miller K, Massie MJ. Depressive disorders. In: Holland J, Breitbart W, Jacobsen P, Lederberg M, Loscalzo M, McCorkle R, editors. Psycho-oncology. New York: Oxford University Press; 2010. p. 311–8.

59. Li M, Fitzgeral P, Rodin G. Evidence-based treatment of depression in patients with cancer. J Clin Oncol. 2012;30(11):1187–96.

60. Levin TT, Alici Y. Anxiety disorders. In: Holland J, Breitbart W, Jacobsen P, Lederberg M, Loscalzo M, McCorkle R, editors. Psycho-oncology. New York: Oxford University Press; 2010. p. 324–31.

61. Doka KJ. Counseling individuals with life-threatening illness. New York: Springer Publishing Company; 2009.

62. Traeger L, Greer JA, Fernandez-Robles C, Temel JS, Pirl WF. Evidence-based treatment of anxiety in patients with cancer. J Clin Oncol. 2012;30:1197–205.

63. Gil F, Grassi L, Travado L, Tomamichele M, Gonzalez JR, The SEPOS Group. Use of distress and depression thermometers to measure psychosocial morbidity among southern European cancer patients. Support Care Cancer. 2005;13:600–6.

64. BrintzenhofeSzoc KM, Kevin TT, Li Y, Kissane DW, Zabora JR. Mixed anxiety/depression symptoms in a large cancer cohort: prevalence by cancer type. Psychosomatics. 2009;50:383–91.

65. Parker PA, Baile WF, de Moor C, Cohen L. Psychosocial and demographic predictors of quality of life in a large sample of cancer patients. Psychooncology. 2003;12(2):183–93.

66. Colleoni M, Mandala M, Peruzzotti G, Robertson C, Bredart A, Goldhirsch A. Depression and degree of acceptance of adjuvant cytotoxic drugs. Lancet. 2000;356(9238):1326–7.

67. DiMatteo MR, Lepper HS, Croghan TW. Depression is a risk factor for noncompliance with medical treatment: Meta-analysis of the effects of anxiety and depression on patient adherence. Arch Intern Med. 2000;160:2101–7.

68. Walker LG, Heys SD, Walker MB, Ogston K, Miller ID, Hutcheon AW, Sarkar TK, Ah-See AK, Eremin O. Psychological factors can predict the response to primary chemotherapy in patients with locally advanced breast cancer. Eur J Cancer. 1999;35(13):1783–8.

69. Watson M, Homewood J, Haviland J, Bliss JM. Influence of psychological response on breast cancer survival: 10-year follow-up of a population-based cohort. Eur J Cancer. 2005;41(12):1710–4.

70. Prieto JM, Atala J, Blanch J, et al. Role of depression as a predictor of mortality among cancer patients after stem-cell transplantation. J Clin Oncol. 2005;23(25):6063–71.

71. Katon W, Lin EH, Kroenke K. The association of depression and anxiety with medical symptom burden in patients with chronic medical illness. Gen Hosp Psychiatry. 2007;29:147–55.

72. Prieto JM, Blanch J, Atala J, Carreras E, Rovira M, Cirera E, Gastó C. Psychiatric morbidity and impact

on hospital length of stay among hematologic cancer patients receiving stem-cell transplantation. J Clin Oncol. 2002;20(7):1907–17.

73. Henriksson MM, Isometsä ET, Hietanen PS, Aro HM, Lönnqvist JK. Mental disorders in cancer suicides. J Affect Disord. 1995;36:11–20.

74. Lazarus RS, Folkman S. Stress, appraisal and coping. New York: Springer; 1984.

75. Lazarus RS. Stress and emotion: a new synthesis. London: Free Association Books; 1999.

76. Antoni MH. Psychosocial intervention effects on adaptation, disease course and biobehavioral processes in cancer. Brain Behav Immun. 2013;30:S88–98. https://doi.org/10.1016/j.bbi.2012.05.009. Epub 2012 May 22

77. Faller H, Schuler M, Richard M, et al. Effects of psycho-oncologic interventions on emotional distress and quality of life in adult patients with cancer: systematic review and meta-analysis. J Clin Oncol. 2013;31(6):782–93.

78. Stanton AL, Rowland JH, Ganz PA. Life after diagnosis and treatment of cancer in adulthood: contributions from psychosocial oncology research. Am Psychol. 2015;70(2):159–74.

79. Matthews H, Grunfeld EA, Turner A. The efficacy of interventions to improve psychosocial outcomes following surgical treatment for breast cancer: a systematic review and meta-analysis. Psycho-oncologyEpub ahead of print. 2017;26(5):593–607.

80. Gudenkauf LM, Ehlers SL. Psychosocial interventions in breast cancer survivorship care. Breast. 2017;38:1–6. https://doi.org/10.1016/j.breast.2017.11.005. Epub ahead of print

81. Zimmerman T, Heinrichs N, Baucom DH. "Does one size fit all?" Moderators in psychosocial interventions for breast cancer patients: a meta-analysis. Ann Behav Med. 2007;34:225–39.

82. Osborn RL, Demoncada AC, Feuerstein M. Psychosocial interventions for depression, anxiety, and quality of life in cancer survivors: meta-analyses. Int J Psychiatry Med. 2006;36:1334.

83. Rehse B, Pukrop R. Effects of psychosocial interventions on quality of life in adult cancer patients: meta analysis of 37 published controlled outcome studies. Patient Educ Couns. 2003;50:225–39.

84. Zainal NZ, Booth S, Huppert FA. The efficacy of mindfulness-based stress reduction on mental health of breast cancer patients: a meta-analysis. Psycho-Oncology. 2013;22:1457–65. https://doi.org/10.1002/pon.3171.

85. Smedslund G, Ringdal GI. Meta-analysis of the effects of psychosocial interventions on survival time in cancer patients. J Psychosom Res. 2004;57:123–35.

86. Barrera I, Spiegel D. Review of psychotherapeutic interventions on depression in cancer patients and their impact on disease progression. Int Rev Psychiatry. 2014;26(1):31–43.

87. Andersen BL, Yan HC, Farrar WB, et al. Psychologic intervention improves survival for breast cancer patients. A randomized clinical trial. Cancer. 2008;113:3450–8.

88. Stagl JM, Lechner SC, Carver CS, et al. A randomized controlled trial of cognitive-behavioral stress management in breast cancer: survival and recurrence at 11-year follow-up. Breast Cancer Res Treat. 2015;154:319–28. https://doi.org/10.1007/s10549-015-3626-6.

89. Carlson LE, Bultz BD. Efficacy and medical cost offset of psychosocial interventions in cancer care: making the case for economic analyses. Psycho-Oncology. 2004;13(12):837–49.

90. The Scientific Evidence of Cost-Effectiveness of Psychological Interventions in Health Care, prepared by the Portuguese College of Psychologists in 2011 (OPP, 2011).

91. Bultz BD, Johansen C. Screening for distress, the 6th vital sign: where are we, and where are we going? Psycho-Oncology. 2011;20:569–71.

92. Jacobsen PB, Wagner LI. A new quality standard: the integration of psychosocial care into routine cancer care. J Clin Oncol. 2012;30(11):1154–9.

93. Bultz BD, Travado L, Jacobsen PB, Turner J, Borras JM, Ullrich AW. 2014 President's plenary international psycho-oncology society: moving toward cancer care for the whole patient. Psycho-Oncology. 2014;24:1587–93. https://doi.org/10.1002/pon.3844.

94. Travado L, Breitbart W, Grassi L, et al. 2015 President's plenary international psycho-oncology society: psychosocial care as a human rights issue—challenges and opportunities. Psycho-Oncology. 2017;26:563–9. https://doi.org/10.1002/pon.4209.

95. Dunn J, Bultz BD, Watson M. Emerging international directions for psychosocial care. In: Holland JC, Breitbart WS, Jacobsen PB, Loscalzo MJ, McCorkle R, Butow PN, editors. Psycho-oncology textbook. 3rd ed. New York: Oxford University Press; 2015. p. 739–44.

96. National Breast Cancer Centre and National Cancer Control Initiative. Clinical practice guidelines for the psychosocial care of adults with cancer. Camperdown, NSW: National Breast Cancer Centre; 2003. http://canceraustralia.gov.au/sites/default/files/publications/pca-1-clinical-practice-guidelines-for-psychosocial-care-of-adults-with-cancer_504af02682bdf.pdf. Accessed 10 Dec 2017

97. Travado L, Dalmas M. Psychosocial oncology care. In: Albreht T, Martin-Moreno JM, Jelenc M, Gorgojo L, Harris M, editors. European guide for quality national cancer control programmes. Ljubljana, Slovenia: National Institute of Public Health; 2015. p. 35–9.

98. Albreht T, Borrás JM, Dalmas M, et al. Survivorship and rehabilitation: policy recommendations for quality improvement in cancer survivorship and rehabilitation in EU Member States. In: Albreht T, Kiasuwa R, Vanden Bulcke M, editors. EUROPEAN guide on quality improvement in comprehensive cancer control. Ljubljana: National Institute of Public HealthBrussels: Scientific Institute of Public Health.

https://cancercontrol.eu/archived/uploads/images/Guide/pdf/CanCon_Guide_FINAL_Web.pdf; 2017.

99. Baken DM, Woolley C. Validation of the distress thermometer, impact thermometer and combinations of these in screening for distress. Psycho-Oncology. 2011;20:609–14.

100. Mitchell AJ. Short screening tools for cancer-related distress: areview and diagnostic validity meta-analysis. J Natl Compr Cancer Netw. 2010;8:487–94.

101. Bultz BD, Travado L, Jacobsen PB, Turner J, Borras JM, Ullrich AW. 2014 President's plenary international psycho-oncology society: moving toward cancer care for the whole patient. Psycho-Oncology. 2015;24:1587–93. https://doi.org/10.1002/pon.3844.

102. Travado L, Reis JC, Watson M, Borràs J. Psychosocial oncology care resources in Europe: a study under the European Partnership for Action Against Cancer (EPAAC). Psycho-Oncology. 2017;26:523–30. https://doi.org/10.1002/pon.4044.

103. Grassi L, Fujisawa D, Odyio P, Asuzu C, Ashley L, Bultz B, Travado L, Fielding R. Disparities in psychosocial cancer care: a report from the International Federation of Psycho-oncology Societies. Psycho-Oncology. 2016;25(10):1127–36. https://doi.org/10.1002/pon.4228.

104. Neamţiu L, Deandrea S, Pylkkänen L, et al. Psycho-oncological support for breast cancer patients: a brief overview of breast cancer services certification schemes and national health policies in Europe. Breast. 2016;29:178–80. https://doi.org/10.1016/j.breast.2016.07.002. Epub 2016 Aug 13

105. Gilbert E, Ussher JM, Perz J. Sexuality after breast cancer: a review. Maturitas. 2010;66:398–407.

106. Lee SJ, Schover LR, Partridge AH, et al. American Society of Clinical Oncology recommendations on fertility preservation in cancer patients. J Clin Oncol. 2006;24:2917–31.

107. Loren A, Mangu PB, Beck LN, et al. Fertility preservation for patients with cancer: American Society of Clinical Oncology clinical practice guideline update. J Clin Oncol. 2013;31:2500–10.

108. Goldfarb SB, Kramer AS, Oppong BA, et al. Fertility preservation for the young breast cancer patient. Ann Surg Oncol. 2016;23:1530–6.

109. Carter J, Lacchetti C, Andersen BL, et al. Interventions to address sexual problems in people with cancer: American Society of Clinical Oncology clinical practice guideline adaptation of Cancer Care Ontario guidelines. J Clin Oncol. 2017;11:492. https://doi.org/10.1200/JCO.2017.75.8995. [Epub ahead of print.

110. Holt-Lumstad J, Smith TB, Layton JB. Social relationships and mortality risk: a meta-analytic review. PLoS Med. 2010;7:e1000316.

111. Weihs KL, Enright TM, Simmens SJ. Close relationships and emotional processing predict decreased mortality in women with breast cancer: preliminary evidence. Psychosom Med. 2008;70:117–24.

112. Kroenke CH, Quesenberry C, Kwan ML, et al. Social networks, social support, and burden in relation-ships, and mortality after breast cancer diagnosis in the Life After Breast Cancer Epidemiology (LACE) study. Breast Cancer Res Treat. 2013;137:261–71.

113. Northouse L, Williams AL, Given B, McCorkle R. Psychosocial care for family caregivers of patients with cancer. J Clin Oncol. 2012;30(11):1227–34. https://doi.org/10.1200/JCO.2011.39.5798. Epub 2012 Mar 12

114. Van Ryn M, Sanders S, Kahn D, et al. Objective burden, resources, and other stressors among informal cancer caregivers: a hidden quality issue? Psychooncology. 2011;20(1):44–52.

115. Cancer Caregiving in the U.S.: An Intense, Episodic and Challenging Care Experience. Report prepared by the National Alliance for Caregiving, in collaboration with the National Cancer Institute and the Cancer Support Community, June 2016. http://www.caregiving.org/wp-content/uploads/2016/06/CancerCaregivingReport_FINAL_June-17-2016.pdf

116. de Moor JHS, Dowling EC, Ekwueme DU, et al. Employment implications of informal cancer caregiving. J Cancer Surviv. 2017;11(1):48–57.

117. Weaver KE, Rowland JH, Alfano CM, NcNeel TS. Parental cancer and the family: a population based estimate of the number of US cancer survivors residing with their minor children. Cancer. 2010;116(18):4395–401.

118. Girgis A, Lambert S, Johnson C, Waller A, Currow D. Physical, psychosocial, relationship, and economic burden of care for people with cancer: a review. J Oncol Pract. 2013;9(4):197–202.

119. Litzelman KI, Green PA, Yabroff KR. Cancer and quality of life in spousal dyads: spillover in couples with and without cancer-related health problems. Support Care Cancer. 2016;24(2):763–71.

120. Frambes D, Given B, Lehto R, Sikorskii A, Wyatt G. Informal caregivers of cancer patients: review of interventions, care activities, and outcomes. West J Nurs Res. 2018;40(7):1069–97. https://doi.org/10.1177/0193945917699364.

121. Badr H, Krebs P. A systematic review and meta-analysis of psychosocial interventions for couples coping with cancer. Psychooncology. 2013;22(8):1688–704.

122. Dorros SM, Segrin C, Badger TA. Cancer survivors' and partners' key concerns and quality of life. Psychol Health. 2017;32(11):1407–27.

123. Weaver KE, Rowland JH, Alfano CM, McNeel TS. Parental cancer and the family: a population-based estimate of the number of US cancer survivors residing with their minor children. Cancer. 2010;116(18):4395–401.

124. Shah BK, Armaly J, Swieter E. Impact of parental cancer on children. Anticancer Res. 2017;37:4025–8.

125. Osborn T. The psychosocial impact of parental cancer on children and adolescents: a systematic review. Psychooncology. 2007;16(2):101–26.

126. Purc-Stephenson R, Lyseng A. How are the kids holding up? A systematic review and meta-

analysis on the psychosocial impact of maternal breast cancer on children. Cancer Treat Rev. 2016;49:45–56.

127. Huizinga GA, Visser A, Zelders-Steyn YE, Teule JA, Reijneveld SA, Roodbol PF. Psychological impact of having a parent with cancer. Eur J Cancer. 2011;47(Suppl 3):S239–46.

128. Morris JN, Martini A, Preen D. The well-being of children impacted by a parent with cancer: an integrated review. Support Care Cancer. 2016;24(7):3235–51.

129. Brown RT, Fuemmeler B, Anderson D, Jamieson S, Simonian S, Hall RK, Brescia F. Adjustment of children and their mothers with breast cancer. J Pediatr Psychol. 2007;32(3):297–308.

130. Wellisch DK, Ormseth SR, Hartoonian N, Owen JE. A retrospective study predicting psychological vulnerability in adult daughters of breast cancer patients. Fam Syst Health. 2012;30(3):253–64.

131. Inhestern L, Bergelt C. When a mother has cancer: strains and resources of affected families from the mother's and father'sperspective – a qualitative study. BMC Womens Health. 2018;18(1):72. https://doi.org/10.1186/s12905-018-0562-8.

132. Coscarelli A. When a parent has cancer: taking care of the children. Informative resource found at: http://www.simmsmanncenter.ucla.edu/index.php/resources/articles-from-the-director/when-a-parent-has-cancer-taking-care-of-the-children/. Accessed 17 Dec 2018.

133. Harpham W. When a parent has cancer: a guide to caring for your children. New York: Harper Collins Publishers; 1997.

134. Heiney SP, Hermann JF. Cancer in our family: helping children cope with a parent's illness. 2nd ed. Atlanta, GA: American Cancer Society; 2013.

135. Ellis SJ, Wakefield CE, Antill G, Burns M, Patterson P. Supporting children facing a parent's cancer diagnosis: a systematic review of children's psychosocial needs and existing interventions. Eur J Cancer Care. 2016;26:e12432.

136. Visser A, Huizinga GA, Van der graaf WT, Hoekstra HJ, Hoekstra-weebers JE. The impact of parental cancer on children and the family: a review of the literature. Cancer Treat Rev. 2004;30(8):683–94.

137. Shea SE, Moore CW. Parenting with a life-limiting illness. Child Adolesc Psychiatr Clin N Am. 2018;27(4):567–78.